Molecular Biology Intelligence Unit

Human B Cell Superantigens

Moncef Zouali, Ph.D.

Institut Pasteur
Paris, France

CHAPMAN & HALL
I(T)P An International Thomson Publishing Company

New York • Albany • Bonn • Boston • Cincinnati • Detroit • London • Madrid • Melbourne • Mexico City • Pacific Grove • Paris • San Francisco • Singapore • Tokyo • Toronto • Washington

R.G. Landes Company
Austin

MOLECULAR BIOLOGY INTELLIGENCE UNIT

HUMAN B CELL SUPERANTIGENS

R.G. LANDES COMPANY
Austin, Texas, U.S.A.

Printed in the U.S.A.

Please address all inquiries to the Publishers:
R.G. Landes Company, 909 Pine Street, Georgetown, Texas, U.S.A. 78626
Phone: 512/ 863 7762; FAX: 512/ 863 0081

North American distributor:
Chapman & Hall, 115 Fifth Avenue, New York, New York, U.S.A. 10003

CHAPMAN & HALL

U.S. and Canada ISBN: 0-412-11981-1

Library of Congress Cataloging-in-Publication Data

Human B-cell superantigens / [edited by] Moncef Zouali.
p. cm. — (Molecular biology intelligence unit)
Includes bibliographical references and index.
ISBN 1-57059-385-X (alk. paper)
1. Superantigens. 2. B cells. I. Zouali, Moncef, 1952–.
II. Series.
[DNLM: 1. Superantigens. 2. B-Lymphocytes. QW 573 H918 1996
QR186.6.S94H85 1996
616.07'92—dc20
DNLM/DLC 96-9598
for Library of Congress CIP

Publisher's Note

R.G. Landes Company publishes six book series: *Medical Intelligence Unit, Molecular Biology Intelligence Unit, Neuroscience Intelligence Unit, Tissue Engineering Intelligence Unit, Biotechnology Intelligence Unit and Environmental Intelligence Unit.* The authors of our books are acknowledged leaders in their fields and the topics are unique. Almost without exception, no other similar books exist on these topics.

Our goal is to publish books in important and rapidly changing areas of bioscience and environment for sophisticated researchers and clinicians. To achieve this goal, we have accelerated our publishing program to conform to the fast pace in which information grows in bioscience. Most of our books are published within 90 to 120 days of receipt of the manuscript. We would like to thank our readers for their continuing interest and welcome any comments or suggestions they may have for future books.

Shyamali Ghosh
Publications Director
R.G. Landes Company

CONTENTS

EDITOR

Moncef Zouali
Département d'Immunologie
Institut Pasteur
Paris, France
Chapter 11

CONTRIBUTORS

Carl A.K. Borrebaeck
Department of Immunotechnology
Lund University
Lund, Sweden
Chapter 8

Jean-Pierre Bouvet
Unité d'Immunocytochimie
Institut Pasteur, CNRS URS 1961
Paris, France
Chapter 12

Jonathan Braun
Department of Pathology
and Laboratory Medicine,
and Molecular Biology Institute
University of California
at Los Angeles
Los Angeles, California, USA
Chapter 10

J. Donald Capra
Molecular Immunology Center
Department of Microbiology
The University of Texas Southwestern
Medical Center
Dallas, Texas, USA
Chapter 16

Mary K. Crow
Division of Rheumatology
The Hospital for Special Surgery
Cornell University Medical College
New York, New York, USA
Chapter 15

Rana Domiati-Saad
Department of Internal Medicine
and Harold C. Simmons Arthritis
Research Center
University of Texas Southwestern
Medical Center at Dallas
Dallas, Texas, USA
Chapter 6

Rick M. Fairhurst
Department of Pathology
and Laboratory Medicine,
and Molecular Biology Institute
University of California
at Los Angeles
Los Angeles, California, USA
Chapter 10

Steven M. Friedman
Division of Rheumatology
The Hospital for Special Surgery
Cornell University Medical College
New York, New York, USA
Chapter 15

CONTRIBUTORS

Christina Furebring
Department of Immunotechnology
Lund University
Lund, Sweden
Chapter 8

Lee Goodglick
Department of Pathology
and Laboratory Medicine
University of California at Los Angeles
Los Angeles, California, USA
Chapter 10

Jörg J. Goronzy
Department of Internal Medicine
Division of Rheumatology
Mayo Clinic & Foundation
Rochester, Minnesota, USA
Chapter 14

Boyd Haley
College of Pharmacy and Markey
Cancer Center
University of Kentucky
Lexington, Kentucky, USA
Chapter 13

Xiaowen He
Department of Internal Medicine
Division of Rheumatology
Mayo Clinic & Foundation
Rochester, Minnesota, USA
Chapter 14

Saleh M. Ibrahim
Department of Neurology
Neuroimmunology Branch
and Clinical Research Group
for Multiple Sclerosis
Julius-Maximilians-University
Würzburg, Germany
Chapter 4

Laure Juompan
Département d'Immunologie
Institut Pasteur
Paris, France
Chapter 11

Saoussen Karray
Département d'Immunologie
Institut Pasteur
Paris, France
Chapter 11

Heinz Kohler
Markey Cancer Center
University of Kentucky Medical Center
Lexington, Kentucky, USA
Chapter 13

Lisa M. Kozlowski
Division of Allergy and Immunology
Department of Medicine
University of Pennsylvania School
of Medicine
Philadelphia, Pennsylvania, USA
Chapter 7

CONTRIBUTORS

Petar Lenert
Louis-Charles Simard
Research Center
Notre-Dame Hospital
University of Montréal
Montréal, Quebec, Canada
Chapter 17

Arnold I. Levinson
Division of Allergy and Immunology
Department of Medicine
University of Pennsylvania School
of Medicine
Philadelphia, Pennsylvania, USA
Chapter 7

Peter E. Lipsky
Department of Internal Medicine
and Harold C. Simmons Arthritis
Research Center
University of Texas Southwestern
Medical Center at Dallas
Dallas, Texas, USA
Chapter 6

Alexander H. Lucas
Children's Hospital Oakland
Research Institute
Oakland, California, USA
Chapter 9

Denise Marcelo
Department of Pathology
and Laboratory Medicine
University of California
at Los Angeles
Los Angeles, California, USA
Chapter 10

Eric C. B. Milner
Virginia Mason Research Center
and the Department of Immunology
University of Washington
Seattle, Washington, USA
Chapter 1

Donald E. Mosier
Department of Immunology
Scripps Research Institute
La Jolla, California, USA
Chapter 10

Mehran Neshat
Department of Pathology
and Laboratory Medicine
University of California at Los Angeles
Los Angeles, California, USA
Chapter 10

Mats Ohlin
Department of Immunotechnology
Lund University,
Lund, Sweden
Chapter 8

Virginia Pascual
Molecular Immunology Center
Department of Microbiology
The University of Texas Southwestern
Medical Center
Dallas, Texas, USA
Chapter 16

Gabriela Pavlinkova
Immpheron Inc.
Lexington, Kentucky, USA
Chapter 13

CONTRIBUTORS

René Pirès
Unité d'Immunocytochimie
Institut Pasteur, CNRS URA 1961
Paris, France
Chapter 12

Kathleen N. Potter
Molecular Immunology Center
Department of Microbiology
The University of Texas
Southwestern Medical Center
Dallas, Texas, USA
Chapter 16

Canh P. Quan
Unité d'Immunocytochimie
Institut Pasteur, CNRS URA 1961
Paris, France
Chapter 12

Eric H. Sasso
Division of Rheumatology
Department of Medicine
University of Washington
Seattle, Washington, USA
Chapter 3

Elaine J. Schattner
Division of Hematology-Oncology
Department of Medicine
The New York Hospital
The Hospital for Special Surgery
Cornell University Medical College
New York, New York, USA
Chapter 15

Gregg J. Silverman
The Sam and Rose Stein Institute
for Research on Aging and the
Theodore Gildred Cancer Center
Department of Medicine-0663
University of California San Diego
La Jolla, California, USA
Chapter 5

Janet Townsley-Fuchs
Department of Pathology
and Laboratory Medicine
University of California
at Los Angeles
Los Angeles, California, USA
Chapter 10

Alfonso Tramontano
IGEN Research Institute
Rockville, Maryland, USA
Chapter 2

Cornelia M. Weyand
Department of Internal Medicine
Division of Rheumatology
Mayo Clinic & Foundation
Rochester, Minnesota, USA
Chapter 14

Dae-Hyun Yoo
Division of Rheumatology
The Hospital for Special Surgery
Cornell University Medical College
New York, New York, USA
Chapter 15

Maurizio Zanetti
Department of Medicine
and the Cancer Center
University of California San Diego
La Jolla, California, USA
Chapter 17

ABBREVIATIONS

AIDS	acquired immune deficiency syndrome
Ab	antibody
Ag	antigen
BcR	B-cell receptor
C	complement
CDR	complementarity-determining region
D_H	Ig heavy chain diversity segment
EBV	Epstein-Barr virus
FR	framework region
HIV-1	human immunodeficiency virus 1
Id	idiotype
Ig	immunoglobulin
J_H	Ig heavy chain joining segment
kb	kilobase
kDa	kilodalton
mAb	monoclonal antibody
MHC	major histocompatibility complex
OD	optical density
PBL	peripheral blood lymphocyte
PBMC	peripheral blood mononuclear cells
PCR	polymerase chain reaction
r	recombinant
RBC	red blood cell
RF	rheumatoid factor
RFLP	restriction fragment length polymorphism
SAg	superantigen
SCID	severe combined immunodeficiency
SLE	systemic lupus erythematosus
SpA	protein A of *Staphylococcus aureus*
TcR	T-cell receptor
V region	variable region of Ig
Vβ	T-cell receptor β-chain variable segment
V_H	Ig heavy chain variable segment
V_L	Ig light chain variable segment

PREFACE

"Nature s'est obligée à ne rien faire qui ne soit dissemblable"
"Nature has committed itself to generating nothing which is dissimilar"
Les Essais, Montaigne, 1580

Throughout evolution the immune system has developed multiple strategies to mount specific responses to virtually all antigens of the environment, and yet avoid destruction of self-components. Central to this unique discriminatory property are the tightly regulated cellular stages that characterize T and B lymphocyte development and the temporally-ordered molecular events that underlie generation of the huge diversity of immune receptors. Upon encounter with "conventional" antigens, B lymphocytes undergo a series of changes which are reminiscent of a choreographed dance, with a succession of movements, such as activation, proliferation and differentiation, each occurring only after completion of the previous one. Although the mechanisms that coordinate these phenomena are not clear, convincing evidence now indicates that antigen triggering of the B-cell receptor is the critical event in generating signals that will be transmitted to downstream intra-cellular effectors. While these transmission pathways are being actively investigated, recent observations have revealed that a group of molecules, called superantigens (SAgs), may interact with B cells in an "unconventional" manner. In contrast to antigens which interact with the six major hypervariable loops of immunoglobulins (Ig) and exhibit a clonal specificity towards B cells, the interaction of SAgs does not conform to this mode of interaction, hence, their propensity to activate a large proportion of B cells. This novel interaction mode has brought these issues into sharp focus by providing an additional B-cell triggering mechanism.

Beginning with advances in defining the molecular basis of Ig interaction with protein A (SpA) of *Staphylococcus aureus* in the late 1980s and the antigenic properties of HIV-1 gp120 in the early 1990s, the B-cell SAg field has now moved into a new active phase, in which significant observations are accumulating. The potent current research relies on a blend of approaches from diverse disciplines, including immunology, molecular biology, cell biology, biochemistry, crystallography and molecular modelling, and the resulting advances are likely to lead to discoveries that could be important not only for understanding B-cell development but also for designing novel means of immunointervention.

This book grew out of a long-standing interest in the mechanisms that control the emergence and the expression of the human antibody repertoire, initially in systemic autoimmunity and then in HIV infection. The picture of B-cell SAg interactions drawn above and the recent description of additional molecules that qualify for this label bring the subject of this volume into focus. This collection of essays as a whole has been designed to show how the concept of B-cell SAgs opens new avenues in understanding B-cell repertoire expression. It aims also to highlight a new tool with which to study B-cell activation and to provide insight into the interactions between the immune system and molecules of endogenous and exogenous origins and their potential pathological consequences.

The recent elucidation of the physical map of the Ig heavy chain (V_H) locus has revealed remarkable properties of human V_H genes. As reviewed in Milner's opening chapter, this progress raises, in turn, several questions with regard to selection of the somatic B-cell repertoire. Notorious among these is the consequence of the high degree of V_H gene polymorphism on expression of V_H segments that are the target of SAg activity, an issue addressed by Sasso in population based-studies of human V_H genes and their potential functional implications on B-cell SAg interactions. Focusing on structural and modelling studies of the Ig variable region and their implications for elucidating SAg binding to the B-cell receptor, Tramontano shows how residues throughout the framework regions provide the infrastructure for the hypervariable regions and can shape the SAg binding site.

Historically, by virtue of its specificity for the Fc part of Igs, SpA of *S. aureus* has been used as an immunopurification reagent. It was realized only recently that V_H3 Igs also interact with the alternative SAg binding site of SpA. This site has been studied in a number of laboratories. For example, Ibrahim finds that it is separate from the antigen binding site and that it is more frequent among IgM than IgA1 and IgG3 antibodies. Using Igs of known sequence, Sasso identified a probable site for SpA binding on framework region, outside the conventional antigen binding site. Silverman used combinatorial expression libraries to determine the molecular correlates of SpA binding and to characterize the site on SpA that binds V_H3 Igs.

In spite of the fact that the interaction of SAgs with B cells is not as fully investigated as that of T cells, there are similarities between the two cell types. Both of them proliferate in response to SAgs, and responses of B and T cells are mediated by the V_H and $V\beta$ domains, with little influence from the coexpressed L or α chain V-regions. Now, Domiati-Saad and Lipsky add another layer of complexity to the field of SAgs. Two staphylococcal enterotoxins (SEA and SED) are well known T-cell SAgs with potent T-cell stimulatory activity, a property responsible for their implication in food poisoning and toxic shock syndrome. The authors show that these toxins might function also as B-cell SAgs and propose a model where SAgs may either induce survival of the target B cells or deliver a death signal.

The human humoral response to the polysaccharide of *Haemophilus influenza* type b represents one of the best characterized protective immune responses to foreign antigens. One of its puzzling characteristics is the dominance of V_H3 heavy chains which may pair with several different light chains to generate the specific paratope. In his review, Lucas suggests that, while the polysaccharide itself probably does not function as a B-cell SAg, it is possible that B-cell SAgs from exogenous sources, such as bacteria colonizing the gut or other mucosal surfaces, or endogenous SAgs could shape the early repertoire by activating V_H3 B cells in a non-clonally restricted manner, thereby biasing the primary repertoire toward V_H3 expression. For their part, Ohlin et al describe a new antibody variable domain-binding component from *Escherichia coli*, with properties pointing to SAg activity.

In addition to SAgs of microbial origin, endogenous molecules may also exhibit this unconventional binding of B cells. One such example is the Fv fragment-binding protein (pFv), a gut-associated endogenous molecule described by Bouvet et al. In addition to being an important factor of mucosal immunity, pFv exhibits potentially important functions: it is a complement activator and a "super-allergen". In collaboration with Silverman, they now show that pFv is also a SAg, and that its binding is closely related to that of SpA. Interestingly, SpA and the endogenous protein Fv recognize overlapping sites in V_H regions. Along the same lines, Kohler et al. describe the intriguing phenomenon in which antibodies exhibit a novel affinity site for nucleotides. The biological role of such a site, however, remains unknown; but the authors assume that it might function as a receptor site for a ligand which could function as a SAg.

The potent functional effects of SAgs on the immune system raise the possibility of their implication in autoimmunity, an issue discussed in three systems. Autoimmune hemolytic anemia is a disease of unknown etiology. Examining the variable region genes used by human antibodies to red blood cells, Potter et al find that a particular V_H gene segment, called VH4-34, is overexpressed and that the first framework region of the antibodies is important in the interaction. Having noted that this gene segment is not frequent in other immune responses, they speculate that polyclonal activation by a SAg followed by antigen selection may be the underlying cause of gammopathies, such as cold agglutinin disease. In other studies, Lenert and Zanetti focus on the CD4 cellular receptor, which has a number of ligands, including major histocompatibility class II molecules and HIV gp120 glycoprotein. Having showed that this receptor also binds Igs through the V_H domain, they speculate that the autoantibodies to CD4 seen in HIV patients and in systemic lupus erythematosus may in fact reflect a B-cell SAg type interaction between CD4 and Igs. The role of B-cell SAgs in rheumatoid arthritis, another systemic autoimmune disease, is discussed by Goronzy et al. Their data suggest that staphylococcal enterotoxin D may directly target V_H3 positive Igs and activate a subset of B cells capable of producing rheumatoid factors.

It has been known for some time that, during the immune response, T-cell triggering by conventional antigens generates signals that are critical for T-cell dependent B-cell responses. In as much as T cells can also be activated by SAgs, Schattner et al analyzed the consequences of this unconventional triggering on the interaction between B and T cells. Since repetitive exposure to certain microbial SAgs can promote T cell-dependent B-cell activation, they propose that interaction of B cells with multivalent self-antigens may lead to their activation and differentiation and, ultimately, to generation of autoantibodies.

Remarkably, B-cell SAgs may have functional consequences. In addition to the multiple properties of pFv, studies by Levinson et al show that SpA may elicit autoantibody production and activation of the complement cascade. Obviously, B-cell SAg activities may have profound clinical consequences, as discussed by Goodglick et al and Karray et al for HIV gp120. Even more provocative are the depletions of V_H3 positive B cells seen during advanced stages of HIV infection, — a potential consequence of the SAg property of gp120.

Thus, recent observations made in vitro and in vivo with B-cell SAgs are highlighted within the current knowledge of B-cell development. Naturally, a number of questions arise. In basic immunology, these Ig variable region-binding proteins are valuable as model systems to study B-cell activation. In this respect, it will be critical to trace the clonal fate of B cells upon interaction with SAgs. In infectious diseases, they are useful in analyzing the mechanisms by which pathogens interact with the human immune system. Here, the challenge at hand, however, is to study the consequences of the SAg properties of HIV gp120. Elucidation of the mechanism of V_H3 positive B-cell depletion seen during this infection may have important consequences with respect to disease management. In autoimmunity, the role of SAgs is particularly intriguing. On the one hand, they may be beneficial to the organism by depleting subsets of B cells whose presence might otherwise put the organism at risk for autoimmune disease. On the other, B-cell triggering by SAgs may provide an unexplored path for the initiation of systemic autoimmune diseases. While this book does not directly answer all these intricately woven questions, it provides a frame of reference for seriously exploring them. Finally, I wish to thank the authors for their contributions to this book and for their patience throughout the various stages of its elaboration.

Moncef Zouali
Paris
March 1996

CHAPTER 1

Organization of the Human V_H Locus and Rearrangement Patterns of the V_H3 Gene Family

Eric C. B. Milner

INTRODUCTION

Antibody genes are formed from discontinuous gene segments (V, D, and J for heavy chains; V and J for light chains) that are physically juxtaposed during B cell development to generate complete transcriptional units.[1,2] Immunoglobulin variable regions have been grouped into families according to amino acid[3,4] or nucleotide similarity.[5-10] Generally, sequence identity is 80% or greater within families, while identity is less than 70% between families. On this basis, seven human V_H gene families have been described. While the murine V_H gene families are thought to be organized into discrete clusters with only a modest amount of interspersion,[6] gene segments comprising the human V_H families are largely interspersed.[7-14]

Early estimates of the size of the region in the human containing the V_H genes ranged from 2500 or 3000 kb based on pulse field gel electrophoresis,[8,11] to 4000 kb based on genetic linkage analysis.[15] Estimates of the size of the V_H repertoire range from 50 to 200 gene segments.[8,16] Two groups have cloned a large fraction of the V_H germline repertoire. Matsuda et al have generated overlapping YAC clones covering 0.8 Mb of the locus and have identified 64 V_H segments.[14] Tomlinson et al have amplified and sequenced 74 germline V_H gene segments using family specific leader primers and recombination signal sequence primers.[17] The latter group has gone on to generate a YAC contig extending the Matsuda map approximately 100 kb.[18] This map extends to the telomere and is thought to

Human B Cell Superantigens, edited by Moncef Zouali. © 1996 R.G. Landes Company.

represent the completion of the map of the V_H locus (Fig. 1.1). Thus, in contrast to the early estimates, the locus occupies only about 1 Mb of DNA.

The completion of the physical map of the V_H locus[14,18] has answered many questions, and has raised a set of new ones. To a large extent, the issue now with respect to gene organization, is to delineate allelic variation among V_H genes and to determine the degree to which variation (or polymorphism) of V_H genes contribute to differences in V gene utilization. Polymorphic variation within the V_H locus takes two fundamental forms. The first is conventional allelic variation in coding region sequences. Putative alleles of a number of genes have been identified by sequence analysis of the same gene isolated from different individuals. The second form of polymorphism and the more problematic to analyze is the result of numerous duplications, insertions, and deletions. This phenomenon leads to the unusual situation in which clearly distinct genes derived by duplication may be absolutely identical but may differ from their respective alleles by one or more nucleotide substitutions.

It is of considerable interest and importance to delineate the alleles of each V_H gene as well as the haplotype structure including the insertion/deletion polymorphisms. In the context of understanding the expressed antibody repertoire, it will be important to know and understand the germline repertoire. To address these issues, we have focused on the identification of specific genes and the discrimination between closely related genes and alleles. We have used synthetic oligonucleotides corresponding to human V_H sequences to analyze sequence variation in human genomic DNA. By employing conditions under which single nucleotide mismatches abrogate hybridization, it has been possible to unambiguously identify individual germline V_H genes and to identify variation in closely related germline genes. We have demonstrated that analysis of the human V_H locus with sequence-specific oligonucleotide probes reveals hybridization patterns of limited complexity and striking heterogeneity.[19,20] Within the framework (FR1) and complementarity-determining-regions (CDR1, CDR2) different oligonucleotide probes are generally "mutually exclusive" by virtue of the nucleotide substitutions that distinguish the probes. Thus, a sequence detected by a given probe will not be detected by any mutually exclusive probe directed to the homologous region of a different V_H gene segment. We have found that the detection of specific sequence motifs by hybridization of restriction enzyme-digested DNA in a modified Southern analysis using short oligonucleotide probes allows the specific identification of germline genes.[19-23] Based on data obtained from genomic hybridization using such probes, it is possible to assign individual genes to specific restriction fragments. By this approach, germline sequences of multiple individuals can be compared with a very high degree of precision.

POLYMORPHISM OF V_H3 GENES

At least 48 V_H3 genes have been mapped to the V_H locus.[13,14,18] Slightly more than half of these have been found to be pseudogenes.[14,18] By assessing the occurrence of specific sequence motifs using oligonucleotide probes it has been possible to identify many of the V_H3 genes and to detect variation in their occurrence. We have analyzed the occurrence of several elements mapping in the vicinity of, or allelic to, V3-30 (designated 1.9III, 56p1, hv3005). The results indicate that all three elements cannot be alleles of the same locus.[21,23] Calculations based on the prevalence of the individual elements 1.9III, 56p1, and hv3005, and considering the known haplotype structures, indicate that 1.9III (V3-30) and hv3005 (V3-30b) are appropriately considered to be alleles and 56p1 (V3-30.3) an insertion/deletion element (Fig. 1.1). Allele frequencies for hv3005 and 1.9III are 0.19 and 0.72, respectively. Because these allele frequencies do not add up to one, it seems likely that an additional haplotype or haplotypes with an allele frequency of .08 which lacks

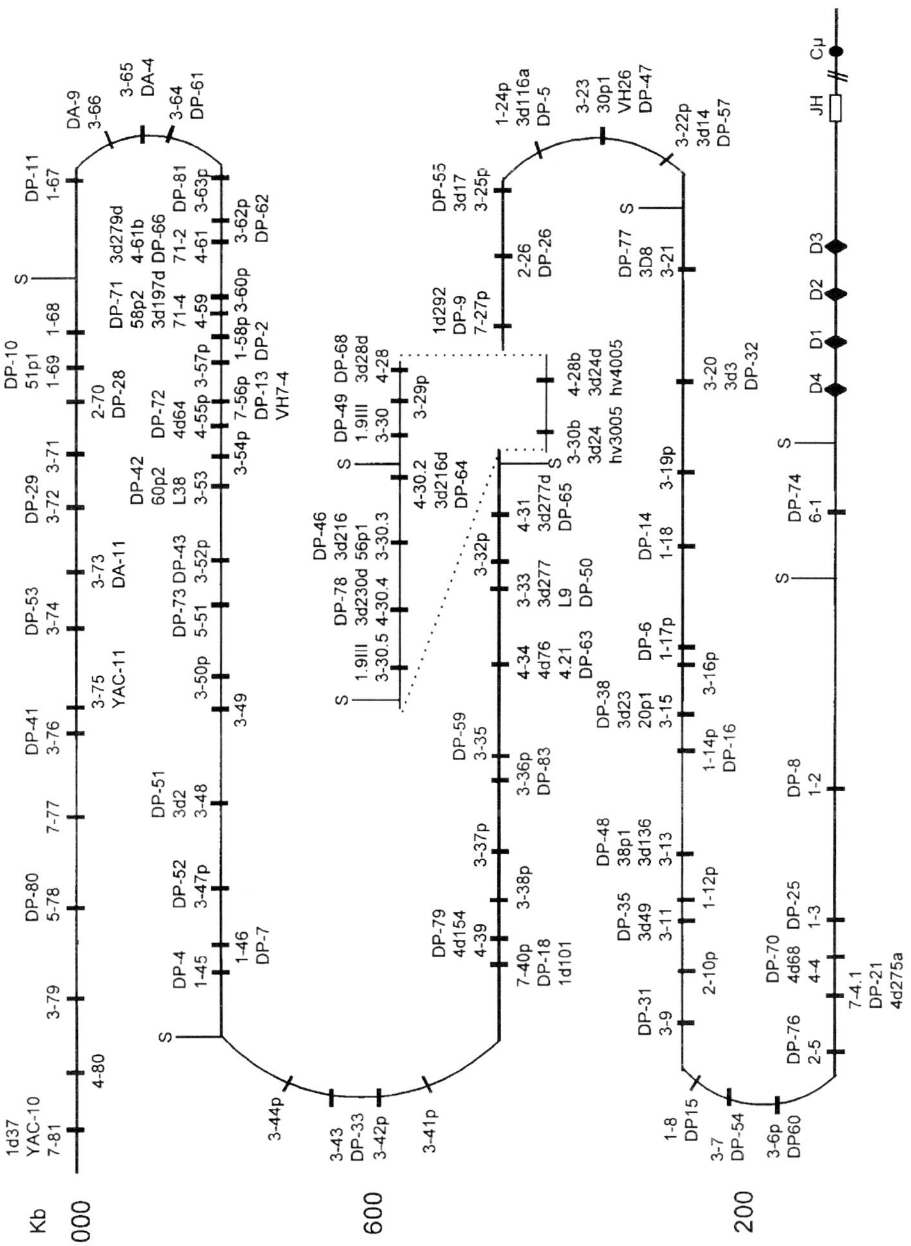

Fig. 1.1. Map of the human V_H locus. The nomenclature of Honjo and colleagues[14] is employed. Other commonly used names of genes are indicated as well. Location of SfiI restriction sites (S) is approximate and was deduced from a pulsed field map of the locus.[21,37] (Modified from data originally reported in refs. 14,18,21,37.)

both 1.9III and hv3005 occurs (i.e., a deletion of V3-30). No additional allelic sequence has been identified, however, suggesting that this putative allele is a blank haplotype. The putative third allele is definitely not 56p1, which in our analysis always occurs on a haplotype carrying one or two copies of 1.9III.

We found that a 50 kb insertion/deletion polymorphism profoundly affected the haplotype structure and allelic relationships in this region and provides a structural explanation for the allelic relationships deduced from the hybridization data.[21] The 50 kb insertion which carries 56p1 and the second copy of 1.9III (V30.5) has been localized to the interval between V3-30 and V4-31 (Fig. 1.1). There is some evidence for heterogeneity in the exact break points among the population. Using a probe adjacent to one of the Sfi1 restriction sites which border the insertion, we have found that approximately 93% of the population carry the insertion, an allele frequency of 0.73. At least six haplotypes can be identified in this region, four of which include the 50 kb insertion. The occurrence of additional haplotypes is likely. Two haplotypes are illustrated in Figure 1.1. As shown, on one haplotype V3-30 has been duplicated to generate the identical element, V3-30.5 (the region of identity includes flanking restriction sites).[20,21] V3-30 is nonetheless allelic to V3-30b (which encodes the hv3005 segment) from which it differs by 5 bp (two amino acid replacements).

A second duplication and insertion/deletion involves the element V3-23, (also known as 30P1 [ref. 10] or VH26 [ref. 24]). All individuals thus far tested carry a copy of V3-23 on a 5 kb Taq I fragment. Approximately 40% of the population carries a duplicated element on a 7 kb Taq I restriction fragment. Phosphorimage analysis of band intensities indicate that the 5 kb band may carry alleles of both loci, only one of which is allelic to the 7 kb band. By deletional analysis in B cell lines, both of the V3-23 loci map to the same interval, suggesting that they may be tandemly arrayed. Additional alleles of V3-23, which exhibit skewed distribution among different ethnic groups, have been delineated by Sasso and colleagues.[25]

Yet another V_H3 duplication involves V3-53, (also known as 60p2[10]). The V3-53 locus occurs on two sets of polymorphic Taq I restriction fragments. The more 3' locus, which we have mapped by deletional analysis to the same interval as V3-53, is carried on Taq I restriction fragments of approximately 3 kb and 4 kb. The second locus which maps 5' to the known V3-53 locus is carried on Taq I restriction fragments of approximately 12 kb and 15 kb. No nucleotide or amino acid substitutions have as yet been associated with these restriction fragment length polymorphisms (RFLP).

HAPLOTYPE STRUCTURE

The existence of numerous insertion/deletion polymorphisms raises the possibility that different haplotypes of the V_H locus may carry substantially different coding information. In addition, we and others have found little evidence for linkage disequilibrium between polymorphic elements in the V_H locus. In several instances where linkage disequilibrium is evident, the elements involved have been physically closely linked; in several instances elements in linkage disequilibrium were carried on the same lambda phage clone placing them within about 15 kb of one another. In an analysis of 11 families in which 42 (of 44) haplotypes could be identified with respect to five loci, four V_H markers and one variable number tandem repeat (VNTR) located 5' to the J_H region, 36 clearly distinct haplotypes could be identified (Milner, E.C.B. of C.M. Alexander, unpublished observations). It seems likely that by analyzing additional markers, all 42 haplotypes would be found to be distinct. We have argued based on similar observations that the haplotype structure in the population is extraordinarily complex.[20,22,26]

PATTERNS OF V_H3 EXPRESSION

One obvious insight made possible by the completion of the physical map of the V_H locus, is that the total number of functional V_H genes is smaller than previously thought. To determine if there was a generally applicable rule to describe V_H3 utilization, the identities of rearranged V region gene segments were determined in unselected peripheral blood B cells from 12 subjects. Although sequence analysis is the most definitive method for ascertaining the identity of any particular rearranged V gene segment, the number of rearrangements that can be analyzed is limited by constraints inherent to sequence analysis. Because we wanted to analyze larger numbers of rearrangements, an alternative approach was used, in which individual V_H gene segments were identified by hybridization to sequence-specific oligonucleotide probes. We have previously described the generation and use of synthetic oligonucleotide probes specifically to identify both germ-line and rearranged individual V_H elements directly in genomic DNA and in libraries of cloned V regions.[19-21,27] This technique is highly specific, in well over 200 sequences that have been determined, no discrepancies between hybridization and sequence have been identified (ref. 27 and unpublished data). Therefore, heavy chain rearrangements were quantitatively amplified from peripheral blood B cells using a V_H3 family-specific 5' primer and a consensus J_H 3' primer. As a control, unrearranged V_H genes were quantitatively amplified using the same family-specific 5' primer and consensus FR3-specific or recombination signal sequence-specific 3' primers. Libraries containing V_H genes were generated by cloning the PCR products into phagemid vectors. The V_H content of the libraries was assessed by hybridization with sequence-specific oligonucleotide probes. Eight V region gene segments were selected for analysis based on two criteria: (1) the gene could be amplified quantitatively from the germline in control experiments, and (2) specific, diagnostic oligonucleotide probes were available for detection of the gene.

By scoring the number of positive wells for the diagnostic oligonucleotide probes and for the family-specific probe, the frequency with which a specific V_H gene segment was present among rearrangements was calculated for each subject. A total of 4568 independent V_H3 rearrangements were obtained from the 12 subjects (an average of 381 clones per subject). As illustrated in Figure 1.2, the striking feature of these results is that the variation seen in the average incidence of rearrangements of each of the genes is remarkably conserved among this population of 12 subjects. Results were stratified according to gender to determine if rearrangement frequency of individual V_H3 gene segments differed between males and females. One-factor analysis of variance indicated that gender did not have a significant effect on the rearrangement frequency of any of the eight V_H3 genes.

For some of the subjects tested, the germline copy number of individual V_H3 genes had been previously determined by independent analysis. It has been found that approximately 25 V_H3 gene segments are quantitatively and equivalently amplified using this combination of primers.[27] In view of this control result, the parsimonious interpretation of any observed differences when rearrangements were amplified would be that these differences were due to actual differences in the frequency of occurrence of that particular V gene segment among rearrangements in peripheral blood B cells.

To determine if age influences the rearrangement frequency of individual V_H3 gene segments, the three most commonly occurring V_H3 genes, V3-23, V3-30 and V3-33 were plotted versus age (Fig. 1.3). Correlation coefficients determined for V3-23, V3-30 and V3-33 were all below 0.6 ($p>0.05$), indicating no correlation between rearrangements of these genes and age of the subject. Correlation coefficients were determined for the remaining V regions as well and no significant correlation was found between gene utilization and adult age for any of the V_H3 gene segments (not shown).

As predicted from previous studies,[27-29] the V3-23 gene segment was the most frequently occurring rearrangement in the majority of subjects. V3-30 and V3-33 are

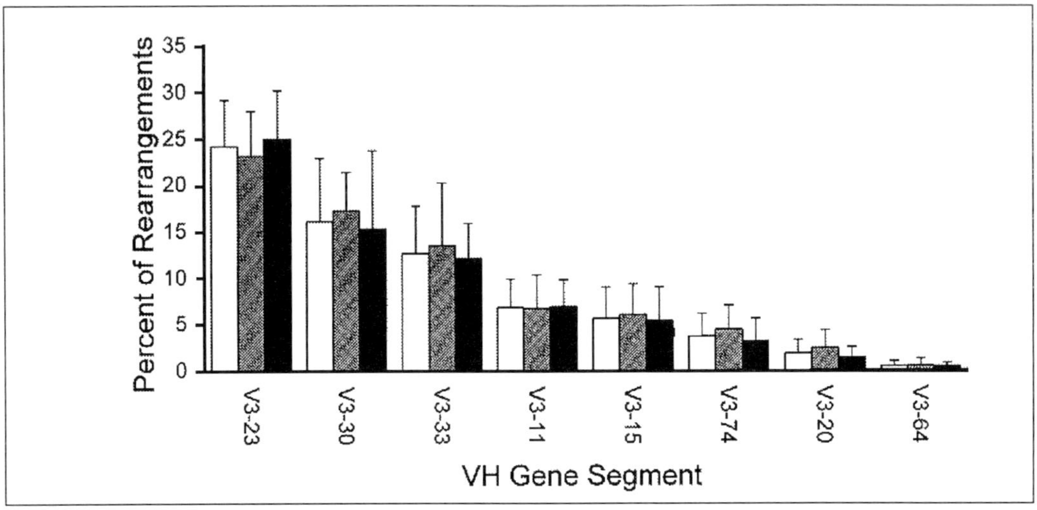

Fig. 1.2. Frequency of occurrence of eight individual V_H3 genes in rearrangements in peripheral blood B cells of 12 adult subjects. Each bar represents the mean percentage of total V_H3 rearrangements contributed by the indicated V_H3 gene for the entire population (open bars), males (light bars), and females (dark bars). A total of 4568 rearrangements were analyzed. Error bars indicate one standard deviation of the means. (Reproduced with permission from Huang et al. Molecular Immunol, in press ©1996.)[38]

also commonly rearranged in most subjects. Four V_H3 genes, V3-11, V3-15, V3-74, and V3-20, made lesser contributions to rearrangements, and the remaining element, V3-64, was rarely represented among rearrangements. Despite this clear-cut pattern of biased utilization seen on a population basis, considerable variation between subjects can be observed in the data presented in Table 1.1. For example, V3-23 accounted for as much as 30.6% to as little as 17.7% of V_H3 rearrangements. Similarly, V3-30 accounted for as much as 31.4% to as little as 7.3% of rearrangements.

The eight gene segments tested in this study accounted for over 70% of all V_H3 rearrangements among the libraries analyzed. The three most commonly found V regions, V3-23, V3-30 and V3-33, accounted for an average of 54% of all V_H3 rearrangements per subject. Results from multiple comparisons of means by Fisher's least significant difference test showed that V3-23 was found most frequently (24.3 ± 4.9%, mean percent ± s.d.), followed by V3-30 (16.1 ± 6.8%), V3-33 (12.7 ± 5.0%), V3-11 (6.8 ± 3.1%), V3-15 (5.6 ± 3.3%). The rest of the V_H3 genes accounted for an average of 0.4% to 3.7% for each gene. The contribution of each individual V region gene segment was a stable property of the gene. Analysis of variance (F-test) showed that, regardless of gender or age of the subjects, differences in the mean frequency of occurrence of rearrangement between V_H3 gene segments were significant ($p < 0.001$).

To assess the clonal diversity of the rearrangements, and to determine if the predominance of V3-23 was an artifactual result due to preferential amplification of a few clones, from 12 to 20 rearrangements of the V3-23 gene were selected at random from each of four subjects for sequence analysis. DNA sequence analysis was performed on a total of 66 such clones. As expected, sequence analysis through the V segments confirmed that all were derived from the V3-23 germ line element, and confirmed the hybridization results. Among the 66 clones, only three pairs of identities were found—two pairs in one subject and one pair in another subject. Two of the pairs were from adjacent wells and probably represent cross contamination during the initial picking of the colonies into the 96 well plate. Thus, the preferential use of V3-23 was not due to preferential amplification of a few clones.

DISCUSSION

The three V regions that were found the most frequently are located within approximately 80 kb of each other near the middle of the V_H locus.[14] Although this close physical location among these most frequently occurring V_H3 genes may be fortuitous, it is possible that the frequent occurrence of these V regions in rearrangements is influenced by their chromosomal location. In this regard, it is noteworthy that the V_H4 gene segment, V4-34 (also known as 4.21 [ref. 30] or 4d76 [ref. 27]), which is the gene most commonly found in V_H4 rearrangements,[27,31] is located approximately 10 kb 5' to V3-33 within this same region.[14] Each of the individuals studied exhibited this pattern of preferential utilization. Similar biased V gene utilization[32] and an association with chromosomal location[33] have been found in the murine antibody repertoire. However, in the mouse, the preference is for elements that map in the D_H-proximal region of the V_H locus,[33] whereas in the human, the preference is for a cluster of elements located near the middle of the locus, with underexpressed elements mapping both more D_H-distal and more D_H-proximal to the preferred cluster. This putative positional variegation is suggestive of the existence of a locus control element which facilitates access of the recombinase to the region.

As there is no convenient means to discriminate among the various germline configurations, it is not possible to determine directly the effect that gene copy number may have on the frequency of occurrence of rearrangements in peripheral blood B cells. It seems likely, however, that individuals who have extra copies of elements will have more rearrangements carrying that element. Thus, from the data in Figure 1.2 and Table 1.1, we predict that the V3-30 locus carries multiple copies in the one individual (donor 4086) who had rearranged V3-30 in 31.6% of V_H3 rearrangements.

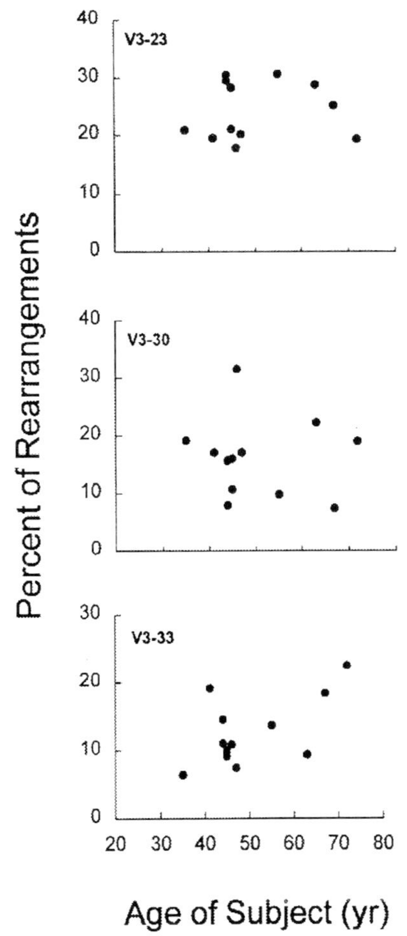

Fig. 1.3. Frequency of occurrence of individual V_H3 genes in rearrangements in peripheral blood B cells is independent of age. Each point represents the percentage of total V_H3 rearrangements contributed by the indicated V_H3 gene from one subject and is plotted according to age of the subject. Ages ranged from 35 to 72 years. Results for the three most commonly rearranged V_H3 genes are shown: V3-23 (top panel), V3-30 (middle panel) and V3-33 (lower panel). (Reproduced with permission from Huang et al. Molecular Immunol, in press ©1996.)[38]

Similarly, we would predict that no duplication of germline V3-30 would be found in the individual (donor 3323) who rearranged V3-30 in only 7.3% of rearrangements. These predictions are supported by gel hybridization analyses which indicate that donor 4086 carries four V3-30 elements while donor 3323 carries a single (probably diploid) V3-30 element (not shown). This suggests that a haploid V3-30 element accounts for approximately 3% to 7% of rearrangements. Nonetheless, as we have previously reported,[27] this does not explain differences in rearrangement frequency between distinct V region loci. For example, two elements, V3-20 and V3-64, consistently accounted for less than 3% of rearrangements, and one element, V3-74, accounted for approximately 3% of rearrangements (Table 1.1). We interpret this to mean that copy number, per se, does not determine efficiency of rearrangement, but that for each individual element, variation between individuals may be influenced by copy number.

In principle, the accumulation of somatic mutations may also contribute to bias in our results. The libraries analyzed in this report were prepared from whole peripheral blood. In healthy subjects, approximately 80% of peripheral blood B cells express surface IgD. This population has virtually no somatic mutation.[34,35] The remaining 20% of peripheral B cells include memory B cells, most of which have acquired somatic mutations.[34] The diagnostic probes used in this study would not detect a gene that had acquired a mutation in the target sequence of the probe. If all V_H genes are equally susceptible to acquisition of somatic mutations, then the relative usage as measured would be unaffected. However, if some V_H

Table 1.1. Frequency of occurrence of rearranged V region genes

Subject	n^a	V3-11	V3-15	V3-20	V3-23	V3-30	V3-33	V3-64	V3-74
		V_H3 Gene Segment							
		percent of total rearrangements							
4038	210	7.1	2.8	2.4	19.5	17.1	19.0	0	2.9
4058	316	7.9	4.4	0.9	30.4	7.9	11.1	0.9	2.5
4080	269	8.6	10.4	0.7	29.4	15.6	14.5	0.4	1.9
3323	191	8.9	9.9	3.1	25.1	7.3	18.3	0.5	2.1
3404	313	5.8	1.3	1.6	21.1	16.0	9.9	0	2.2
4105	336	2.1	6.0	2.4	30.6	9.8	13.7	0.3	8.6
3326	441	10.2	9.8	1.4	19.3	19.0	22.4	0.2	2.3
4086	434	4.4	2.5	0.7	17.7	31.6	10.8	0	1.8
4078	338	1.8	5.3	0	28.7	22.2	9.5	1.8	8.6
3116	913	10.1	9.1	5.1	28.3	10.7	9.1	0.2	3
4112	346	4.3	2.9	2.9	20.2	17.1	7.5	Δ^b	5.2
4087	461	10.6	3.0	Δ	20.8	19.1	6.5	0.4	2.8
mean		6.8	5.6	1.8	24.3	16.1	12.7	0.4	3.7
s.d.		3.1	3.3	1.5	4.9	6.8	5.0	0.5	2.5

[a] *n*, number of rearrangements studied;
[b] Δ, subject has a germ-line deletion of the indicated gene segment;
(Reproduced with permission from Huang et al. Molecular Immunol, in press ©1996.)[38]

genes are better substrates for the mutator mechanism than others, then such genes would be undercounted in these assays. This has been addressed in other studies by determining the complete sequences of randomly picked clones. Although numerous rearrangements that had been blank by hybridization as a result of mutation could be assigned to the appropriate germline source by sequence analysis, no significant change in V_H usage was found (A.M. Glas, S.-C. Huang, R. Jiang, and E.C.B. Milner, unpublished data).

The results presented here indicate that predominance of particular V_H3 genes is a product of molecular or selective processes favoring these elements. Because we have analyzed only a subset of the V_H3 gene family, it is possible that additional V_H3 genes also make predominant contributions to the repertoire. However, other experiments have not revealed the presence of additional, predominantly expressed V_H3 genes.[36]

Acknowledgments

I wish to express my gratitude and indebtedness to current and former members of my laboratory who have contributed so much to these studies: Shu-Cai Huang, Ronghua Jiang, Ko Willems van Dijk, Eric H. Sasso, Silvére van der Maarel, Andrew Bull, Catherine Alexander, Ivy Suzuki, Wendy Hufnagle, George Pinchuk, and Sambasiva P. Rao. Supported in part by NIH grants AR39918 and CA18221.

References

1. Honjo T. Immunoglobulin genes. Annu Rev Immunol 1983; 1:499-528
2. Tonegawa S. Somatic generation of antibody diversity. Nature 1983; 302:575-581.
3. Kabat EA, Wu TT, Perry HM et al. Sequences of proteins of immunological interest. (U.S. Dept. of Health and Human Services, Bethesda), 1991; 5th Edition.
4. Dildrop R. A new classification of mouse Vh sequences. Immunol Today 1984; 5:84-86
5. Riblet R, Brodeur P. Polymorphism and evolution of Igh-V gene families. Curr Top Microbiol Immunol 1986; 127:167-72.
6. Brodeur PH, Riblet R. The immunoglobulin heavy chain variable region (Igh-V) locus in the mouse. I. One hundred Igh-V genes comprise seven families of homologous genes. Eur J Immunol 1984; 14:922-30.
7. Shen A, Humphries C, Tucker P et al. Human heavy-chain variable region gene family nonrandomly arranged in familial chronic lymphocytic leukemia. Proc Natl Acad Sci USA 1987; 84:8563-7.
8. Berman JE, Mellis SJ, Pollock R et al. Content and organization of the human Ig VH locus: definition of three new VH families and linkage to the Ig CH locus. EMBO J 1988; 7:727-38.
9. Lee KH, Matsuda F, Kinashi T et al. A novel family of variable region genes of the human immunoglobulin heavy chain. J Mol Biol 1987; 195:761-8.
10. Schroeder HW, Jr., Hillson JL, Perlmutter RM. Early restriction of the human antibody repertoire. Science 1987; 238:791-3.
11. Matsuda F, Lee KH, Nakai S et al. Dispersed localization of D segments in the human immunoglobulin heavy-chain locus. EMBO J 1988; 7:1047-51.
12. Kodaira M, Kinashi T, Umemura II et al. Organization and evolution of variable region genes of the human immunoglobulin heavy chain. J Mol Biol 1986; 190:529-41.
13. Walter MA, Surti U, Hofker MH et al. The physical organization of the human immunoglobulin heavy chain gene complex. EMBO J 1990; 9:3303-13.
14. Matsuda F, Shin EK, Nagaoka H et al. Structure and physical map of 64 variable segments in the 3' 0.8-megabase region of the human immunoglobulin heavy-chain locus. Nature Genetics 1993; 3:88-94.
15. Johnson MJ, Natali AM, Cann HM et al. Polymorphisms of a human variable heavy chain gene show linkage with constant heavy chain genes. Proc Natl Acad Sci USA 1984; 81:7840-4.
16. Walter MA, Cox DW. Analysis of genetic variation reveals human immunoglobulin VH-region gene organization. Am J Hum Genet 1988; 42:446-51.
17. Tomlinson IM, Walter G, Marks JD et al. The repertoire of human germline VH sequences reveals about fifty groups of VH

segments with different hypervariable loops. J Mol Biol 1992; 227:776-98.

18. Cook GP, Tomlinson IM, Walter G et al. A map of the human immunoglobulin VH locus completed by analysis of the telomeric region of chromosome 14q. Nature Genetics 1994; 7:162-8.
19. Willems van Dijk K, Schroeder HW Jr, Perlmutter RM et al. Heterogeneity in the human immunoglobulin VH locus. J Immunol 1989; 142:2547-54.
20. Sasso EH, Willems van Dijk K, Milner ECB. Prevalence and polymorphism of human VH3 genes. J Immunol 1990; 145: 2751-7.
21. Willems van Dijk K, Milner LA, Sasso EH et al. Chromosomal organization of the heavy chain variable region gene segments comprising the human fetal antibody repertoire. Proc Natl Acad Sci USA 1992; 89:10430-4.
22. van der Maarel SM, Willems van Dijk K, Alexander CM et al. Chromosomal organization of the human VH4 gene family: Location of individual gene segments. J Immunol 1993; 150:2858-68.
23. Sasso EH, Willems van Dijk K, Bull A et al. VH genes in tandem array comprise a repeated germline motif. J Immunol 1992; 149:1230-6.
24. Matthyssens G, Rabbitts TH. Structure and multiplicity of genes for the human immunoglobulin heavy chain variable region. Proc Natl Acad Sci USA 1980; 77:6561-5.
25. Sasso EH, Buckner JH, Suzuki LA. Ethnic differences in polymorphism of an immunoglobulin VH3 gene. J Clin Invest 1995; 96:1591-600.
26. Willems van Dijk K, Sasso EH, Milner ECB. Polymorphism of the human immunoglobulin VH4 gene family. J Immunol 1991; 146:3646-51.
27. Suzuki I, Pfister L, Glas A et al. Representation of rearranged VH gene segments in the human adult antibody repertoire. J Immunol 1995; 154:3902-11.
28. Guillaume T, Rubinstein DB, Young F et al. Individual VH genes detected with oligonucleotide probes from the complementarity-determining regions. J Immunol 1990; 145:1934-45.
29. Stewart AK, Huang C, Stollar BD et al. High-frequency representation of a single VH gene in the expressed human B cell repertoire. J Exp Med 1993; 177:409-18.
30. Sanz I, Kelly P, Williams C et al. The smaller human VH gene families display remarkably little polymorphism. EMBO J 1989; 8:3741-8.
31. Kraj P, Friedman DF, Stevenson F et al. Evidence for the overexpression of the VH4-34 (VH4.21) Ig gene segment in the normal adult human peripheral blood B cell repertoire. J Immunol 1995; 154:6406-20.
32. Gu H, Tarlinton D, Muller W et al. Most peripheral B cells in mice are ligand selected. J Exp Med 1991; 173:1357-71.
33. Sheehan KM, Mainville CA, Willert S et al. The utilization of individual VH exons in the primary repertoire of adult BALB/c mice. J Immunol 1993; 151:5364-75.
34. Suzuki I, Milner ECB, Glas AM et al. Immunoglobulin heavy chain variable region gene usage in bone marrow transplant recipients: lack of somatic mutation indicates a maturational arrest. Blood 1996; 87: 1873-80.
35. Pascual V, Liu Y-J, Magalski A et al. Analysis of somatic mutation in five B cell subsets of human tonsil. J Exp Med 1994; 180:329-39.
36. Hufnagle WO, Huang S-C, Suzuki II et al. A complete preimmune human VH3 repertoire. Ann N Y Acad Sci 1995; 764:293-5.
37. Willems van Dijk K, Milner LA, Milner ECB. Mapping of human H chain V region genes (VH4) using deletional analysis and pulsed field gel electrophoresis. J Immunol 1992; 148:2923-31.
38. Huang S-C, Jiang R, Milner ECB. Nonstochastic utilization of Ig V region genes in unselected human peripheral B cells. Mol Immunol 1996; in press.

CHAPTER 2

Framework Structures of Immunoglobulin Variable Domains: Implications for Antigen and Superantigen Binding

Alfonso Tramontano

INTRODUCTION

Antibody (Ab) molecules and B cell receptors (BcR) are comprised of a set of homologous modules, known collectively as immunoglobulin (Ig) domains. Four domains of the heavy chain and two of the light chain of Abs reiterate a characteristic antiparallel β-barrel structural motif. The structure's inherent versatility is evident in the display of binding sites in Abs for effector functions on the constant (C) domains whereas specificity for antigen (Ag) is encoded on the variable (V) domains. The uniform structural architecture of V domains belies the virtually unlimited Ag-binding specificities expressed by Ab molecules. Sequences at these domains of the heavy (V_H) and light (V_L) chain polypeptides reveal the process by which diversity is permitted within the context of a single folding motif. Short hypervariable sequences are localized at three defined regions on the heavy chain (H1, H1, H3) and three on the light chain (L1, L2, L3). Highly conserved framework (FR) sequences bracket each variable sequence within V_H and V_L. The Ag-binding site is assembled by V_H-V_L domain association with FR regions forming the sides and core of the structure and the hypervariable regions converging at one end as a set of loop structures also called complementarity determining regions (CDR). As their name implies, FR sequences provide a

Human B Cell Superantigens, edited by Moncef Zouali. © 1996 R.G. Landes Company.

scaffold to support the Ag-binding site, with their termini serving as anchor points for CDRs. An FR ensemble could be regarded as a universal template for CDR loops, an inference that derives from the structural uniformity of Ab molecules of diverse specificities as well as of diverse species. V domains have traditionally been studied as part of the Ag-binding fragment (Fab) produced by proteolytic cleavage of the heavy chains. Monoclonal antibodies (mAb) have contributed greatly to the elucidation of the structural basis for antigenic specificity. The Protein Data Bank now includes a number of Fab three-dimensional structures resolved by X-ray crystallography, including several structures of Ag-complexed Fab molecules.[1] The three-dimensional homology among Fab structures is exploited in molecular-replacement methods facilitating structure determination by X-ray diffraction studies,[2] and in computational modeling of Ag binding site structures.[3,4]

Ab diversification is established by various mechanisms which include genetic recombination of short discontinuous gene segments, somatic mutations in the hypervariable regions of the fully assembled V region genes, and combinatorial association of the heavy and light chain polypeptides.[5,6] Genetic segments for the V regions of heavy chain (V_H, D_H, and J_H) and light chain (V_L and J_L) are inherited in their germ-line configurations. Early recognition of sequence similarities within FR regions provided a basis for the categorization of V_H and V_L polypeptide sequences into a small number of families.[7] The evolutionary conservation of these sequences reflects primarily the contribution of the encoded FR polypeptides to the preservation of protein function and stability, while the diversity among families could suggest more specialized functions of FR sequences.

V region binding interactions outside of the traditional Ag combining site are described or implicated in an expanding context which includes regulation of the B lymphocyte repertoire, reactivity with autoantigens, and anti-idiotypic networks. A variety of proteins, both foreign and endogenous, have been reported to bind Ig through unconventional interactions with V domains. Mounting evidence of their ability to stimulate a broad population of B cells without the normal clonal restriction suggests their designation as B cell superantigens (SAg). By analogy with established T cell superantigens and their interaction with the T cell receptor (TcR) new immunological mechanisms may be anticipated for SAg in the B cell compartment. These developments need further clarification from a structural perspective. Unconventional binding implicates molecular determinants that should include FR structures. In this setting an appreciation for the molecular recognition potential of Ig molecules is of value. This chapter summarizes recent insights from structure and modeling studies that contribute to the understanding of FR determinants in relation to variability at the Ab paratopes and to the deduced unconventional binding sites on the V region.

FR CONTRIBUTIONS TO AG BINDING

To a first approximation one might expect that any specific binding site structure could be constructed on a set of FR sequences. Recently the CDR structures have been classified according to a limited variety of main-chain conformations found in the known X-ray structures.[4,8] Each "canonical structure" is defined by a pattern of specific residues within the local sequence and the length of the loop. A procedure is thus available to determine from sequence data alone the structures of five of the six CDRs, which can be combined to construct a model of an Ag-binding site. Variable domains of known structures with similar FR sequences are used as the starting point for building a model. Several new crystallographically determined CDR structures were accurately predicted.[8] However, high resolution structures and engineering of Ab molecules have revealed latent contributions of FR elements to the Ig paratope. Apart from providing the infrastructure for CDRs, FR residues can help to shape the binding site by participating in direct contact with bound Ag or as part of a second shell of residues that make tertiary contacts with the CDRs. The original distinction of hypervariable and FR residues was based on homologies among the known Ig sequences.[9] This does not necessarily imply a clear boundary between residues that participate in Ag contact and those that are prohibited. In actual structures of Ab-Ag complexes determined by X-ray crystallography the number of contacts vary with the size of the interface and some CDRs may not be involved. With larger ligands a number of contacts between FR residues and the bound Ag are observed. All of these residues are confined to the FR regions immediately flanking the CDRs.[10-15] In a second category, numerous residues dispersed over the FR regions can have short-range or long-range effects on CDR conformations. Differences have been observed in the relative positions or orientations of shared canonical CDR structures when comparing X-ray structures[4] or X-ray and modeled structures[8] by superposition of FR regions. These displacements were attributed to the cumulative influence of many FR residues that differed in the two structures. Chothia et al ultimately acknowledge that sequence variations within the FR regions can shift the canonical structures relative to each other by small but significant amounts.[8] In a recent comparison of high resolution X-ray structures, framework coordinates were least-squares superposed to illustrate increasing relative displacements towards the FR/CDR junctions (Fig. 2.1).[16] These positions may be considered as anchoring points for the conformationally defined CDR structures. Minor shifts or main-chain divergence at several FR termini can thus be magnified into significant overall differences between two Ag-binding sites. These observations strongly suggest that numerous residues

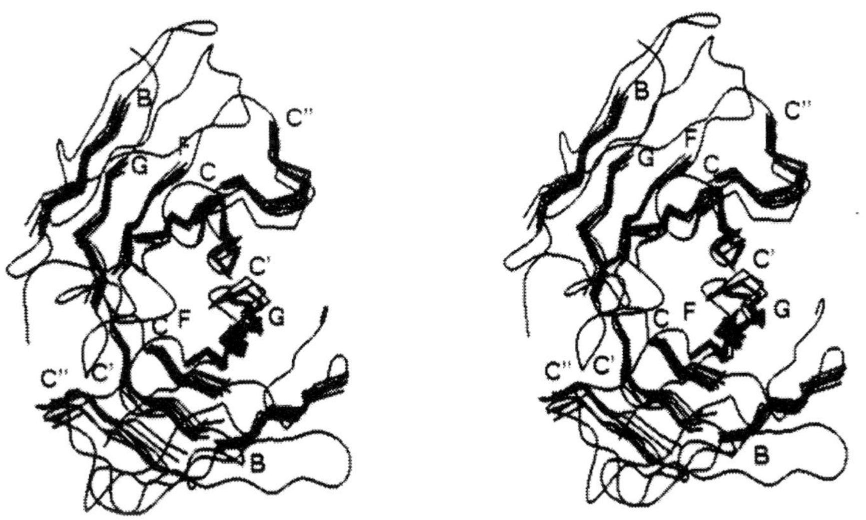

Fig. 2.1. Comparison of seven V_H and V_L framework regions and their endpoints by superposition of short segments of main-chain in core strands FR2 and FR3 of V_H and V_L. Systematic deviations in FR termini connected by CDR loops (C/B, CDR1; C'/C", CDR2; F/G, CDR3) and β-strand main-chain atoms (α-carbon traces) are apparent in both V_L (top) and V_H (bottom) chains as viewed facing down the antigen binding sites. The complete backbone of an Fv (4-4-20) is shown as smooth lighter trace. (Reproduced with permission from: Bajorath J, et al. J Biol Chem 1995; 270: 22081-84. ©1995 The American Society for Biochemistry and Molecular Biology.)

throughout FR regions can be critical to the shape of the Ag-binding site. Somatic mutations at certain FR positions may be important in clonal selection for affinity maturation. However it is also possible that certain FR-canonical CDR combinations are incompatible.

The prediction of canonical loop conformations has been refined by accommodating the apparent steric constraints between certain CDR structures and their proximal FR residues. In particular the observed structures of CDR H2 loops have not conformed to expected canonical conformations defined by sequence patterns in the loop. Variations in the main-chain conformations and the relative position of CDR H2 appeared to depend on the size of an underlying residue in the FR3 region. It has been anticipated that for a majority of V_H sequences, the size of the residue at position 71 is a principal determinant of the H2 loop structure.[17] The coupling of FR residue identity to binding site specificity has been unraveled in the course of engineering chimeric molecules combining FR and CDR segments from diverse species. The technique of CDR "grafting" introduced by Winter and co-workers promises a method for transferring the Ag-binding function of a murine mAb to a human FR structure.[18,19] In the process of "humanizing" the Ab acquires useful effector functions and sheds its foreign epitopes, making it less antigenic in human therapeutic applications. Essential improvements to the approach included introduction of selected mutations in the V_H and V_L FR regions to match the residues in the donor molecule. In the absence of three-dimensional structure information, the rational choice of sites for mutation has been made on the basis of a related structure or model indicating proximity of FR residues with critical CDR structures. Positions within both V_L and V_H domains have been investigated and found to influence ligand binding properties.[20,21] In the future, knowledge of the interspecies FR structure compatibilities could assist in the choice of appropriate human V genes used to humanize specific rodent Abs.

FUNCTIONAL CORRELATES FOR FR STRUCTURES OF V DOMAINS

The functional significance of V domain structures outside the classical Ag-binding site is a matter of emerging interest. Anomalous binding activity of various antigenically naive or immature Ig species could suggest that conserved V gene-encoded structures participate in unconventional interactions. The newborn mouse immune system expresses a high proportion of autoreactive and polyspecific Ig.[22,23] DNA-binding activity is associated with monoclonal representatives from the human fetal repertoire[24] and autoantibodies utilizing germ-line-encoded or unmutated V_H elements.[25,26] Structural relationships among Ig in the early B cell repertoire, rheumatoid factors (RF), and unique anti-DNA mAbs associated with autoimmune disease are suggested by shared reactivities toward anti-idiotypic Abs (anti-Id)[27-29] and by preferential usage of V gene elements with high segmental sequence homologies.[30]

Anti-Ids are directed against the V region of Ab molecules and so identify determinants (idiotopes) that contain sequences contributed from CDR or FR of the heavy or light chain. Idiotopes that overlap the conventional binding site constitute a novel subset as the anti-Id may present an internal image of the Ag structure.[31] More commonly idiotopes are outside, or only partially overlap the Ag-binding site. Anti-Id mAbs can define idiotopes that have three-dimensional structures composed of discontinuous sequences or that are confined to short linear sequences. Conformational idiotopes can also depend on remote FR structures or V_H-V_L combination. For example, upon grafting of a presumed CDR-encoded idiotope of a mouse anti-TNFα mAb to a human framework, anti-Id reactivity was reduced five to sevenfold. Several heavy chain residues in FR1, FR2, and FR3 were substituted with the cognate residues from the mouse sequence to restore the idiotope as well as TNF-binding activity.[32] Similarly, an idiotope within FR1 of certain human V_H4 family-encoded Abs is indirectly affected by light chain-association, with a preference for $V_L\kappa$-pairing.[33] Shared idiotopes of autoAbs could suggest the presence of structures that help to determine autoreactivity. Certain FRs are natural candidates for such "public" structures as they are present at accessible surfaces of the V domain and are encoded by a limited number of conserved gene elements.

Immobilized synthetic peptide arrays have been used to identify linear elements of idiotopes. Anti-Id antisera were found to react with sequences that mapped to FR2/H2, FR3 and FR1 sequences in V_H and similar regions on V_L domains of a DNA-binding murine mAb whose idiotope is associated with the pathological process leading to systemic lupus erythematosus (SLE) in mice.[34] Using the same technique, anti-Id reactivity to eight-residue peptides representing overlapping sequences of light chains of RF and other Ab identified sites in FR3 and FR1 sequences of V_L.[35,36] Immunoreactivity of these sequences is consistent with the surface-exposed orientation of residues at the homologous sites in V_H or V_L. Similar results were obtained in an earlier study using a panel of mAbs of known sequence to map an anti-V_H specificity.[37]

Cross-reactive anti-Id responses can be directed to simple continuous sequences containing residues from FR or CDR. Such is the case for a dominant idiotope of human IgM RFs.[38] Cross-reactive idiotopes of polyreactive and autoimmune Ig and of certain anti-hapten Abs[39] suggest restricted V_H or V_L gene usage in these species. This phenomenon is a hallmark of autoreactive Ig and RF in particular.[29,40-42] Intriguingly, a shared idiotope in human mAbs elicited against HIV-1 was identified as a heavy chain sequence spanning over FR3/H3 as deduced from an apparently complementary sequence in an anti-Id mAb.[43] A synthetic peptide with the same sequence was recognized by the anti-Id. Immunoassay revealed the presence of antibodies in HIV-1 infected sera which mimic the anti-Id in binding the FR3/H3 peptide, implying an autoAb response triggered by the virus. The potential biological role of the autoAb is of interest in understanding the regulation of the immune response to HIV-1. A number of studies now indicate that the immune response to infectious agents preferentially utilizes a small set of V_H genes that also encode autoAb. This shared V_H gene usage could implicate an important function for these genes in the adult repertoire.[44,45]

UNCONVENTIONAL V DOMAIN BINDING

Unconventional V region-mediated specificity appears also to account for the capacity of some proteins to bind a large fraction of the Ig repertoire, suggesting a B cell counterpart to the T lymphocyte superantigens.[46,47] Several examples of V region-directed activities that circumvent normal clonal specificities of the B cell repertoire have now been reported.[48,49] Whereas a particular antigenic specificity could represent less than 0.1% of the total expressed Igs, a small group of defined proteins are recognized by as much as 50% of Ig at their V domains. Their interactions are typically not competitive with the binding of a conventional antigen, and can be manifested in a naive or unimmunized Ig repertoire. Proteins interacting with Ig in this manner may be able to skew the humoral immune response by their activity on B cells or circulating Ig. Sites outside the Ag-binding site that are common to Ig molecules selected for binding have been deduced on the basis of homologies in the V_H sequences. Determinants of these specificities are apparently conferred by particular V_H genes. Structural details of these unconventional binding interactions are otherwise quite limited. Characterization of the Ig interaction with putative SAg molecules may help elucidate new B cell regulatory mechanisms.

Fab-binding and B cell mitogenic activity of staphylococcal protein A (SpA) have been known for some time.[50,51] Sasso et al have demonstrated a specific utilization of V_H3 gene products in antibodies that bind SpA.[52,53] These include many Abs in the human fetal repertoire that express the germ-line configuration[54] and in an unselected human Fab library.[55] SpA-binding capacity is high in early development and appears to diminish with age, leading to speculation that this activity represents a primitive function of the preimmune repertoire.[56] Sequences unique to SpA-reactive V_H molecules have been mapped to FR3 and FR1, which coincide with family-specific gene elements of human V_H3.[54,57] The conservation of these sequences in many mouse V_H genes and their correspondence with determinants of the V_HIII clan could also account for the common occurrence of SpA binders in other species.[58] These properties define a likely prototype for a B cell SAg.

It has been proposed that a bacterial product like SpA is not a unique ligand for the unconventional binding site of Ig.[59] A factor identified in the human gut, protein Fv (pFv), demonstrates Fab-binding properties with similarities to SpA.[60] It is thought to enhance immune defense in association with secretory Ig.[61] Although Ig-binding correlated with V_H3 gene usage, the restriction is not exclusive of other V_H families.[62] Affinities of pFv for monoclonal IgM of up to 6.7×10^8 M^{-1} are comparable or better than those reported for SpA-binding. Recently binding of HIV gp120 with B cells and serum Ig expressing V_H3 gene products suggests a determinant similar to that for SpA.[63] The affinity for a monoclonal IgM was estimated at 1×10^8 M^{-1}. As a candidate SAg HIV gp120 has been suggested to account for oligoclonal depletion of V_H3^+ B cells in individuals with AIDS.[64] The progressive loss of V_H3^+ B cells would appear to follow their normal or enhanced expansion in early infection. Thus gp120 may act initially in a manner similar to SpA, by stimulating V_H3 B cells, but ultimately contribute to anergy or apoptosis.[48,65]

V_H FAMILY HOMOLOGIES AND FR

Nucleotide sequence similarities of the germ-line V_H gene segments allow the classification of families of Ig genes within mammalian species.[7,66,67] Diversification of germ-line V_H genes into numerous family members provides evidence that evolutionary selection does not favor any particular V_H sequence. However, striking homologies in short V_H FR elements are noted within families and among different mammalian species.[68,69] These similarities allow the designation of three clans that perhaps represent a set of ancestral Ig genes. The two determinants of this classification define coding regions for V_H FR1 and FR3. The conservation of these segments would appear to reflect selection of some attribute of the encoded protein. The sequences are juxtaposed on V_H to define a uniform surface feature that is well removed from the antigen-binding site (Fig. 2.2). The structural definitions of the three V_H clans is consistent with the description of three V_H structure patterns depending on FR1 and FR3 residues as reported by Saul and Poljak.[70] A presumed environmental pressure acting to preserve these structures across phylogenetic development of the vertebrate immune system has provocative connotations. Conserved structures on the surface of V_H molecules could define functional determinants that impart a survival advantage to the organism. Observations that the mouse and human V_H repertoires are restricted in fetal development, with the overrepresentation of V_H3-like elements[30,71,72] could similarly implicate specificities encoded in family-specific FRs that are important to the early B cell development.

The detection of certain V_H and V_L family-associated idiotopes in autoAbs found in rheumatoid arthritis, SLE and other autoimmune or infectious diseases has stimulated keen interest in the functional correlates of these structures. Speculation that specific germ-line gene segments, together with unspecified mutations or D-J combinations, encode distinct surface-exposed FR structures in V domains provides a molecular rationale for potential immunoregulatory activity or other unconventional binding activity of disease-related Ig species. Recent analysis of a murine mAb sequence derived from mice with lupus nephritis suggested that a structure composed of V_H FR1, FR3 together with a sequence from the H3/FR4 junction may define a unique three-dimensional determinant that is characteristic of a subset of autoAbs expressed only in mice with lupus.[73] This site was proposed as a target for a hypothetical B cell SAg. Speculation along these lines is supported by recent work indicating analogous unconventional binding sites in Ig for candidate SAg proteins.

CONSERVED STRUCTURES AND SURFACE TOPOLOGY

A growing archive of Fab three-dimensional structures provides a basis for detailed comparisons of the configurations at Ag-binding sites and other V region features. FRs comprise a set of highly conserved tertiary structures irrespective of the species, antigenic specificity or isotype of Abs being compared. A more stringent analysis shows that the buried residues and those that form the interface between V_H and V_L domains are the most spatially invariant. The interface residues are primarily at sequences of β-sheet in FR2 and in FR3/FR4 sequences flanking CDR3 in both the heavy and the light chain. These units form the core of the V_HV_L structure which is coherently arranged as a third β-barrel motif. The FR2 sequences of V_H and V_L are in effect the least accessible regions in the V_HV_L structure. The coordinates of a small set of core residues (35-38 in FR2 and 86-88 in FR3 of V_L, and 36-39 in FR2 and 90-92 in FR3 of V_H) were used for superposition to generate a comparison of different high resolution X-ray structures.[16] The cumulative deviations (rms deviations) for all FR main-chain atoms calculated in pairwise comparisons are small (less than 1 Å) with the residues forming FR termini contributing proportionately larger values of 1 Å or more. Displacements are observed not only at the junctions of the CDRs but also at positions opposite the Ag-binding site and in main-chain coordinates of sur-

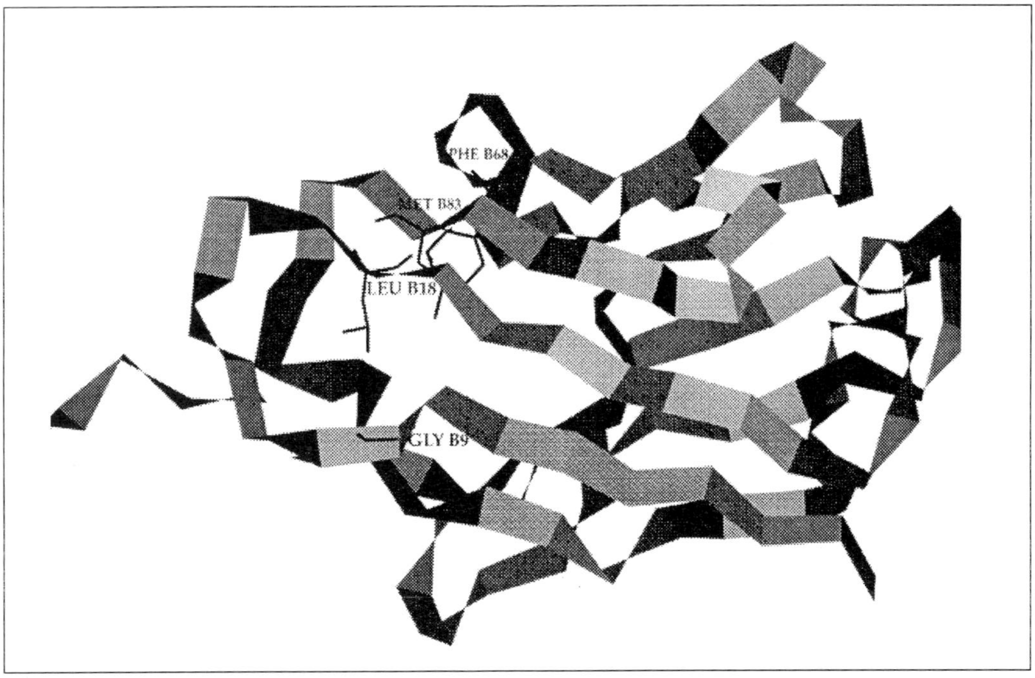

Fig. 2.2. Contiguous surface of β-sheet defined by FR1 and FR3 residues of V_H. The α-carbon trace is displayed as a ribbon and viewed from the side of the β-barrel motif. The model is based on coordinates of V_H3-Fab Hil (Brookhaven Protein Data Bank, PDB code 8FAB) and MacImdad® software (Palo Alto, CA). Conformation-defining residues 9, 18, 67 and 82 are indicated as stick figures. Numbering at positions 67 and 82, (68 and 83 in figure) differs from that in text due to sequential numbering of CDR H2 insert residues in the PDB file.

face-exposed regions which correspond to FR1 and FR3 sequences.

Defined sequence-dependent patterns in FR structure were discerned by the careful comparison of main-chain and side-chain conformations in V_H FR of human and mouse Fab crystal structures.[70] For example, the structures of Fab New and Fab Hil show systematic differences in the packing of β-sheet formed from FR1 and FR3. Residues 9 and 67, located within FR1 and FR3 respectively, along with the adjacent residues 18 and 82 on the intervening β-strands, comprise a cluster that interact in a coordinated fashion to define the variable conformation at the surface of the V_H domain. The systematic displacements at these residues is a structural consequence of the inward-pointing side-chains of residues 18, 67 and 82 which enforces their steric interaction in the compact interior of the protein. The volume of the buried side-chain of residue 67 is complemented by pairing with a suitable residue at position 9 (Fig. 2.2). V_H sequences of the human subgroup III would appear to share the same structure, represented by Fab Hil (Fig. 2.3A) and Fab Kol (Fig. 2.3B), with the preferential pairing of Gly9 with Phe67. The Fab New structure (Fig. 2.3C) appears to represent a group of molecules, prevalent in the human subgroup II and mouse subgroups IA, IB and IIA, in which a Pro9 is associated with a nonaromatic residue at position 67. A third class, displaying Ala or Ser at position 9 and a nonaromatic residue at position 67, occurs frequently in human subgroup I and mouse subgroups IIB and IIC. These are presumed to have a distinct structure, with examples seen in the anti-arsonate Fab 19.9 (Fig. 2.3D) and the anti-lysozyme Fab HyHEL-5. The residues at the four key positions in the structures illustrated in Figure 2.3 are given in Table 2.1.

Conformational patterns in the FR main-chain can also be expected to reflect on the local surface features. The solvent-accessibility of FR side-chains in the variable domains of Fab Kol have been calculated by Padlan.[74] A representation of fractional exposure (Fig. 2.4) shows that numerous solvent-exposed side-chains are concentrated at FR1 and FR3 sequences whose residues contribute to the regular surface of β-sheet seen in Figure 2.2. The only other pronounced contiguous sequence of accessible FR residues is at positions 40-44 in FR2. However, this sequence forms the turn region at the V domain surface that interfaces with the constant domain in the Fab. The illustration of residue exposure also serves to emphasize the buried sequences corresponding to the interior sheet structures at the V_H-V_L interface, as previously noted.

Table 2.1. Amino acid residue identity at positions 9, 18, 67 and 82 of the V_H structures illustrated in Figures 2.3A-D

		Structure/Residue Position						
(Fig. 2.3 label)		**9**	**18**	**67**	**82**	species	subgroup	clan
Hil	(A)	G	L	F	M	human	III	III
Kol	(B)	G	L	F	M	human	III	III
New	(C)	P	L	V	L	human	II	II
R19.9	(D)	A	V	T	L	mouse	VA	I

Subgroup designations are as reported in ref. 7. Clan designations are as defined in refs. 68 and 69.

IMPLICATIONS FOR SAG RECOGNITION

The conserved V_H3 family-specific structures may be expected to encompass the determinants for unconventional ligands for V_H3-encoded Ig. Structural motifs of V_H FR to a first approximation describe topological features of the binding site. Variable affinities of a SAg ligand for monoclonal Igs suggest that permissible mutations in FR or CDR can attenuate or even abrogate the interaction, even though the three-dimensional changes to the FR structures are probably minimal. Ig subsets may thus be able to discriminate diverse SAg structures. The binding of SpA and of HIV gp120 to a variety of nonimmune or germ-line V_H3-encoded Ig could indicate a direct correlation of the binding site with the characteristic structure pattern represented in Fab Hil and Fab Kol, both of the human V_H3 family (Fig. 2.3A,B). However, additional surface-exposed residues must be involved since some V_H3-derived Ig, possessing the pattern-defining FR residues at positions 9, 18, 67 and 82, do not bind SpA.[55,59] While systematic mutational studies will be required to precisely delineate the binding site, evidence for the contribution of a single residue, Lys57 at a nonconserved position in H2, to SpA binding has been reported.[57] How this non-FR residue is related to the family-specific structure is unknown, and it may not represent a defined SpA contact residue as this position is not invariant in SpA binders. Sasso et al speculate that the FR3 loop adjacent to H2 presents a plausible SAg interaction site as SpA-specific clones retain the germ-line configuration in this region (residues 74-77).[53] This structure is also significant because it projects away from the surface created by main-chain atoms of the β-sheet of FR1/FR3. Residues 72-77 make up one of two contiguous sequences of heavy chain FR regions that are solvent-exposed in the Fab (Fig. 2.4). The orientation of this loop in the V_H3-encoded structures (Fig. 2.3A,B) may differ significantly from that seen in structures from other families (Fig. 2.3C,D). Tilting of the loop main-chain atoms over the FR1/FR3 surface could obstruct binding with the surface residues in the latter structures. Residues within the sequence 74-77 could contribute to complementarity at the periphery of interfacing surfaces in an Ig-SAg complex. Furthermore, packing against the CDR H2 loop could allow a reciprocal influence of H2 residues on the FR3 loop conformation just as CDR H2 canonical structure is dependent on residue identity at H71 in FR3.[17] Differences between the SpA-binding and nonbinding molecules in the FR1 main-chain conformation near residues 9 and 18 are also apparent in the perspectives shown in Figure 2.3. In both examples of the V_H3-defined structure the surface is distinctly convex, with the interior FR1 strand forming the crest. The FR3 loop is tilted away from this peak. In structures representing human V_H2 (and clan II) the surface is nearly flat, while in the third type of structure, representing human V_H1 and clan I, a downward shift in FR1 near residue 9 creates a sharp discontinuity. Position 9 identity has been noted to be critical in clan designation and in defining these structural patterns.[69,70]

Superficial inspection of the available models is not likely to reveal characteristics of a binding site such as those formed by the CDRs. The β-sheet comprised of FR1/FR3 residues is relatively flat or convex such that side-chains emanating from the surface have roughly similar orientations or diverge from the center. This may indicate that the interaction with SpA or other ligands involves docking over a large surface area rather than the convergence of side-chains into a cavity or pocket. This type of interfacing is characteristic of some Ab-Ag complexes,[75] and may be expected when relatively inflexible epitopes are involved. The FR structures that are presumed to interact with SAg are probably quite rigid and unlikely to undergo conformational changes to accommodate the ligand. Conversely, structural analysis of the ligand may reveal a complementary flat or concave surface for modeling of a complex. Three-dimensional structure characterization

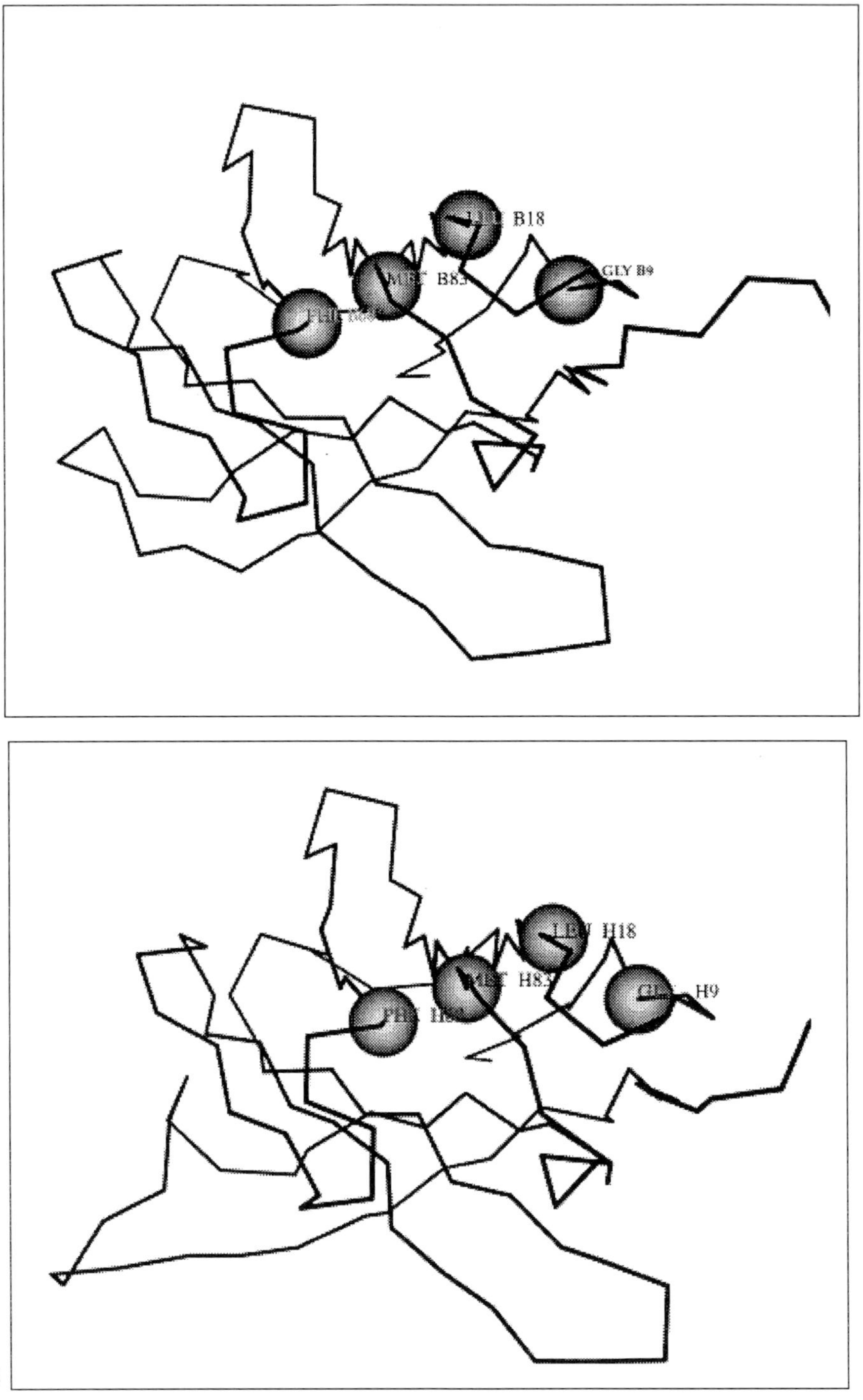

A

B

Fig. 2.3. Three conformational patterns of the V_H framework surface illustrated by four Fab structures. The α-carbon traces of V_H domains show the surface features of FR1/FR3 β-strands viewed on edge. Three patterns, defined by highlighted residues,[70] are illustrated by (A,B): Fab Hil and Fab Kol respectively, both of human V_H3 family, representing clan III, (C) Fab New, representing clan II and (D): Fab 19.9, representing clan I. The SAg-binding V_H3 structure (A,B) is distinguished by the convex shape of the surface, as indicated by the relative positions of highlighted residues, and by downward tilt of the FR3 loop shown at the top of each figure (see text). Structures with conformation of Fig. 2.3D (on next page) have a characteristic displacement of up to 5.2 Å at position 9 relative to structures with other patterns.[70] Residue numbering and graphic modeling are as noted in Fig. 2.2 (PDB files: A, 8FAB; B, 2FB4; C, 7FAB; D, 2F19).

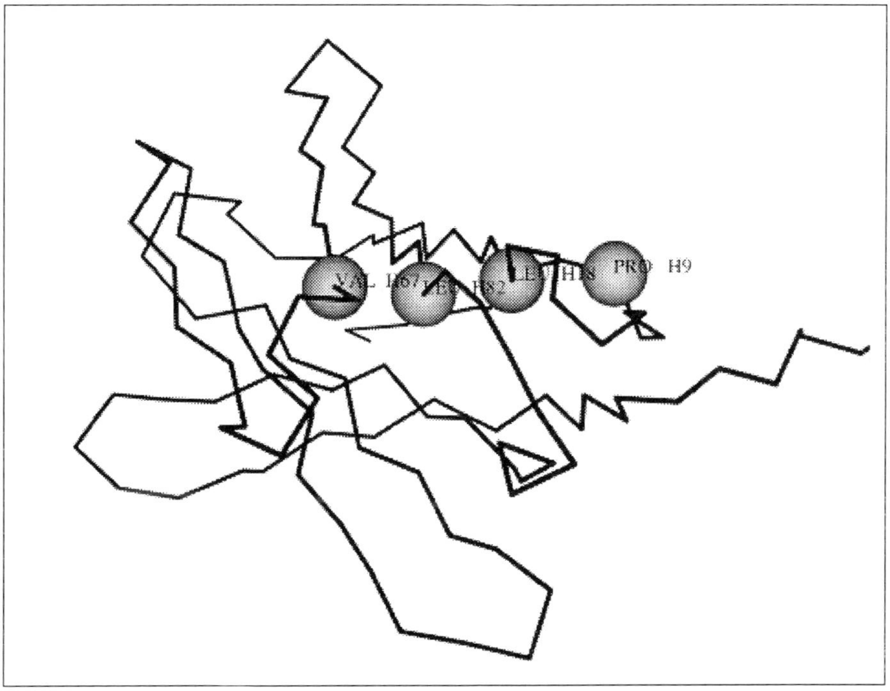

C

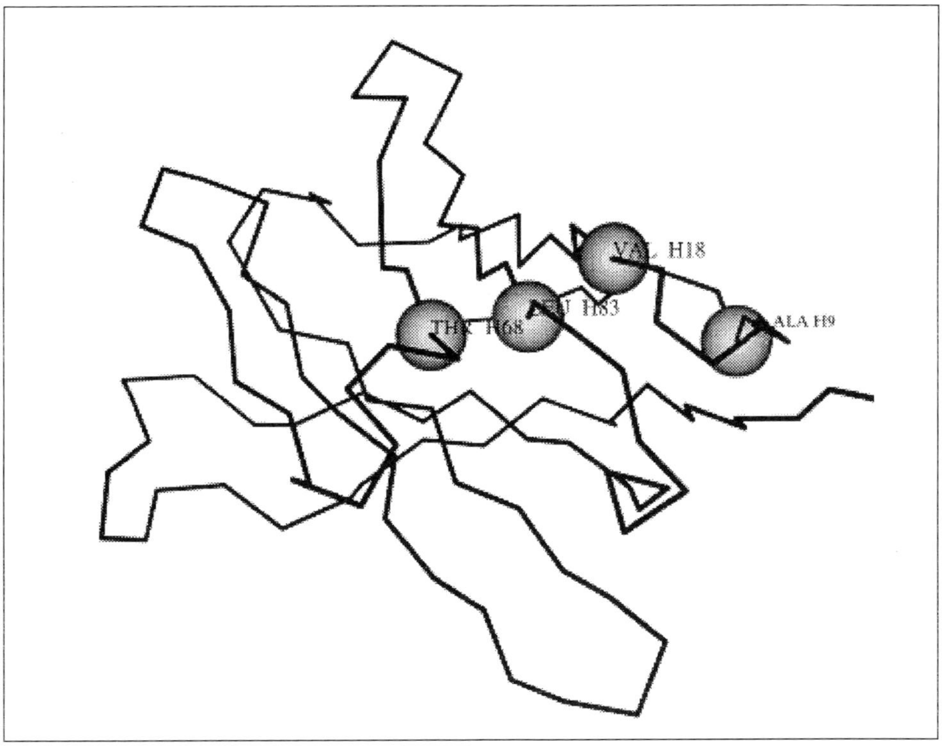

D

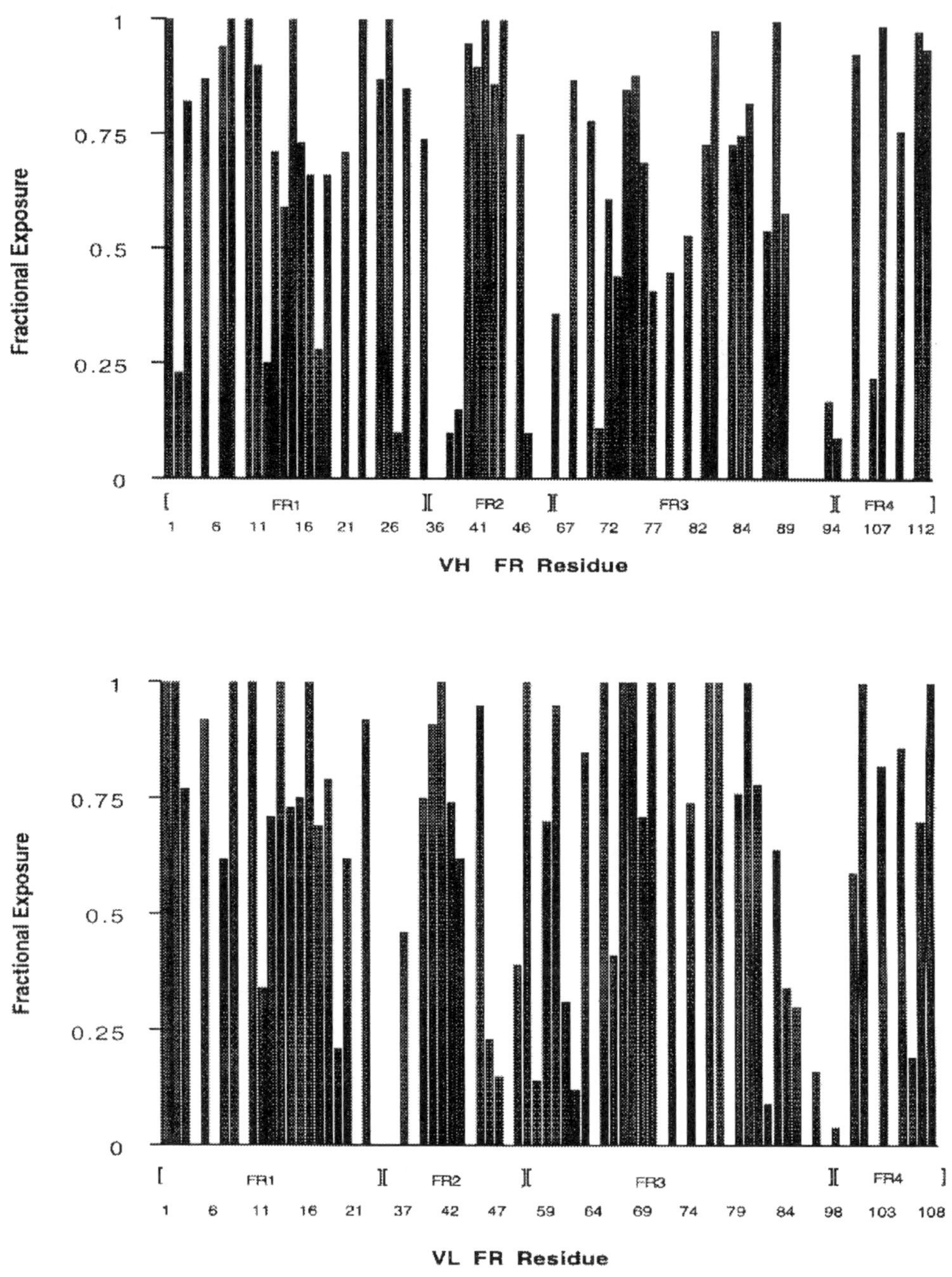

Fig. 2.4. Solvent exposures of FR residue side-chains in V_H and V_L of Fab Kol. Exposures are expressed as fractional accessibility according to definitions in ref. 74. Uninterrupted sequences of exposed residues, excepting those in FR2 of V_H and V_L that are at domain interfaces, correspond to residues at the FR1/FR3 surface, and also suggest determinants of an anti-Id response (see text).

of the relevant SpA domains or other putative V_H ligands will be essential for a further understanding of the functional significance of these ligands as B cell SAgs. In the absence of such information useful corollaries could be found in the structural analysis of other known Ig-binding proteins. Structural details of light chain-binding protein of *Peptostreptococcus magnus*, protein L, have been reported which may reveal commonalty among proteins that recognize conserved features of Ig molecules.[76] Because Ig domains duplicate the β-barrel motif, proteins interacting with FR structures in V or C domains could entail docking to surfaces with similar shapes. NMR studies of protein L identified sites on its tertiary structure that are affected on complexation.[77] Refinement of the structure to higher resolution should resolve details of the molecular shape of the binding site and the mode of interaction. It has been suggested that various bacterial proteins that bind Ig may have evolved from common structures. Protein L appears to share the global fold and other surface features of protein G, which is derived from related streptococci and binds Ig at C_H1.[78,79]

Ig and TcR V Region Analogy and SAg Recognition

Well-established similarities between the structures of V domains of Ig and the VαVβ domains of the TcR invite further comparisons of their ligand-binding functions. Conserved nucleotide sequences of Vα and Vβ gene elements indicate a similar organization as in Ig V genes. The protein fold at the V domains of the TcR is therefore anticipated to closely match that found in Ig. A nearly identical FR scaffold in the TcR and Ig V regions was assumed in engineering of a disulfide bridge between Vα and Vβ domains in a TcR Fv based on the known interchain disulfide linkage in Ig molecules.[80] Furthermore grafting of presumptive CDRs, based on Ig definitions, from Vα and Vβ chains of a given TcR to a second set of TcR frameworks, with the successful transfer of Ag and MHC specificity, provide additional strong evidence of the structural correspondence between the TcR V domains and V regions in Ig.[81] T cell Ag and SAg recognition determinants in the Vβ portion of the TcR were predicted on the basis of mutational studies.[82-84] In particular, a loop region analogous to FR3 74-77 in V domains is implicated in SAg specificity. Conformity of the two systems is reinforced by observed V_H and $V_β$ family-restricted specificity of B cell and T cell SAgs with their respective targets. These data corroborate the tentative analogy between models for SAg interaction with FR sequences in V_H and in $V_β$ domains. It may therefore be valid to extend this analogy to infer structural attributes of a candidate B cell SAg from the recent three-dimensional structure characterizations of T cell SAgs, staphylococcal enterotoxin B (SEB) and toxic shock syndrome toxin-1 (TSST-1) and their complexes with MHC molecules.[85-88] The structures of SEB and TSST-1, together with evidence from mutation studies, implicate apparently similar binding sites for complexation of TcRs. Because these proteins must first form complexes with class II MHC molecules before reacting with TcRs the putative Vβ-specific sites are perhaps more relevant in the MHC-complexed rather than in uncomplexed states. The TcR-interaction domain is evident in the MHC-complexed TSST-1 molecule.[88] This displays a broad concave surface facing away from the MHC-binding site. Residues implicated in TcR binding sit in a depression at the center of the surface while secondary structural elements protrude on either side (Fig. 2.5). Features of the sites may be indicative for binding to V_H-like determinants on the TcR. The shape of the site is consistent with a surface that would complement the model site suggested in Figures 2.3A,B. With a Fab oriented such that the C domain is directed away from the bound MHC molecule, as would be expected for the membrane-anchored Vβ domain, a V_H-like structure could fill the saddle-like upper surface of TSST-1 using the convex FR1/FR3 surface. This orientation also allows the V_H FR3 loop (corresponding to predicted hypervariable loop 4 in Vβ)[82] to insert into the center of TSST-1 where it may make direct contact with some of the residues critical for TcR binding.

While these models are purely speculative, they may provide a basis for further studies. Mutations in V_H domains directed at defining the unconventional binding site for SpA or other ligands might consider some of the residues implicated in the models. Previous analysis of V_H sites that recommends residues for mutagenesis to potentially alter immunogenicity[74] would also indicate appropriate sites within the proposed surface for SAg-binding. If the V_β-V_H analogy is valid the TcR V_β-TSST-1 model could suggest specific residues on V domains that project into the binding site of a SAg to pair with critical sites. Ultimately, three-dimensional structure analysis by X-ray crystallography or other methods will be required to elucidate the structure-function relationships in Ig-B cell SAg interactions.

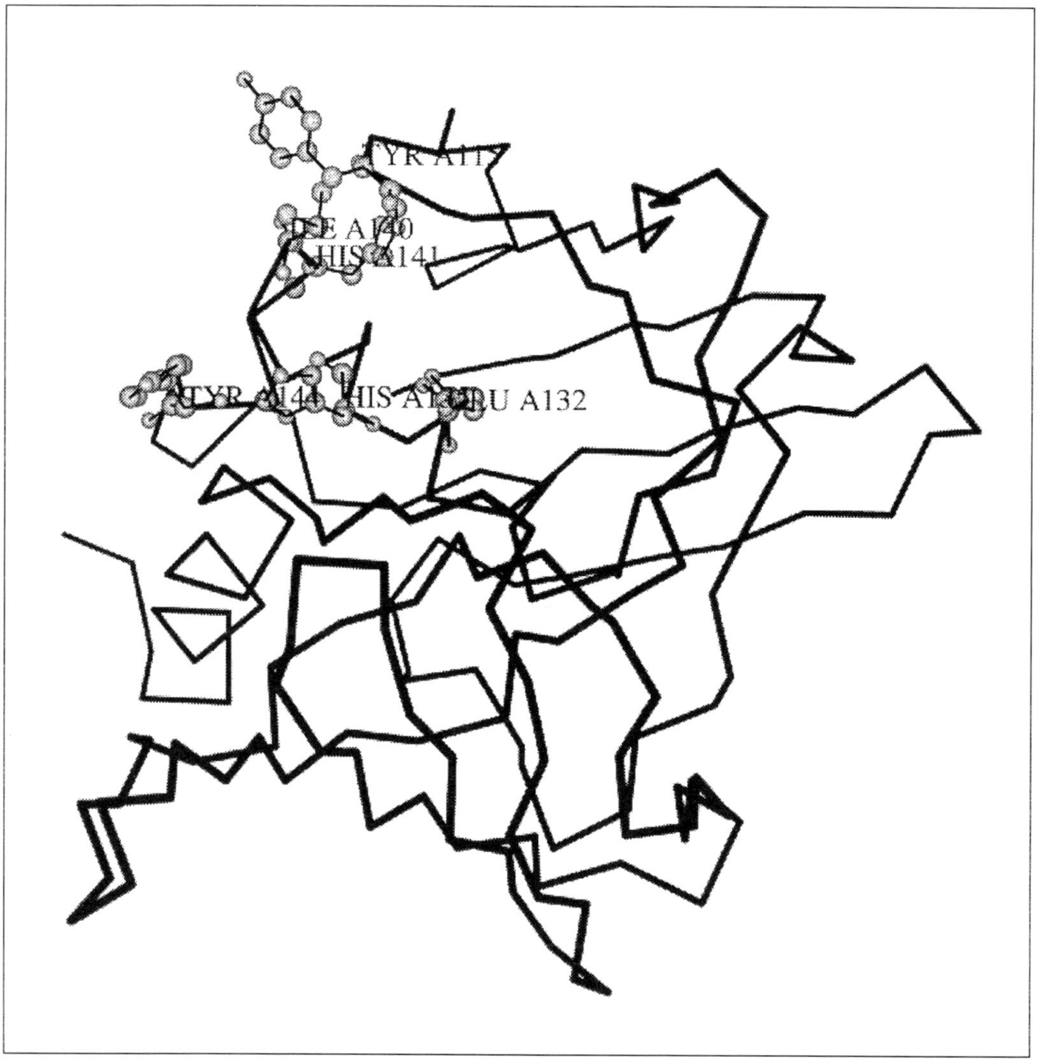

Fig. 2.5. Structure of toxic shock syndrome toxin-1. The presumed Vβ-binding region is suggested by the surface at the top of the figure. Residues that have been implicated in TcR specificity are represented as ball-and-stick models. The shape of this surface is consistent with the complementary to a Vβ surface that is modeled by the FR regions of V_H implicated in SAg binding. MHC binding occurs at the bottom groove as shown.[88] The illustration was produced as described for Fig. 2.2 (PDB code 1TSS).

B cell SAgs may reveal another arm of the immune system interface with its environment. It has been proposed that conserved surface features in V_H could specify structural determinants that confer an advantageous immunological function.[68,69] Evidence supporting a functional rôle of V_H FR structures in B cell regulation was reported in a study of B lymphocyte development in the rabbit. Unique V_Ha allotypic specificities are associated with certain structures in FR1 and FR3. Pospisil et al found that B cells expressing surface Ig with the V_Ha2 allotype were preferentially expanded and positively selected in the rabbit appendix. B cells of V_Ha-mutant rabbits that do not express the allotypic FR structures suffered extensive apoptosis and little proliferation.[89] The authors hypothesize that an unidentified foreign or endogenous SAg may signal B cell proliferation and development through V_H FR1/FR3-mediated interaction with the BcR. It is not clear whether candidate SAgs, derived from bacterial or viral sources, benefit the pathogens or the immune defense. As targets for the preimmune repertoire, SAg could allow an otherwise vulnerable host to mount a primitive immune response.[59] On the other hand the SAg activity of gp120 would appear to contribute a mechanism for immune impairment by HIV-1. According to one theory the coevolution of the vertebrate immune system and evasive mechanisms of a cytopathic agent gives rise to complementary facets that ensure the mutual survival of both organisms.[90] Superantigens may be cooperative in the balance between survival of the virus and survival of the host.

References

1. Padlan EA. Anatomy of the antibody molecule. Molec Immunol 1994; 31:169-217.
2. Sheriff S, Padlan EA, Cohen GH, et al. Molecular-replacement structure determination of two different antibody-antigen complexes. Acta Crystallogr B 1990; 46:418-25.
3. Chothia C, Lesk AM, Levitt M, et al. The predicted structure of immunoglobulin D1.3 and its comparison with the crystal structure. Science 1986; 233:755-58.
4. Chothia C, Lesk AM. Canonical structures for the hypervariable regions of immunoglobulins. J Mol Biol 1987; 196:901-17.
5. Tonegawa S. Somatic generation of antibody diversity. Nature 1983; 302:575-81.
6. Honjo T. Immunoglobulin genes. Annu Rev Immunol 1983; 1:499-528.
7. Kabat EA, Wu TT, Perry HM et al. Sequences of proteins of immunological interest, 5th edn. Bethesda: U. S. Department of Health and Human Services, Public Health Service, National Institutes of Health, 1991.
8. Chothia C, Lesk AM, Tramontano A, et al. Conformations of immunoglobulin hypervariable regions. Nature 1989; 342:877-83.
9. Wu TT, Kabat EA. An analysis of the sequences of the variable regions of Bence Jones proteins and myeloma light chains and their implications for antibody complementarity. J Exp Med 1970; 132:103-19.
10. Amit AG, Mariuzza RA, Phillips SEV, et al. Three-dimensional structure of an antigen-antibody complex at 2.8 Å resolution. Science 1986; 233:747-53.
11. Sheriff S, Silverton, EW, Padlan EA, et al. Three-dimensional structure of an antibody-antigen complex. Proc Natl Acad Sci USA 1987; 84:8075-79.
12. Padlan EA, Silverton EW, Sheriff S, et al. Structure of an antibody-antigen complex: crystal structure of the HyHEL-10 Fab-lysozyme complex. Proc Natl Acad Sci USA 1989; 86:5938-42.
13. Bentley GA, Boulet G, Riottot MM, et al. Three-dimensional structure of an idiotope-anti-idiotope complex. Nature 1990; 348:254-57.
14. Fischmann TO, Bentley GA, Bhat TN, et al. Crystallographic refinement of the three-dimensional structure of the Fab D1.3-lysozyme complex at 2.5 Å resolution. J Biol Chem 1991; 266, 12915-20.
15. Tulip WR, Varghese JN, Laver WG, et al. Refined crystal structure of the influenza virus N9 neuraminidase-NC41 Fab complex. J Mol Bio 1992; 227:122-148.
16. Bajorath J, Harris L, Novotny J. Conformational similarity and systematic displacement of complementarity determining region loops in high resolution antibody X-ray structures. J Biol Chem 1995; 270:22081-84.

17. Tramontano A, Chothia C, Lesk AM. Framework residue 71 is a major determinant of the position and conformation of the second hypervariable region in the V_H domains of immunoglobulins. J Mol Biol 1990; 215:175-82.
18. Jones PT, Dear PH, Foote J, et al. Replacing the complementarity-determining regions of a human antibody with those from a mouse. Nature 1986; 321:522-24.
19. Verhoeyen M, Milstein CM, Winter G. Reshaping human antibodies: grafting an anti-lysozyme activity. Science 1988; 239:1534-36.
20. Riechmann L, Clark M, Waldmann H, et al. Reshaping human antibodies for therapy. Nature 1988; 332:323-27.
21. Foote J, Winter G. Antibody framework residues affecting the conformation of the hypervariable loops. J Mol Biol 1992; 224:487-499.
22. Dighiero G, Lymberi P, Holmberg D, et al. High frequency of natural autoantibodies in newborn mice. J Immunol 1985; 134:765-71.
23. Hillson J, Perlmutter RM. Autoantibodies and the fetal antibody repertoire. Int Rev Immunol 1990; 5:215-29.
24. Watts RA, Hillson J, Oppliger IR, et al. Sequence analysis and idiotypic relationships of BEG-2, a human fetal antibody reactive with DNA. Lupus 1991; 1:9-17.
25. Chen P, Liu M, Sinha S, et al. A 16/6 idiotype-positive anti-DNA antibody is encoded by a conserved V_H gene with no somatic mutations. Arthritis Rheum 1988; 31:1429-31.
26. Dersimonian H, Schwartz RS, Barrett KJ, et al. Relationship of human variable region heavy chain germ-line genes to genes encoding anti-DNA autoantibodies. J Immunol 1987; 139:2496-501.
27. Isenberg D, Williams W, Axford J, et al. Comparison of DNA antibody idiotypes in human sera: an international collaborative study of 19 idiotypes from 11 different laboratories. J Autoimmun 1990; 3:393-414.
28. Isenberg DA, Staines NA. DNA-antibody idiotypes: an analysis of their role in health and disease. J. Autoimmun 1990; 3:339-55.
29. Kipps TJ, Robbins BA, Carson DA. Uniform high frequency expression of autoantibody-associated cross-reactive idiotypes in the primary B cell follicles of human fetal spleen. J Exp Med 1990; 171:189-96.
30. Schroeder Jr. HW, Wang JY. Preferential utilization of conserved immunoglobulin heavy chain variable gene segments during human fetal life. Proc Natl Acad Sci USA 1990; 87:6146-50.
31. Pan Y, Yuhasz SC, Amzel LM. Anti-idiotypic antibodies: biological function and structural studies. FASEB J 1995; 9:43-9.
32. Corti A, Barbanti E, Tempesti PR, et al. Idiotope determining regions of a mouse monoclonal antibody and its humanized versions. Identification of framework residues that affect idiotype expression. J Mol Biol 1994; 235:53-60.
33. Potter KN, Li YC, Capra JD The cross-reactive idiotopes recognized by the monoclonal antibodies 9G4 and LC1 are located in framework region 1 of two non-overlapping subsets of human VH4 family encoded antibodies. Scand J Immunol 1994; 40:43-9.
34. Staines NA, Ward FJ, Denbury AN, et al. Primary sequence and location of idiotopes of V-88, a DNA-binding monoclonal autoantibody, determined by idiotope scanning with synthetic peptides on pins. Immunology 1993; 78:371-8.
35. Hay FC, Soltys AJ, Tribbick G, et al. Framework peptides from kappa IIIb rheumatoid factor light chains with binding activity for aggregated IgG. Eur J Immunol 1991; 21:1837-41.
36. Marchalonis JJ, Dedeoglu F, Kaymaz H, et al. Antigenic mapping of a human lambda light chain: correlation with three dimensional structure. J Protein Chem 1992; 11:129-37.
37. Black A, Padlan EA, Givol D, et al. Two Ig framework II epitopic specificities recognized by a rabbit antiserum and a monoclonal antibody to mouse V_H chains. J Immunol 1990; 144:2620-6.
38. Chen PP, Goni F, Fong S, et al. The majority of human monoclonal IgM rheumatoid factors express a primary structure-dependent cross-reactive idiotype. J Immunol 1985; 134:3281-5.
39. Nahmias C, Cazaubon S, Strosberg D. A rabbit antiserum detects a V_H J558 subgroup

marker highly expressed among anti-alprenolol antibodies. J Immunol 1989; 142:871-6.

40. Chen PP, Albrandt K, Orida NK, et al. Genetic basis for the cross-reactive idiotypes on the light chains of human IgM anti-IgG autoantibodies. Proc Natl Acad Sci USA 1986; 83:8318-22.

41. Chen PP, Robbins DL, Jirik FR, et al. Isolation and characterisation of a light chain variable region gene for human rheumatoid arthritis. J Exp Med 1987; 166:1900-5.

42. Carson DA, Chen PP, Kipps TJ, et al. Molecular basis for the cross-reactive idiotopes on human anti-IgG autoantibody. Ciba Found Symp 1987; 129:123-34.

43. Wang QL, Wang HT, Blalock E, et al. Identification of an idiotypic peptide recognized by autoantibodies in human immunodeficiency virus-1-infected individuals. J Clin Invest 1995; 96:775-80.

44. Adderson EE, Shackelford PG, Quinn A, et al. Restricted immunoglobulin V_H usage and VDJ combinations in the human response to *Haemophilus influenzae* type b capsular polysaccharide. Nucleotide sequences of nonspecific anti-Haemophilus antibodies and polyspecific antibodies cross-reacting with self antigens. J Clin Invest 1993; 91:2734-43.

45. Huang DF, Olee T, Masuho Y, et al. Sequence analyses of three immunoglobulin G anti-virus antibodies reveal their utilization of autoantibody-related immunoglobulin V_H genes, but not V lambda genes. J Clin Invest 1992; 90:2197-208.

46. Herman A, Kappler JW, Marrack P, et al. Superantigens: mechanism of T cell stimulation and role in immune responses. Annu Rev Immunol 1991; 9:745-72.

47. Kotzin BL, Leung DY, Kappler J, et al. Superantigens and their potential role in human disease. Adv Immunol 1993; 54:99-166.

48. Zouali M. B cell superantigens: implications for selection of the human antibody repertoire. Immunol Today 1995; 16:400-7.

49. Silverman GJ. Superantigens and the spectrum of unconventional B cell antigens. Immunologist 1994; 2:57-64.

50. Inganas M. Comparison of mechanism of interaction between protein A of *Staphylococcus aureus* and human monoclonal IgG, IgA and IgM in relation to classical Fc and the alternative $F(ab')_2$ protein A interactions. Scand J Immunol 1981; 13:343-352.

51. Romagnani S, Giudizi MG, del Prete G, et al. Demonstration on protein A of two distinct immunoglobulin-binding sites and their role in the mitogenic activity of *Staphylococcus aureus* Cowan I on human B cells. J Immunol 1982; 129:595-602.

52. Sasso EH, Silverman GJ, Mannik M. Human IgM molecules that bind staphylococcal protein A contain V_HIII H chains. J Immunol 1989; 142:2778-83.

53. Sasso EH, Silverman GJ, Mannik M. Human IgA and IgG $F(ab')_2$ that bind to staphylococcal protein A belong to the V_HIII subgroup. J Immunol 1991; 147:1877-83.

54. Hillson JL, Karr NS, Opplinger IR, et al. The structural basis of germ-line-encoded V_H3 immunoglobulin binding to staphylococcal protein A. J Exp Med 1993; 178:331-6.

55. Sasano M, Burton DR, Silverman GJ. Molecular selection of human antibodies with an unconventional bacterial B cell antigen. J Immunol 1993; 151:5822-39.

56. Silverman GJ, Sasano M, Wormsley SB. Age-associated changes in binding of human B lymphocytes to a V_H3-restricted unconventional bacterial antigen. J Immunol 1993; 151:5840-55.

57. Randen I, Potter KN, Li Y, et al. Complementarity-determining region 2 is implicated in the binding of staphylococcal protein A to human immunoglobulin V_HIII variable regions. Eur J Immunol 1993; 23:2682-6.

58. Seppala I, Kaartinen M, Ibrahim S, et al. Mouse Ig coded by V_H families S107 or J606 bind to protein A. J Immunol 1990; 145:2989-93.

59. Silverman GJ. Unconventional B cell antigens and human immune repertoires. Ann NY Acad Sci 1995; 764:342-55.

60. Bouvet JP, Pires R, Quan C, et al. Nonimmune V_H-binding specificity of human protein Fv. Scand J Immunol 1993; 33:381-386.

61. Bouvet JP, Pires R, Iscaki S, et al. Nonimmune macromolecular complexes of Ig in human gut lumen. Probable enhancement

of antibody function. J Immunol 1993; 151:2562-71.

62. Silverman GJ, Roben P, Bouvet JP, et al. Superantigen properties of a human sialoprotein involved in gut-associated immunity. J Clin Invest 1995; 96:417-26.
63. Berberian L, Goodglick L, Kipps TJ, et al. Immunoglobulin V_H3 gene products: natural ligands for HIV gp120. Science 1993; 261:1588-91.
64. Berberian L, Valles-Ayoub Y, Sun N, et al. A V_H clonal deficit in human immunodeficiency virus-positive individuals reflects a B cell maturation arrest. Blood 1991; 78:175-9.
65. Goodglick L, Braun J. Revenge of the microbes. Superantigens of the T of B cell lineage. Am J Pathol 1994; 144:623-36.
66. Rechavi G, Bienz B, Ram D, et al. Organization and evolution of immunoglobulin V_H gene subgroups. Proc Natl Acad Sci USA 1983; 79:4405-9.
67. Ollo R, Sikorav JL, Rougeon F. Structural relationships among mouse and human immunoglobulin V_H genes in the subgroup III. Nucl Acids Res 1983; 11: 7887-97.
68. Schroeder Jr. HW, Hillson JL, Perlmutter RM. Structure and evolution of mammalian V_H families. Int Immunol 1989; 2:41-50.
69. Kirkham PM, Mortari F, Newton JA, et al. Immunoglobulin V_H clan and family identity predicts variable domain structure and may influence antigen binding. EMBO J 1992; 11:603-9.
70. Saul FA, Poljak RJ. Structural patterns at residue positions 9, 18, 67 and 82 in the framework regions of human and murine immunoglobulins. J Mol Biol 1993; 230:15-20.
71. Perlmutter RM, Kearney JF, Chang SP, et al. Developmentally controlled expression of immunoglobulin V_H genes. Science 1985; 227:1597-601
72. Schroeder Jr HW, Hillson JL, Perlmutter RM. Early restriction of the human antibody repertoire. Science 1987; 238:791-3
73. Zack DJ, Wong AL, Weisbart RH. Novel structural features of autoantibodies in murine lupus: a possible superantigen binding site? Immunol Cell Biol 1994; 72: 513-20.
74. Padlan EA. A possible procedure for reducing the immunogenicity of antibody variable domains while preserving their ligand-binding properties. Mol Immunol 1991; 28:489-98.
75. Davies DR, Sheriff S, Padlan EA. Antibody-antigen complexes. J Biol Chem 1988; 263:10541-4.
76. Wikstrom M, Drakenberg T, Forsen S, et al. Three-dimensional solution structure of an immunoglobulin light chain-binding domain of protein L. Biochemistry 1994; 33:14011-7.
77. Wikstrom M, Sjobring U, Drakenberg T. Mapping of the immunoglobulin light chain-binding site of protein L. J Mol Biol 1995; 250:128-33.
78. Derrick JP, Wigley DB. Crystal structure of a streptococcal protein G domain bound to an Fab fragment. Nature 1992; 359: 752-4.
79. Lian LY, Barsukov IL, Derrick JP, et al. Mapping the interactions between streptococcal protein G and the Fab fragment of IgG in solution. Nature Struct Biol 1994; 6:355-357.
80. Reiter Y, Kurucz I, Brinkmann U, et al. Construction of a functional disulfide-stabilized TcR Fv indicates that antibody and TcR Fv frameworks are very similar in structure. Immunity 1995; 2:281-7.
81. Katayama CD, Eidelman FJ, Duncan A, et al. Predicted complementarity determining regions of the T cell antigen receptor determine antigen specificity. EMBO J 1995; 14:927-38.
82. White J, Pullen A, Choi K, et al. Antigen recognition properties of mutant V beta 3^+ T cell receptors are consistent with an immunoglobulin-like structure for the receptor. J Exp Med 1993; 177:119-25.
83. Pullen AM, Wade T. Marrack P, et al. Identification of the region of T cell receptor beta chain that interacts with the self-superantigen MIs-1a. Cell 1990; 61: 1365-74.
84. Cazenave PA, Marche PN, Jouvin-Marche E, et al. V beta 17 gene polymorphism in wild-derived mouse strains: two amino acid substitutions in the V beta 17 region greatly

alter T cell receptor specificity. Cell 1990; 63:717-28.

85. Swaminathan S, Furey W, Pletcher J, et al. Crystal structure of staphylococcal enterotoxin B, a superantigen. Nature 1992; 359:801-5.
86. Prasad GS, Earhart CA, Murray DL, et al. Structure of toxic shock syndrome toxin-1. Biochemistry 1993; 32:13761-6.
87. Jardetzky TS, Brown JH, Gorga JC, et al. Three-dimensional structure of a human class II histocompatibility molecule complexed with superantigen. Nature; 1994; 368:711-8.
88. Kim J, Urban RG, Strominger JL, et al. Toxic shock syndrome toxin-1 complexed with a class II major histocompatibility molecule HLA-DR1. Science 1994; 266:1870-4.
89. Pospisil R, Young-Cooper GO, Mage RG. Preferential expansion and survival of B lymphocytes based on V_H framework 1 and framework 3 expression: "positive" selection in appendix of normal and V_H-mutant rabbits. Proc Natl Acad Sci USA 1995; 92:6961-5.
90. Zinkernagel RM. Immunology taught by viruses. Science 1996; 271:173-8.

CHAPTER 3

Functional Implications of Immunoglobulin V_H Germline Genes—V_H3 Superantigen Staphylococcal Protein A and V_H Gene Polymorphism

Eric H. Sasso

INTRODUCTION—IMMUNOGLOBULIN V_H GENES

The binding specificities of immunoglobulin (Ig) molecules are determined primarily by the amino acid sequences of their heavy (H) and light (L) chain variable (V) regions. In some instances, specificity resides predominantly in one V region, most often, that of the H chain. The V_H protein, usually about 110 to 120 amino acids long, is encoded by V_H, D, of J_H gene segments that are juxtaposed from their respective multigene clusters by developmentally regulated gene rearrangement events. The V_H gene segment encodes about 98 codons, which comprise most of the V_H protein, and include framework regions (FR) 1, 2, and 3, and complementarity-determining regions (CDR) 1 and 2. It is the major determinant of H chain V region tertiary structure, and a significant contributor to the antigenic specificity of the hypervariable loops.

Human Ig V_H genes are classified into seven families, with members of the same family sharing at least 80% nucleotide sequence homology.[1-4] The largest V_H gene family, V_H3, accounts for 51 of 95 V_H gene loci identified on chromosome 14.[5,6] The next largest families, V_H1 and V_H4, contribute 17 and 13 gene loci, respectively. While the V_H3 family also has the largest portion of pseudogenes, it still accounts for nearly half of all functional V_H elements.[5-7] Ig V_H genes appear to differ greatly in their intrinsic propensity for expression, such that certain members of

Human B Cell Superantigens, edited by Moncef Zouali. © 1996 R.G. Landes Company.

the V_H1, V_H3, and V_H4 families are often "overexpressed" relative to other V_H genes. Most human V_H gene loci (and essentially all that have been found expressed) have been mapped within a region spanning 1100 kb, in the subtelomeric band q32.3, on the long arm of chromosome 14.[5-7] While this V_H gene map was derived from study of two genomes, it enables the identification of most V_H genes from other genomes as well.

The V_H gene map provides an essential point of reference for two important questions in humoral immunity: (1) What binding specificities are encoded by the various germline V_H genes? and (2) How and to what extent do V_H germline gene repertoires differ? The first question ought logically to focus on intergenic variations in the CDR, which encode the hypervariable loops involved in classical antigen (Ag) binding. Classical Ag-specific responses in which one or two V_H genes predominate have been described, including the responses to immunization with phosphorylcholine or p-azophenylarsonate in the mouse, and *H. influenza* type B capsular polysaccharide in humans. Thus far, however, the only examples of antigenic specificities that are encoded by many or all members of a large V_H gene family involve nonclassical interactions, between Ig and the B cell superantigens. As will be discussed below, the interactions of Ig with nonclassical and classical ligands have different molecular bases. The second question, that of V_H gene polymorphism, also considers locus-to-locus variations in the CDR, but it emphasizes the variations seen when a single V_H locus is examined in many different individuals. The study of V_H polymorphism also considers the flanking regions and gene copy numbers, both of which can influence V_H gene expression. Polymorphisms of Ig V_H genes thus have the potential to influence the quantity and complexity of binding specificities expressed in the antibody (Ab) repertoire.

The presentation that follows will review work done in both of these areas. The novel specificity that human V_H3 Ig have for Staphylococcal protein A (SpA) will be discussed first. This correlation of Ig structure and function has established SpA as the prototype B cell superantigen (SAg). Next, population-based studies of polymorphism of several functionally important V_H genes will be discussed. The emerging picture of Ig V_H polymorphism reveals that individual V_H germline repertoires differ from the established V_H map. These differences may have significant functional implications.

STAPHYLOCOCCAL PROTEIN A—THE PROTOTYPE B CELL SUPERANTIGEN

THE ALTERNATIVE BINDING SITE OF SPA

SpA is a membrane protein, sometimes secreted, that is produced by most strains of *Staphylococcus aureus*. The SpA molecule has a three dimensional structure that resembles a string of beads, in which five highly homologous 7 kDa domains, E, D, A, B and C,[8] are followed by a 20 kDa transmembrane anchor, domain X.[9] SpA has two distinct types of Ig-binding specificities (Table 3.1). One, for the Fc region of IgG, has been intensively studied, and is the basis for the routine use of SpA as an immunopurification reagent. An Fc-binding site is present on all five homology units,[8] enabling free SpA molecules to complex with IgG Fc in a 1 to 2, or 2 to 4 ratio.[10] X-ray crystallography has demonstrated close contact between a site on SpA domain B that involves its single tyrosine residue and a site on an IgG Fc fragment that includes amino acids on both sides of the Cγ2-Cγ3 interface region.[11] This Fc site resembles that bound by many rheumatoid factors[12] and by another microbial Fc-binding molecule, streptococcal protein G.[13] It is distinct from, but may overlap, the Cγ2 site bound by C1q.[14,15]

The other SpA specificity is for the Fab region of some IgM, IgA, IgG, IgE, and presumably IgD. Termed the "alternative binding site" of SpA,[16] it has received less scientific attention than the Fc-binding

Table 3.1. SpA has two types of Ig-binding sites

	Ig-Binding Site On SpA	
	Conventional	**Alternative**
Ig region bound	Fc	Fab
Ig site bound	Cγ2-Cγ3 interface	H chain V region
Ig classes/subclasses bound	IgG1, 2, 4, some 3	IgM, IgA, IgG, IgE, IgD (some of each)
Sites per SpA molecule	5	≥2
Activity in Tyr-mod SpA*	absent	present
Binding to rabbit IgG	Yes	No
Human V_H gene association	None	V_H3

*SpA that has been chemically modified by iodination of tyrosines.

sites. SpA has at least two alternative binding sites, on domains B of D.[12,17,18] The maximum number per SpA molecule is uncertain, and the location of the alternative site within any single homology unit has yet to be solved crystallographically. Nevertheless, two lines of evidence prove the Fab-binding sites on SpA to be distinct from the Fc-binding sites. First, binding of IgM to SpA is inhibited by $F(ab')_2$, but not by Fc fragments of IgG.[19] Second, SpA molecules in which tyrosines have been chemically modified by iodination, termed Tyr-mod SpA, bind normally to Ig Fab, but not at all to IgG Fc.[19] On Ig Fab, the site that binds to SpA has been shown by immunochemical studies to be independent of the Ig L chain, and present on protein fragments containing the H chain V region.[20] The SpA-binding site is outside the conventional Ag-binding site of the hypervariable loops, however, because Fab fragments from a mouse hybidoma Ab were able to bind simultaneously to SpA and to the immunizing hapten.[21] Further evidence that Ig Fab specificity for SpA is structurally and functionally distinct from conventional Ab specificities comes from the finding that Fab activity for SpA is often a property of Ag-specific Ab.[22,23]

These reports suggest that the ability of some Ig molecules to bind the SpA alternative site is a genetically determined phenotype. The following section summarizes work that established that this specificity is a property of Ig encoded by V_H3 genes.

Human IgM that Bind SpA Are Encoded by V_H3 Genes

IgM Paraproteins

To examine the molecular basis for Ig Fab-mediated binding to SpA, a panel of 24 human monoclonal IgM was studied.[24] Most IgM were cryoglobulins, and 16 had rheumatoid factor (RF) activity. Each IgM paraprotein was tested for: (1) ability to bind to SpA, in a solid phase radioimmunoassay (RIA), and (2) V_H and V_L subgroup, using a Western blot assay in which H and L chains were detected with subgroup-specific anti-peptide antisera. Binding to SpA was seen with 10 of the 11 V_HIII IgM, but none of the 7 V_HI or 6 V_HII IgM (Table 3.2).[24] L chain class, V_κ subgroups, and RF activity were similar among SpA binders and nonbinders. V_HIII IgM bound equally well to SpA and Tyr-mod SpA, further confirming that the Fc-binding site of SpA had no role in these results.[24] Because the employed anti-peptide antisera targeted FR1 consensus peptides, V_HI subgroup proteins could have derived from V_H1, V_H5, or V_H7 genes, and V_HII subgroup proteins from V_H2 or V_H4 genes.[25] Detected V_HIII subgroup proteins should have all have derived from genes of

Table 3.2. The SpA alternative site binds to IgM, IgA and IgG encoded by V_H3 genes

Specimen Tested (Ref.)	Source	N	SpA-binding Ig	SpA-nonbinding Ig	% of V_H3 Ig that bind to SpA
Monoclonal IgM (24)	paraproteins	24	10 V_H3	13 non-V_H3, 1 V_H3	91%
Monoclonal IgM (33)	fetal B cells	27	15 V_H3	9 V_H1, 1 each: V_H4, 5, 6	100%
Polyclonal IgM (24)	serum isolate*	1	47%‡	34%	~90%
Polyclonal IgA (46)	serum isolate*	1	22%‡	78%	~69%
Polyclonal IgG $F(ab')_2$ (46)	serum isolate*	1	15%‡	85%	~50%
Polyclonal IgM RF (12)	serum isolates†	11	2-30%§	N.D.	N.D.

* a commercial preparation from multiple donors.

† IgM RF, each affinity isolated, and size purified under dissociating conditions, from sera of 9 patients with RA, one with hypergammaglobulinemic purpura, and one with no identified illness.

‡ For polyclonal IgM, IgA, and IgG $F(ab')_2$, values are the portion of a single test sample eluted from SpA-Sepharose. Of total IgM fractionated, 34% fell through, 47% was eluted, and 19% was unrecovered. IgA and IgG $F(ab')_2$ were 100% recovered.

§ Estimates, where for each ^{125}I-labeled IgM RF isolate, the % bound to SpA at equilibrium in radio-immunoassay (RIA) was divided by 0.71. (In a separate experiment, polyclonal IgM eluted from SpA-Sepharose subsequently bound to SpA in RIA at a level of 71%.)

N.D. Not determined.

the V_H3 family.[25] These results established that among human IgM paraproteins, binding to SpA is a specific functional marker for IgM encoded by V_H3 genes, and nearly all such V_H3 IgM bind to SpA.

Polyclonal Human IgM

The above finding suggested that the V_H3 restriction of IgM binding to SpA is not unique to paraproteins, but is a property of human IgM in general. To demonstrate this point, a preparation of polyclonal human IgM purified from pooled sera of multiple donors was studied. When fractionated by SpA-Sepharose affinity chromatography, 34% of the total IgM fell through, and 47% bound and was subsequently eluted (Table 3.2).[24] The remainder was unrecovered. Western blot analysis of the eluant and fall-through fractions showed a nearly complete partition of V_HIII IgM into the SpA-binding fraction, and nearly all V_HI and V_HII IgM into the fall-through.[24] This result recapitulated that of the IgM paraproteins. Thus, binding to SpA is a highly sensitive and specific marker for both monoclonal and polyclonal circulating V_H3 IgM.

Unmutated IgM of the Pre-Immune Fetal Repertoire

The high prevalence of IgM that bound to SpA implied that this specificity does not require somatic mutations, which are relatively infrequent in circulating IgM. In addition, SpA binding has been seen with IgM of chronic lymphocytic leukemia (CLL) B cells,[26] which are usually unmutated.[27,28] From these considerations, it was predicted that specificity for SpA must be encoded by the unmutated germline sequences of most commonly expressed V_H3 genes. These same V_H3 genes have been found to predominate in the fetal B cell repertoire, where they are expressed with essentially no somatic mutation.[2,29-32] Therefore, to demonstrate that Fab-mediated specificity for SpA is encoded by germline V_H3 genes, 27 monoclonal IgM derived from human fetal B lymphocytes were studied.[33] Nucleotide sequence analysis showed each to have V_H sequences in definite or probable germline configuration. Binding to SpA in ELISA occurred with 15 of 15 V_H3 IgM, but none of 12 IgM from the V_H1 (nine), V_H4, V_H5, or V_H6 families (one each) (Table 3.2).[33] Use of D, J_H, and C_L genes was similar among V_H3 and non-V_H3 IgM. The SpA binders derived from 11 different V_H3 germline genes which, because two were probably alleles, represent 10 different V_H3 germline gene loci. Included were VH26, which is one of the most frequently expressed V_H genes, and 56p1, 1.9III, and hv3019b9, which are closely related V_H elements that appear frequently in fetal and adult repertoires. These results directly demonstrated that SpA specificity is encoded by the germline sequence of one third of functional V_H3 gene loci. Combining results of other reports, specificity for SpA can be attributed to an additional 7 V_H3 gene loci.[18,23,34-36] Although these latter V_H3 sequences were in most cases mutated, their associated specificities for SpA were probably germline-encoded, and specific for the alternative binding site. Thus, at least 17, or about 57%, of the functional V_H3 loci have been demonstrated to encode proteins with binding specificity for SpA (Table 3.3). It can be concluded that specificity for the alternative binding site of SpA is encoded by the unmutated germline sequences of the majority, and perhaps all, functional V_H3 gene loci.

Human Polyclonal Rheumatoid Factors

That SpA binding activity is a specific marker for nearly all V_H3 IgM, whether or not they are RF, means SpA can be used to estimate the V_H3 composition of IgM RF in patients. In a study of IgM RF binding specificities, polyclonal IgM RF were isolated and purified from sera of nine patients with rheumatoid arthritis (RA), one with hypergammaglobulinemic purpura and one without diagnosed disease.[12] Each isolate was tested for binding to SpA and to a panel of human and rabbit IgG, and IgG fragments. In addition, to determine whether the IgM RF bound to the same Cγ2-Cγ3 interface site as that bound by SpA, the 7 kDa fragment D of SpA was used as a site-specific inhibitor of RF activity. It was found that all IgM RF had some direct binding to SpA in RIA, but the degree varied from almost

Table 3.3. V_H3 gene loci that encode SpA-binding Ig

V_H3 Germline Genes		SpA-Binding V_H3 Sequence	
Locus	Other Names	Clone Name	Reference*
3-7	DP-54	2E8	33
3-9	DP-31	SV-21	34
3-11	DP-35, 22-2B	5D4	33
Novel (3-11)	(DP-35, 22-2B)	2E5	33
3-13	DP-48, 13-2	4D5, 2B10	33
3-15	1.9I, 20p1	SV-19	34
3-20	DP-32	6H9	33
3-23	DP-47, VH26, 30p1, 18/2	2D10, 2B8, 2E7	33
3-30	DP-49,1.9III	6H7	33
3-30.3	DP-46, 56p1	5D11, 6C8, 6H12	33
3-33	DP-50, hv3019b9	5A10	33
3-43	DP-33	SV-18	34
3-53	DP-42, 60p2	SV-17, IW-34	34, 35
3-64	DP-61	3G11	33
3-73	MGTL	Hum2-3	18
3-74	DP-53, H11	Spa1-14, Hum14-3	36,18
Novel	DP-45	Ab #28	23

(*) Several V_H genes appear in more than one report. For the sake of economy, preference is given to a report of SpA-binding Ig having unmutated V_H sequences, or to a first report. Gene 2E5 is novel, but closest to the V3-11 gene. Locus names are from references 5-7, in which the map location of the DP-45 gene is not described.

none, to a maximum level (21% bound, at equilibrium) equal to half that seen with the nonimmune polyclonal IgM described above (42% bound) (Table 3.2).[12] This result indicates that about 2% to 30% of the IgM RF molecules had specificity for SpA (by adjusting for the fact that SpA-binding IgM do not bind 100% in RIA). With one of the polyclonal IgM RF isolates, and one of 12 similarly studied monoclonal IgM RF (of which 4 were SpA-binders), fragment D actually improved binding to solid phase IgG, due to a Fc-fragment D-IgM RF sandwich effect.[12] These same two IgM RF were also the only ones to bind strongly to isolated SpA fragment D in the absence of IgG.[12] Thus, these data indicated that: (1) the V_H3 content of circulating IgM RF appears to vary greatly between RA patients, (2) domain D of SpA has a V_H3-specific alternative binding site, (3) the Fc-binding and Fab-binding sites of a single SpA domain can be simultaneously engaged by separate Ig molecules, and (4) V_H3 IgM that bind well to the complete SpA molecule differ in their relative ability to bind the alternative site on isolated domain D. The relatively low levels of SpA-binding found in most of the polyclonal IgM RF isolates are at odds with an observed V_H3 predominance in synovial IgM RF[37-39] and might reflect biased retention of V_H3 RF in the synovial compartment or a high prevalence in RA patients of V_H3 IgM RF that fail to bind SpA. This latter effect could result if circulating IgM RF tend to be unusually highly mutated, as has been described for the IgM of circulating and synovial B cells in RA.[35,40,41]

Human IgA and IgG F(ab')$_2$ that Bind SpA Are Encoded by V_H3 Genes

Polyclonal Human IgA and IgG F(ab')$_2$

The above evidence, plus reports of Fab-mediated SpA binding by human myloma proteins and by serum isolates of IgA or IgG,[22,42-45] indicated that the V_H3 restriction seen with IgM should occur with other Ig classes as well. To demonstrate this point, polyclonal human IgA and IgG (Fab')$_2$ fragments were fractionated on SpA-Sepharose, and the V_H composition of the obtained fractions was determined by the Western blot assay described above.[46] The employed Ig were isolates from multiple-donor pools and, as such, were expected to be representative of human Ab in general. Results paralleled those seen with polyclonal IgM in that the SpA-binding fractions were dominated by V_H3 Ig and contained little (in IgA) or no (in IgG F(ab')$_2$) non-V_H3 Ig.[46] Some interesting differences were seen, however (Table 3.2). First, the eluted SpA-binding fractions were smaller—22% of IgA and 15% of IgG F(ab')$_2$ versus 47% of the IgM.[24,46] Other investigators found a similar difference in the sizes of SpA-binding fractions obtained from polyclonal IgM, IgA, and IgG.[47] Second, the subsets of V_H3 molecules that failed to bind SpA were much larger—about one-third of the V_H3 IgA, and one half of the V_H3 IgG F(ab')2, versus only about 10% of the V_H3 IgM (Table 3.2).[24,46] Third, the estimated portion of total Ig represented by the V_H3 family, i.e., SpA-binding V_H3 Ig plus SpA non binding V_H3 Ig, was larger in the IgM sample than the IgA or IgG F(ab')$_2$.[24,46] Thus, Fab binding to SpA is both restricted to and highly prevalent among human Ig encoded by V_H3 genes, regardless of C_H class. However, the strongest association occurs with IgM, of which nearly all V_H3 molecules bind to SpA.

Implications of the V_H3-Restriction of Ig Fab Binding to SpA

SpA is a Superantigen

These data have several direct implications, many of which have been confirmed or refined by subsequent research (Table 3.4). First, the V_H3 restriction of Fab binding to SpA strongly suggests that the V_H3 site bound by SpA is one that distinguishes V_H3 genes from genes of other V_H families, but not from each other. A binding site in FR1 and/or FR3 is thus implicated in a binding interaction analogous to that of microbial superantigens and T cell receptor β chains.[48,49] On this basis, it was proposed that SpA be considered an Ig superantigen.[46] Work described in the next section expands upon this conclusion.

Polyclonal B Cell Activation by SpA is V_H3 Restricted

SpA, either on Sepharose beads or on the surface of the Cowan I strain of *Staphylococcus aureus* (SAC), has been widely used as polyclonal activator of human B cells. This activity is due principally to SpA binding to the Fab region of cell surface Ig and has been shown to be absent among normal and CLL B cells whose membrane Ig fail to bind SpA.[19,26] The data presented above predicted that SpA-induced polyclonal B cell activation should be highly selective for V_H3-expressing B cells.[24] Several reports have demonstrated this V_H3 restriction, thereby expanding the analogy between SpA and the T cell SAg.[35,50,51] It is likely, however, that this restriction is not absolute[52] and may depend upon the B cell population employed.[19] In addition, because *Staphylococcus aureus* strains lacking SpA have also been found to activate B cells,[53] activation with SAC might involve a second mechanism, one that could be independent of SpA, and not restricted to V_H3 B cells.

SpA as an Immunopurification Reagent

It is apparent that the concept of SpA as an immunopurification reagent must be changed. In the past, it has been routine to regard SpA as specific for human IgG1, IgG2 and IgG4, and to overlook its binding to some IgM, IgA, IgE, and IgG3. Since upwards of half of circulating IgM, and smaller but significant portions of IgA and IgG (and probably IgE), are bound by the SpA alternative site, purification or isolation with SpA should predictably result in a partition of V_H3 Ig molecules into the "IgG1+2+4" fraction. This fact indicates that it may be appropriate to reread the literature of experiments in which SpA was used without concern for the alternative binding site.

Murine Ig that Bind to SpA are Restricted to V_H3-like Gene Families

Mammalian Ig V_H gene sequences are highly conserved, and sequence homology is greater between genes from equivalent V_H families of different species, such as human and mouse, than between genes from different V_H families of the same species.[54] Accordingly, it has been found that among murine IgG and IgM, two of the four V_H3-like families, S107 and J606, encode Fab-mediated specificity for SpA (Sasso, Kearney, and Mannik, unpublished data).[55] Genes from the other two murine V_H3-like families, X24 and 7183, do not encode specificity for SpA, even though a 7183 gene, 81x, is homologous to the human V_H3 gene 56p1, which does.[33] As expected, Ab encoded by genes of murine V_H families that are not V_H3-like, J558, 36-60, 3609, VGAM3-8, and Q52, did not encode SpA-binding Ab (Sasso, Kearney, and Mannik, unpublished data).[55] The modest contribution the S107 and J606 gene families make to the murine peripheral B cell repertoire is consistent with the small portions of murine IgM that are

Table 3.4. Implications of the V_H3 restriction of Ig Fab binding to SpA

1. SpA is a superantigen.
2. Polyclonal B cell activation by SpA is V_H3-restricted.
3. Immunopurification with SpA is not specific for human IgG1, IgG2 and IgG4.
4. Murine IgM that bind to SpA are encoded by V_H3-like genes.
5. V_H3 Ig binding to SpA is not a typical preimmune Ig specificity.
6. SpA binds to an unconventional site on V_H3 Ig.

bound by SpA[56,57] and might explain why SpA has not been widely used as a polyclonal activator of murine B cells.

V_H3 Ig Binding to SpA is Not a Typical Preimmune Specificity

V_H3 gene-encoded specificity for SpA is fundamentally different from the specificities of preimmune polyreactive Ab, even though both are encoded by unmutated germline V genes. In general, unlike the V_H3-encoded specificity for SpA, the specificities associated with polyreactive Ab are neither restricted to nor broadly characteristic of genes from any single V_H gene family.[58-62] Furthermore, Ab often lose polyreactivity as they accumulate somatic mutations, especially upon becoming high-affinity IgG of Ag-selected B cell clones.[61-63] In contrast, SpA binding is largely unaffected by the modest mutational load characteristic of IgM and is often present in Ag-specific IgG. Nevertheless, it is likely that somatic mutation sometimes abrogates V_H3 Ig specificity for SpA, as suggested by the finding that the SpA-nonbinding subsets of V_H3 molecules are larger in IgA and IgG, than IgM[24,46] and as demonstrated in a report of mutated V_H3 IgM that do not bind SpA.[64] These findings are consistent with the model that SpA binds to an unconventional site involving the FR, where the mutation density is relatively low, rather than a classical site centered in the CDR where the density of mutations is highest.

Localizing the Site on V_H3 Ig that is Bound by SpA

V_H3 IgM All Target the Same Site on SpA

To determine whether IgM bind to more than one type of site on SpA, inhibition studies were performed.[24] In an RIA with SpA on the solid phase, a V_H3 monoclonal IgM (Erik) completely inhibited binding to SpA by polyclonal human IgM, and by a second monoclonal V_H3 IgM (Buc).[24] Allowing for minor binding site differences that might exist between the SpA domains, this result demonstrates that the V_H3 molecules represented in the polyclonal IgM all bind to approximately the same site(s) on SpA. It also implies that different V_H3 IgM bind to SpA via the similar V_H determinants, since it seems unlikely that different epitopes on V_H3 Ig would all target the same site on SpA.

The SpA Binding Site is Dependent Upon V_H3 Determinants in FR1 and/or 3' CD2/FR3

To further define the Ig V_H region bound by SpA, the amino acid sequences of 15 fetally expressed V_H3 monoclonal IgM were compared to those of 9 SpA-nonbinding IgM from the V_H1 family, and one each from V_H4, V_H5, and V_H6.[33] All of the IgM were definitely or probably unmutated. At 24 amino acid positions (8 in FR1, 2 in FR2, 3 in 3' CDR2, and 11 in FR3), all V_H3 sequences had a conserved residue from which all V_H1 sequences differed by a nonconservative change. Excluding the FR2 residues, which are inaccessible to solvent, these residues localized a candidate SpA-binding site to two peptides, one in FR1 (amino acid positions 9 to 27), the other in 3' CDR2/FR3 (positions 62 to 84).[33] In an intact, folded Ig molecule, these peptides form two closely adjacent, solvent-exposed β-pleated sheets in a V_H region that is removed from the hypervariable loops (Fig. 3.1). This V_H structure includes the prominent FR3 loop, and is analogous to the region on TcR β chains that is bound by T cell superantigens.[48,49]

Additional insight into the SpA-binding site on V_H3 Ig was gained by considering two SpA-nonbinding IgM that derived from the V_H3 gene 1.9III, whose germline sequence encodes specificity for SpA.[33] One of these IgM, RF-SJ1,[66,67] differs from the 1.9III germline sequence by six amino acids, of which those at FR3 positions 76, 82a, and 84 are the most likely causes of SpA-non binding. The other IgM, RF-TS2[66,67] differs from 1.9III by four amino acids—at positions 57 and 59 in mid-CDR2, and positions 75 and 80, in FR3. The FR3 substitutions identified in these SpA non-binding Ig (at positions 75, 76, 80, 82a, and 84) were also highlighted by the above analysis of V_H3 germline sequences, suggesting that the FR3 peptide 75-84 contains a determinant that is critical for binding to SpA. If, as is likely, several amino acids contribute to a conformational V_H binding site for SpA, other determinants could also be involved. In fact, evidence that CDR2 residues can influence SpA binding was provided by an experiment with a third SpA non-binder, RF-SJ3.[64] The only sequence differences between the V_H region of RF-SJ3 and the 1.9III gene are at position 57 (the same substitution present in RF-TS2), and position 4, in FR1. RF-SJ3 specificity for SpA was restored by using site-directed mutagenesis to revert the position 57 glutamic acid to the 1.9III germline-encoded residue, lysine.[64] Thus, the glutamic acid at CDR2 position 57 was sufficient to abrogate specificity for SpA in RF-SJ3, and probably in RF-TS2 as well.

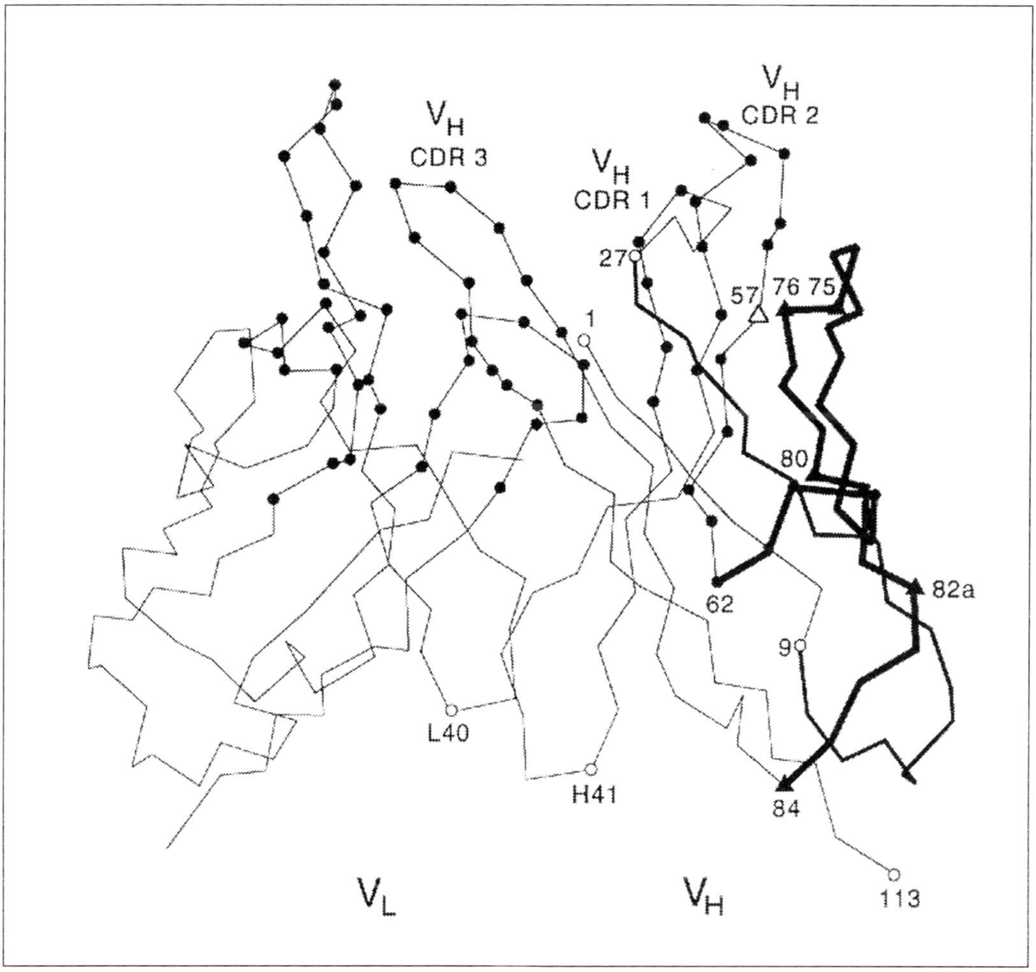

Fig. 3.1. V_H3 residues implicated in the Fab site that binds to SpA. Shown is an α carbon backbone model of an Ig V_L-V_H pair. (Left) *V_L polypeptide,* (right) *V_H;* (Filled dots) *V_L and V_H CDR residues. V_H CDR loops are labeled. V_H regions containing residues associated with binding to SpA are indicated by a medium line in FR1 (9-27) and a heavy line in 3' CDR2 (62-65) and FR3 (66-84).[33]* (Filled triangles) *V_H FR3 residues at which a nonconservative substitution is associated with loss of specificity for SpA.[33]* (Open triangle) *Residue 57, at which a lysine to glutamic acid substitution abrogates binding to SpA.[64] Also indicated* (open circles) *are the first and terminal V_H residues (1 and 113), and a FR2 residue on the V_L (L40) and V_H (41) chains. Figure is modified from that of McPC603 in Kabat et al.[65]*

This result with RF-SJ3 indicates that SpA binding may require contact with residue 57 in CDR2. It does not exclude the possibility that, in RF-TS2, binding to SpA might also have been abrogated by its FR3 substitutions at positions 75 and/or 80. Furthermore, it is consistent with an unconventional binding site centered on FR determinants because residue 57 is exposed to solvent and sits in proximity to FR3 (Fig. 3.1). Nevertheless, several comparative sequence analyses have failed to clearly identify any individual FR residues that make contact with SpA.[23,33,34,68,69] Thus, although substantial evidence implicates determinants in FR3, FR1 and/or 3' CDR2 as necessary to the SpA binding site and spotlights the 75–84 peptide in FR3 as a likely site for SpA contact, only residue 57 in mid-CDR2 has been directly shown to alter specificity for SpA. As this puzzle awaits solution, it remains highly probable that SpA binds to a relatively lateral site on the V_H protein, removed from the classical Ag-binding pocket and the apices of the hypervariable loops (Fig. 3.1).

Summary—SpA and V_H3 Ig

The above discussion demonstrates that SpA is a B cell superantigen by virtue of its ability to bind to the Fab region of Ig encoded by many if not all functional genes from the largest human Ig V_H family, V_H3. This correlation is independent of the Ig class, the L chain, and the D or J_H genes. The V_H3 site bound by SpA is unconventional, in that it is likely centered on FR determinants outside the hypervariable loops and might extend to include position 57 in CDR2 (Fig. 3.1). It is probably rare for somatic mutations to significantly improve the affinity of V_H3 Ig for SpA, but they can sometimes abrogate it. This effect might explain why the percentages of V_H3 molecules which fail to bind SpA are larger among IgA and IgG than among IgM. B cells activated by SpA predominantly express V_H3 genes. The biological importance of this bias remains to be determined. Since the effect of molecular binding to B cell surface Ig depends upon the stage of B cell development, the input of other signaling molecules, and the concentration, avidity, and crosslinking ability of ligand, it is conceivable that in vivo staphylococcal infections might induce anergy, deletion, or activation of Ig^+ V_H3 B cells.[70] In this light, it will be of great interest to examine the impact SpA-bearing staphylococci have on humoral immunity both in normal and autoimmune states.

Polymorphism of Ig V_H Genes—Implications for Superantigen Effects

The Spectrum of Ig V_H Gene Polmorphism

Ig V_H Loci Differ in Types and Prevalence of Polymorphisms

In the last several years, it has become apparent that many Ig V_H genes are polymorphic. Several types of polymorphism are possible. At a given V_H locus, allelism can occur as: (1) variation in the V_H coding region sequence due to point mutations or gene conversion events, (2) a null allele, due to gene absence by deletion, or (3) a two-gene or multigene cluster due to gene duplication or insertion. Sometimes, deletions and insertions involve gene blocks of several adjacent V_H gene loci. Polymorphisms, in the form of restriction fragment length variations (RFLP), can also result if these evolutionary events occurred in flanking regions, upstream or downstream of the gene. For a given V_H locus, the consequences of flanking region changes are probably insignificant, if due to an isolated change in a restriction enzyme cutting site. They can have functional impact, however, if important regulatory sites are modified. As will be described below, Ig V_H alleles often reflect combinations of these evolutionary mechanisms. In addition, the alleles of a given locus can result from different mechanisms. The overall amount of heterogeneity of Ig V_H repertoires is due not only to these types of allelic variation, but also to haplotype scrambling. Across the 1100 kb of the V_H cluster, linkage disequilibrium is largely absent, except among closely adjacent V_H loci.[7,71] Thus, the complexity of V_H gene heterogeneity is such that neither the types nor prevalence of alleles at a V_H gene locus can be completely predicted from knowledge of another V_H locus.[71] To know, one must look.

Defining the Alleles of Ig V_H Loci

A clear understanding of V_H polymorphism requires identifying the alleles of a locus in question, and knowing for each allele its coding region sequence, gene copy number, RFLP, and prevalence. In addition, unnoticed variations might differentially influence the intrinsic propensity of alleles to be rearranged. Population-based studies, supplemented by analysis of gene segregation in families and allele-specific sequence data, are essential to convincingly demonstrate allelism among Ig V_H genes. A high-resolution view of V_H allelism has been slow to emerge because, when similar V_H sequences are cloned from unrelated individuals, it is routinely not possible to know whether they are alleles or from distinct V_H loci. Furthermore, the limited specificity of RFLP analysis by conventional Southern hybridization means that the identity of detected V_H genes is usually not known, and discrimination between comigrating allelic sequence variants is usually not possible.

These constraints have been overcome by studying V_H polymorphism with synthetic oligonucleotide probes, usually 21 bp in length.[71,72] Using a modified Southern hybridization technique and postwashes with tetramethylammonium chloride, oligonucleotide RFLP analysis is exquisitely specific, and is sufficiently sensitive to detect single-copy germline genes in genomic DNA. The nucleotide sequences of target regions in detected V_H genes can be exactly predicted, and homologous genes can be readily distinguished.[73-76] A critical advantage of sequence-specific RFLP analysis is that the data obtained are comprehensive. A positive result identifies all genes having sequence identical to that of the oligomer probe. A "blank" hybridization result is a definitive negative, in that no gene with the sequence of the employed probe can exist in that genome. Several V_H gene loci have been studied in depth by this approach. They are discussed in the following sections.

Polymorphism of Ig V_H3 Genes

The 56p1 Gene—a Polymorphic Member of Tandemly Arrayed V_H3/V_H4 Gene Pairs

The 56p1 gene was originally reported as the most frequently expressed V_H element in a fetal library.[2] Subsequent reports have confirmed its high frequently in some fetal and adult expressed repertoires.[29,31,77] In addition, hybridization studies with a flanking region probe that codetects 56p1 and hv3005, which differ by only two silent nucleotide substitutions, found them to be simultaneously absent in about 20% of lupus and RA patients, versus only 2% of normals.[78] To elucidate the germline representation of 56p1, hv3005, and two closely related V_H3 genes, a hybridization study of normal, predominantly Caucasian subjects was performed with oligonucleotide probes.[71] The 56p1 gene was detected in 62%, hv3005 in 35%, 1.9III in 92% and hv3019b9 in 96%.[71] Simultaneous absence of 56p1 and hv3005 occurred in 19%.[71] The distribution of these genes in the population indicated that: (1) 56p1, 1.9III and hv3019b9 occupy three (or more) separate loci, (2) 56p1, when present, was usually linked to 1.9III, and (3) hv3005 appeared to be allelic to both 1.9III and 56p1. Furthermore, in some haplotypes, 1.9III and hv3019b9 were duplicated, meaning that diploid genomes can have up to four copies of either.[71] At least five different 56p1/hv3005/1.9III haplotypes were found. The relatively high gene prevalence of the four V_H3 genes (35% to 96%) indicated that individual V_H loci are commonly dominated by only one to four alleles. It was concluded that V_H gene heterogeneity derives, in large part, from the diversity of haplotypes in the population, and not only from allelic variation.[71]

Table 3.5. Polymorphism of 56p1 and related V_H3 genes

1. Four related V_H3 elements- 56p1, hv3005, 1.9III (V3-30), hv3019b9 (V3-33). Prevalences: 62%, 35%, 92%, 96%.
2. 56p1 (V3-30.3) occurs on a 5-gene, 50 kb insertion, with a duplicated 1.9III (V3-30.5), and three V_H4 genes (V4-30.1, 4-30.2, 4-30.4).
3. hv3005 is allelic to the 50 kb insertion, occupying 56p1-negative haplotypes.
4. hv3019b9 is a distinct locus (V3-33), outside the 50 kb insertion, that is sometimes duplicated.
5. Null alleles exist for each of these V_H3 elements. Simultaneous absence of 56p1 and hv3005 was seen in 19% of normal Caucasians.
6. The V_H3 genes are interspersed with V_H4 genes.
7. Ethnic differences exist.

Subsequent study of these V_H3 genes in an Afro-American population found lower prevalence than in Caucasians for hv3005, 1.9III and hv3019b9.[79] This ethnic difference was partly due to the existence in Afro-Americans of novel alleles of hv3005 and hv3019, each of which has an RFLP and coding region sequence distinct from those of its allelic counterpart (Sasso and Suzuki, unpublished data). Preliminary data suggest that in Afro-Americans these two alleles might be more prevalent in lupus patients than normals.[79]

To further clarify the germline relation of 56p1, hv3005, 1.9III, and hv3019b9, a lambda phage library of genomic DNA was studied.[73] Four clones were found, each containing one of the V_H3 genes, each of which was linked to one of four homologous V_H4 genes. Family segregation data indicated that two of these V_H3/V_H4 gene pairs, 56p1/3d216d and 1.9III/1.9II, occupied one haplotype, and another, hv3005/hv4005, occupied the other haplotype. The fourth V_H3/V_H4 pair, hv3019b9/3d277, could have derived from either.[73] Another report has confirmed these findings, and shown that linked 56p1 and 1.9III genes are part of a 50 kb 5-gene insertion.[80] When present, this insertion occurs between the V_H3/V_H4 gene pairs 3019b9/3d277d (also known as V3-33/V4-31) and 1.9III/1.9II (also known as V3-30/V4-28). Thus, duplication events have interspersed V_H3 and V_H4 genes, such that in places, they appear in tandemly arrayed gene pairs (Table 3.5).

Ethnic Differences in Polymorphism of the VH26 Gene

The VH26 gene is one of the most frequently expressed human Ig V_H genes.[81,82] Also known as 18/2,[83] 30p1,[2] DP-47,[84] or V3-23,[5] it was the first human V_H3 gene to be cloned.[85] (Subsequently, a corrected nucleotide sequence was designated VH26c).[86] VH26 has been found to encode autoantibodies, including anti-DNA Ab and RF,[39,83,87] as well as Ab to a number of microbial Ag, including rabies virus,[62] *Haemophilus influenza* type b polysaccharide,[88,89] SpA,[33] and HIV gp120.[90] VH26 also encodes the 16/6 idiotype, which has been associated with systemic lupus erythematosus.[91,92] The VH26 gene was mapped to a region over 300 kb upstream of the most 3' V_H gene, V_H6,[93] then localized to the V3-23 locus, 320 kb 5' of V_H6.[5] VH26 occupies two loci, however, because RFLP analysis with oligonucleotide probes identified two nonallelic VH26 hybridization bands, designated the A and B loci, on Taq I fragments of 7.0 kb and 5.0 kb, respectively.[93] In some haplotypes, the 7.0 kb band of locus A is absent.[93,94]

To better understand the germline representation of VH26, oligonucleotide probes targeting VH26 CDR were used in sequence-specific RFLP analysis of DNA from 72 Caucasians, 52 Asians, 35 American blacks, and members of six families (Fig. 3.2).[76] The A locus was detected in 89% of Caucasians, 75% of Asians and 26% of Blacks ($p < 0.0005$). The B locus was detected on a 5.0 kb Taq I restriction fragment in nearly all subjects, but additional bands, whose distribution in the population and segregation in families indicated they are B locus alleles, occurred at 6.8 kb in 10% of Asians and 3% of Blacks ($p < 0.025$), and at 3.7 kb in 1.4% of Caucasians, 21% of Asians, and 9% of blacks ($p < 0.025$) (Table 3.6). In Asians only, the 3.7 kb restriction fragment occurred as a multiple-duplication unit containing three or four gene copies based on its markedly increased hybridization band intensity. Examples of duplications of other VH26 alleles, and null alleles of the B locus, were also seen. The number of different VH26 alleles identified was three at locus A, and 8 at locus B.[76]

Cloning of germline V_H genes indicated that the locus B allele at 5.0 kb contains an exact VH26 sequence, as might the alleles at 7.0 and 6.8 kb. In contrast, the sequence cloned from the 3.7 kb allele of locus B differed from VH26 by 9 nucleotides, encoding 5 amino acid changes in CDR2 (Fig. 3.3).[76] This novel sequence variant appears to have evolved by a gene conversion event, in which a CDR2 segment was donated by either of the upstream V_H3 genes 60p2 or 8-1B (loci V3-53 or V3-66, respectively). As such, the 3.7 kb VH26 allele belongs to a different CDR2 canonical structure group than VH26 and could encode different antigenic specificities.[95] In the population studied, the total gene doses at locus A plus locus B ranged from one to as many as six copies of VH26-containing genes and from zero to

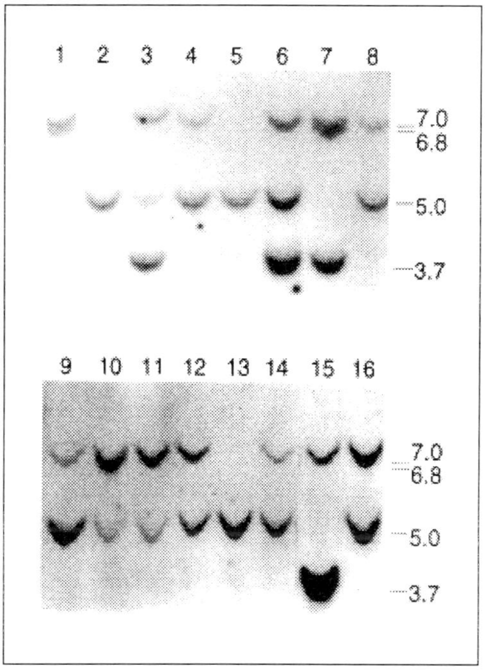

Fig. 3.2. Detection of VH26 and related germline genes by oligonucleotide hybridization. Aliquots of DNA extracted from peripheral blood leukocytes from 16 unrelated donors were digested with TaqI and separated on 1% agarose gels, 12 μg per lane. Gels were dried down and hybridized with [^{32}P] end-labeled probe M8 which targets VH26 in CDR1. VH26-related hybridization bands appear on fragments of 7.0 kb (locus A), and 6.8, 5.0, and 3.7 kb (all locus B). Hybridization results in lanes 8 and 14 resemble those of a control subject known to have one gene copy at 7.0 kb, and two gene copies at 5.0 kb. Lanes 1, 7, and 10 depict the 6.8 kb locus B allele. Lane 15 shows a subject who is homozygous for the 3.7 kb multi-duplication allele of locus B. Lane 16 shows a subject with a total of 6 copies of VH26 genes. Restriction fragment sizes, in kb, appear to the right. (Reprinted with permission from Sasso EH et al. J Clin Invest 1995; 96: 1591-00. ©1995 American Society for Clinical Investigation.)

Table 3.6. Prevalences of VH26 hybridization bands detected in three ethnic groups

Taq I band	White (n=72)	Asian (n=52)	Black (n=35)	P value
7.0 kb, locus A64 (89%)	39 (75%)	9 (26%)	<0.0005	
6.8 kb, locus B	0	5 (10%)	1 (3%)	<0.02
5.0 kb, locus B	72 (100%)	50 (96%)	34 (97%)	N.S.
3.7 kb, locus B	1 (1.4%)	11 (21%)	3 (9%)	<0.001

The numbers and percentages of subjects possessing hybridization bands detected with VH26 probe M8 are indicated by TaqI restriction fragment size and ethnicity. P values are derived from chi square analysis with two degrees of freedom. N.S., not significant (P>0.05). (Reprinted, with modifications, with permission from: Sasso EH et al. J Clin Invest 1995; 96: 1591-00. ©1995 American Society for Clinical Investigation.)

A

```
          50        52  a   53                 CDR2                 60                                                     70
VH26    GCT ATT AGT GGT AGT GGT GGT AGC ACA TAC TAC GCA GAC TCC GTG AAG GGC CGG TTC ACC ATC TCC AGA GAC
5.0 kb  --- --- --- --- --- --- --- --- --- --- --- --- --- --- --- --- --- --- --- --- --- --- --- ---
3.7 kb  -T- --- TA- A-C G-- --- A-- --- --- --- --T --- --- --- --- --- --- --- --- --- --- --- --- --T
8-1B*   -T- --- TA- A-C G-- --- A-C(   )--- --- --- --- --- --- --- --- --- --- --- --- --- --- ---
8-1B    -T- --- TA-(   )--C --- --- --- --- --- --- --- --- --- --- --- --- --- --- --- --- --- ---
60p1    -T- --- TA-(   )--C --- --- --- --- --- --- --- --- --- --- --- --- --- --- --- --- --- ---
```

B

```
            50  CDR2    60           70
VH26        A ISGSGGSTYYA DSVKGRFTIS RD
5.0 kb      - ----------- ---------- --
3.7 kb      V -YSG-S----- ---------- --
8-1B*       V -YSG-S.---- ---------- --
8-1B        V -Y.-------- ---------- --
60p1        V -Y.-------- ---------- --
```

Fig. 3.3. Sequence analysis of VH26 locus B alleles. (A) Nucleotide sequences cloned from 5.0 kb and 3.7 kb TaqI restriction fragments are shown beneath the VH26 reference sequence (limited to all of CDR2 and part of FR3). Shown underneath for comparison are the sequences of the V_H3 germline genes 8-1B (V3-66) and 60p2 (V3-53). Asterisk (*) indicates an alternative alignment of the 8-1B CDR2, to facilitate comparison with the 3.7 kb gene sequence. The coding region sequences of the 5.0 kb and 3.7 kb genes are identical to VH26 at all positions not shown. (B) Amino acid sequences translated from the nucleotide sequences shown in (A). Absence of a codon or amino acid, respectively, is indicated by a blank space in parentheses, or a dot (.). Codon numbering is according to Kabat et al.[65]

as many as 6 to 8 copies of the 3.7 kb allele (Fig. 3.2).[76] A proposed evolutionary relationship among the VH26 alleles is depicted in a phylogenetic tree, in Figure 3.4. In summary, these results demonstrate that VH26 occupies two polymorphic loci. The A locus was absent most often in Blacks, whereas novel alleles of the B locus occurred most often in Asians. These differences could influence VH26 expression because they involve the gene copy number and coding region sequences of VH26 alleles.

Polymorphism of a Frequently Expressed Ig V_H1 Gene—51p1

The 51p1 Locus is Highly Polymorphic

51p1 is an immunoglobulin V_H1 gene that is frequently expressed in B cell CLL[96] and early in B cell ontogeny[2] and is a major source of paraprotein rheumatoid factors.[97] The 51p1 gene locus, also known as V1-69,[6] is highly polymorphic. Thirteen alleles have been identified by genomic hybridization, each being distinguishable by its restriction fragment size, coding region sequence, or both.[75] The alleles were cloned and sequenced from genomic DNA, revealing differences of up to seven coding

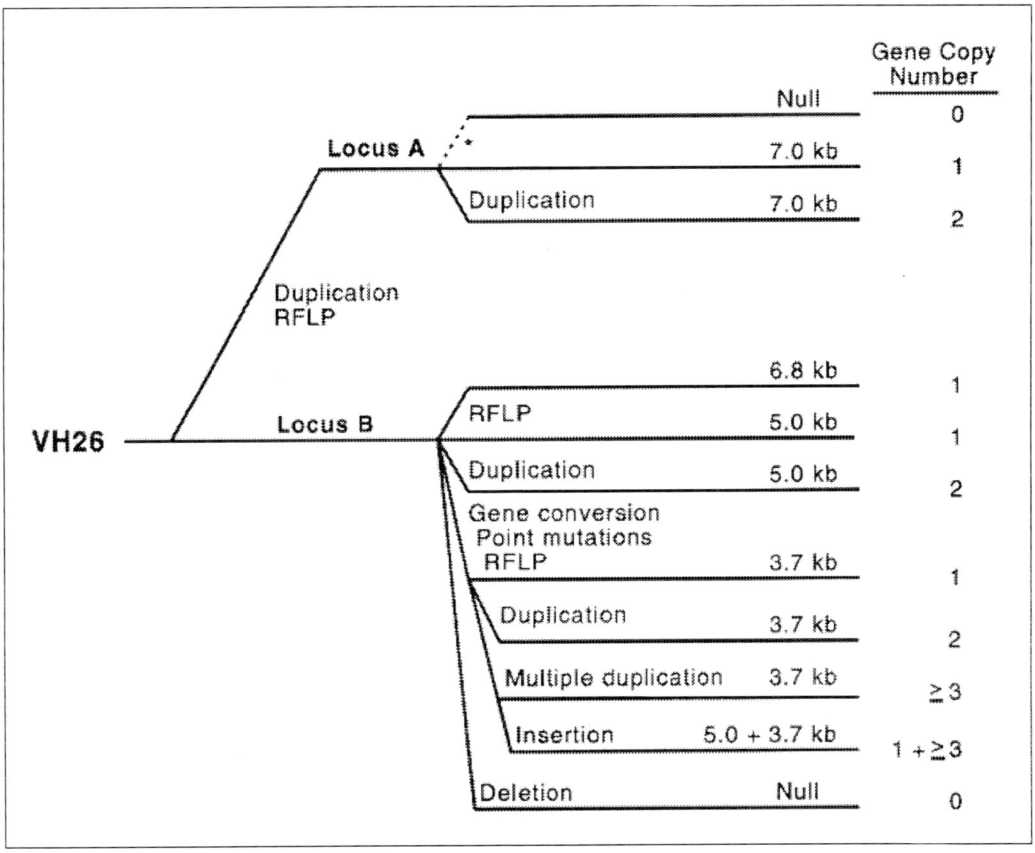

Fig. 3.4. Phylogenetic tree of VH26 genes. The two VH26 loci, A and B, could have arisen from duplication of a prototype VH26 locus, followed by subsequent germline events creating the 11 alleles shown to the right. Alleles containing more than one gene copy, as indicated to the extreme right, presumably represent haplotypes of closely linked loci. Asterisk (*) indicates that locus A null alleles could hypothetically occur in haplotypes that lack the initial VH26 duplication or in haplotypes from which locus A was deleted. (Reprinted with permission from: Sasso EH et al. J Clin Invest 1995; 96: 1591-00. © 1995 American Society for Clinical Investigation.)

region nucleotides that encode up to five amino acid changes, four of which are in the CDR.[75] These genes, therefore, could encode different preimmune Ab specificities. Based on their distinctive CDR2 sequence motifs, the 13 alleles were classified in either of two gene subsets—51p1-related, or hv1263-related. Two of the 51p1-related genes (on 7.5 kb and 4.0 kb Taq I fragments) usually occurred as a linked pair on the same haplotype, resulting from gene duplication.[75] Other duplications were rare, and null alleles were not seen. Consequently, all people had a total of two to four gene copies from the 51p1 locus, of which zero to four were 51p1-related, and zero to two were hv1263-related. In a predominantly Caucasian population, the prevalence of 51p1-related and hv1263-related alleles were 85% and 58%, respectively.[75] These data showed that the 51p1 locus consists of a complex set of alleles (Table 3.7). As seen with VH26 and the genes related to 56p1, 51p1 polymorphism affects both the V_H coding region sequence and the gene copy number.

Expression of the 51p1 Gene is Proportional to its Germline Gene Copy Number

Quantitative studies of 51p1 gene expression have been possible through use of G6, a murine anti-idiotypic mAb. G6 specifically detects Ig encoded by nonmutated genes of the 51p1-related subset, but not genes from the hv1263-related subset or other V_H genes.[98,99] In adult human tonsils, almost all G6 reactivity occurs in IgD$^+$/IgM$^+$ B lymphocytes, found in the mantle zone.[98] Flow cytometric analysis found that up to 12% of IgD-bearing tonsillar B cells were G6-reactive, although most subjects had fewer, and some had no G6-reactive B cells.[98] Since a haploid V_H gene accounts for about 1% of functional V_H loci, this result was striking, both for the high values measured in some subjects and the wide variation seen in the population. It was hypothesized that polymorphism at the 51p1 locus might underlie this variation. Therefore, 35 human tonsils were studied to compare the number of 51p1-related germline gene copies with the proportion of G6-reactive IgD-bearing tonsillar B cells.[99] All subjects who had no copy of 51p1-related genes lacked any G6-reactive B cells, whereas those with four copies of 51p1-related genes had the highest proportions of G6-positive IgD B cells—up to 11.4%. Over the entire data set, the percentage of IgD-bearing B cells that reacted with G6 was proportional to the 51p1-related gene copy number ($R = 0.92$, $p < 0.001$), with each copy accounting, on average, for 2.4% to 4.0% of the IgD-bearing B cells.[99] This result indicates that 51p1-related genes are expressed by a relatively large percentage of IgD-bearing tonsillar B cells. The percentage reflects a high intrinsic propensity for expression by 51p1-related genes, and is proportional to their germline gene copy number. IgD$^+$/IgM$^+$ B lymphocytes are predominately preimmune, unmutated, mature B cells, from which memory B cells and plasma cells are derived.[100] Thus, the data identify a mechanism by which V_H gene copy number may play a significant role in shaping the humoral immune repertoire.

Table 3.7. The 51p1 locus - a complex set of alleles

1. At least 13 alleles.
2. At least 9 different nucleotide sequences (> 97.7% coding region homology). Up to 4 amino acid changes in the CDR.
3. Two gene subsets: 51p1-related (85% prevalence) and hv1263-related (58%).
4. Two prevalent 51p1-related genes usually occur as linked gene pair, due to gene duplication.
5. Null alleles are rare or nonexistent.
6. Diploid copy number of 51p1-related genes ranges from 0 to 4.
7. Frequency of 51p1-related gene expression in preimmune tonsillar B cells (IgD$^+$, IgM$^+$) can be high (from 0% up to 12%) and is proportional to the germline gene copy number (R=0.92).

Implications of Ig V_H Polymorphism for the Effects of Superantigen SpA

Ig V_H gene polymorphism might affect B cell expression in two principal ways. First, it can influence the proportion of primary B cells that express a particular V_H gene. Second, it has the potential to alter the mosaic of preimmune antigenic specificities generated in primary B cells. Consequently, V_H gene polymorphism might also influence the representation of V_H genes in secondary B cells, and the composition of circulating Ig. The first, quantitative effect, can result from polymorphism of V_H gene copy number, and be further modulated by polymorphism of V_H gene regulatory regions. Thus, duplication of functional V_H3 loci, as can occur with the 1.9III, hv3019b9, VH26, and other genes, would be expected to expand the subset of primary B cells whose surface Ig can bind SpA.[81] Similarly, deletions of functional V_H3 loci may reduce it.[31] The fact that V_H haplotypes are very heterogeneous means that the actual number and proportion of functional V_H3 genes must vary considerably between people—from the low extreme of repertoires dominated by V_H3 gene deletions to the high extreme of repertoires dominated by V_H3 gene duplications. The quantitative impact of a V_H3 superantigen on B cells or circulating Ig generated by these opposite repertoire types might be quite different.

Regarding the second effect, polymorphism of V_H coding region amino acids has the potential to influence the B cell response to conventional Ag by altering the specificities of surface Ig receptors. Studies described above show that V_H germline sequence variations often encode nonconservative amino acid substitutions in CDR1 and CDR2. Thus, the composition of the B cell subpopulation engaged by a classical Ag might be governed, in part, by the available repertoire of V_H genes. The same is probably not true for the nonclassical interaction of B cells with SpA. Specificity for SpA is a property of nearly all circulating V_H3 IgM and is encoded by most, if not all commonly expressed V_H3 germline genes. Thus, V_H gene sequence polymorphisms (as recognized thus far) are not expected to greatly affect the size of the SpA-responding subset of V_H3 B cells. This conclusion reflects the extreme conservation of FR residues among V_H3 genes, and the apparent paucity (or absence) of V_H3 genes whose germline CDR abrogate specificity for SpA.

It is conceivable, however, that B cell responses to classical Ag may be modulated by superantigens. For example, by being present during immune development or during immunization, SpA might alter the size, tempo, or V_H gene content of Ag-specific responses, especially those that characteristically use a restricted set of V_H genes. Furthermore, since increasing evidence implicates Ag-specific clonal selection in the production of autoAb, SpA might be able to influence the timing or pathological impact of autoimmune responses. These speculations offer an outline for future studies.

Acknowledgments

The preparation of this manuscript was supported by National Institutes of Health grant AR 40561.

References

1. Kodaira M, Kinashi T, Umemura I. Organization and evolution of variable region genes of the human immunoglobulin heavy chain. J. Mol. Biol. 1986; 190:529-41.
2. Schroeder, H Jr, Hillson JL, Perlmutter RM. Early restriction of the human antibody repertoire. Science 1987; 238:791-93.
3. Berman JE, Mellis SJ, Pollock R et al. Content and organization of the human Ig V_H locus: definition of three new V_H families and linkage to the Ig C_H locus. EMBO J 1988; 7:727-38.612-17.
4. Mortari F. J. Newton J. Wang, and H. Schroeder. 1992. The human cord blood antibody repertoire. Frequent usage of the V_H7 gene family. Eur J Immunol 22:241-245.
5. Matsuda F, Shin EK, Nagaoka H et al. Structure and physical map of 64 variable

segments in the 3' 0.8-megabase region of the human immunoglobulin heavy-chain locus. Nature Genetics 1993; 3:88-94.
6. Cook, G P, Tomlinson IM, Walter G et al. A map of the human immunoglobulin V_H locus completed by analysis of chromosome 14q. Nature Genet 1994; 7:162-68.
7. Cook GP, Tomlinson IM. The human immunoglobulin V_H repertoire. Immunol Today 1995; 16:237-42.
8. Moks T, Abrahmsén L, Nillson B et al. Staphylococcal protein A consists of five IgG-binding domains. Eu J Biochem 1986. 156:637-43.
9. Guss B, Uhlén M, Nilsson B et al. Region X, the cell-wall-attachment part of staphylococcal protein A. Eur J Biochem 1984; 138:413-20.
10. Hanson DC, Phillips ML, Schumaker VN. Electron microscopic and hydrodynamic studies of protein A-immunoglobulin G soluble complexes. J. Imunol. 1984; 132:1386-96.
11. Deisenhofer J. Crystallographic refinement and atomic models of a human Fc fragment and its complex with a fragment B of protein A from staphylococcus aureus at 2.9- and 2.8 A resolution. Biochemistry 1981; 20:2361-70.
12. Sasso EH, Barber CV, Nardella FA et al. Antigenic specificities of human monoclonal and polyclonal IgM rheumatoid factors. The Cγ2-Cγ3 interface contains the major deteminants. J Immunol 1988; 140: 3098-07.
13. Stone G, Sjöbring U, Bjork L et al. The Fc binding site for streptococcal protein G is in the Cγ2-Cγ3 interface region of IgG and is related to the sites that bind staphylococcal protein A and human rheumatoid factors. J Immunol 1989; 143:565-70.
14. Laky M, Sjöquist J, Moraru II et al. Mutual inhibition of the binding of C1q and protein A to rabbit IgG immune complexes. Mol Immunol 1985; 22:1297-302.
15. Duncan AR, Winter G. The binding site for C1q on IgG. Nature 1988; 332:738-40.
16. Inganäs M. Comparison of mechanisms of interaction between protein A from *Staphylococcus aureus* and human monoclonal IgG, IgA, and IgM in relation to the classical Fc and the alternative $F(ab')_2$ protein A interactions. Scand J Immunol 1981; 13:343-52.
17. Inganäs M, Johansson, SGO, Sjöquist J. Further characterization of the alternative protein-A interaction of immunoglobulins: demonstration of an Fc-binding fragment of protein A expressing the alternative reactivity. Scand J Immunol 1981; 14:379-88.
18. Roben PW, Salem AN, Silverman GJ. V_H3 family antibodies bind domain D of stpahylococcal protein A. J Immunol 1995; 154:6437-45.
19. Romagnani S, Grazia Giudizi M. del Prete G et al. Demonstration on protein A of two distinct immunoglobulin-binding sites and their role in the mitogenic activity of *Staphylococcus aureus* Cowan II on human B cells. J Immunol 1982; 129:596-02.
20. Vidal MA, Conde FP. Altenative mechanism reactivity of Protein A-immunoglobulin interaction: the V_H-associated reactivity of a monoclonal human IgM. J Immunol 1985; 135:1232-38.
21. Young WW Jr., Tamura Y, Wolock DM et al. Staphylococcal protein A binding to the Fab fragments of mouse monoclonal antibodies. J Immunol 1984; 133:3163-66.
22. Field PR, Shanker S, Murphy AM. The use of protein A-sepharose affinity chromatography for separation and detection of specific IgM antibody in acquired rubella infection: a comparison with absorption by staphylococci containing protein A and density gradient ultracentrifugation. J Immunol Methods 1980; 32:59-70.
23. Akerström B, Nilson, BHK, Hoogenboom HR et al. On the interaction between single chain Fv antibodies and bacterial immunoglobulin-binding proteins. J Immunol Methods 1994; 177:151-63.
24. Sasso EH, Silverman GJ, Mannik M. Human IgM molecules that bind to Staphylococcal protein A contain V_HIII chains. J Immunol 1989; 142:2778-83.
25. Kirkham PM, Mortari F, Newton JA. Immunoglobulin VH clan and family identity predicts variable domain structure and may influence antigen binding. EMBO J 1992; 11:603-09.
26. Romagnani S, Giudizi MG, Almerigogna F et al. Protein A reactivity on IgM and

IgD-bearing lymphocytes from patients with chronic lymphocytic leukemia. Clin Immunol Immunopathol 1981; 19:139-48.

27. Meeker TC, Grimaldi JC, O'Rourke J et al. Lack of detectable somatic hypermutation in the V region of the Ig H chain gene of a human chronic B lymphocytic leukemia. J Immunol 1988; 141:3994-98.
28. Kipps TJ, Tomhave E, Pratt LF et al. Developmentally restricted immunoglobulin heavy chain variable region gene eexpressed at high frequency in chronic lymphocytic leukemia. Proc Natl Acad Sci USA 1989; 86:5913-17.
29. Schroeder HW, Wang JY. Preferential utilization of conserved immunoglobulin heavy chain variable gene segments during fetal life. Proc Natl Acad Sci, USA 1990; 87:6146-50.
30. Raaphorst F, Timmers E, Kenter M et al. Restricted utilization of germ line V_H3 genes and short diverse third complementarity-determining regions (CDR3) in human fetal B lymphocyte immunoglobulin heavy chain rearrangements. Eur J Immunol 1992; 22:247-51.
31. Hillson JL, Opplinger IR, Sasso EH. et al. Emerging human B cell repertoire, influence of developmental stage and interindividual variation. J Immunol 1992; 149:3741-52.
32. Cuisinier AM, Gauthier L, Boubli L. et al. Mechanisms that generate human immunoglobulin diversity operate from the 8th week of gestation in fetal liver. Eu J Immunol 1993; 23:110-18.
33. Hillson JL, Karr NS, Oppliger IR. et al. The structural basis of germline-encoded V_H3 immunoglobulin binding to staphylococcal protein A. J. Exp. Med 1993; 178:331-36.
34. Sasano M, Burton DR, Silverman GJ. Molecular selection of human antibodies with an unconventional bacterial B cell antigen. J Immunol 1993; 151:5822-39.
35. Vasquez Kristiansen S, Pascual V, Lipsky PE. Staphylococcal protein A induces biased production of Ig by V_H3-expressing B lymphocytes. J Immunol 1994; 153:2974-82.
36. Hokada M, Hayashimoto A, Yamanaka H et al. Molecular basis for the interaction between human IgM and staphylococcal protein A. Clin Immunol Immunopath 1994; 72:394-401.
37. Thompson KM, Randen I, Borretzen M et al. Variable region gene usage of human monoclonal rheumatoid factors derived from healthy donors following imunization. Eur J Immunol 1994; 24:1771-78.
38. Sasso E. Immunoglobulin V genes in rheumatoid arthritis. Rheumatic Disease Clinics of North America 1992; 18:809-36.
39. Ermel R., Kenny T, Chen PP et al. Molecular analysis of rheumatoid factors derived from rheumatoid synovium suggests an antigen-driven response in inflamed joints. Arthritis and Rheum 1993; 36: 380-88.
40. Huang, S-C, Hufnagle WO, Glas A et al. Analysis of the V_H repertoire in RA patients reveals an elevated antigen-driven component and a markedly diminished preimmune component. Arthritis Rheum 1994; 37:S287.
41. Bridges SL Jr, Lee SK, Koopman WJ et al. Analysis of immunoglobulin gamma heavy chain expression in synovial tissue of a patient with rheumatoid arthritis. Arthritis Rheum 1993; 36:631-41.
42. Saltvedt E, Harboe E. Binding of IgA to protein-A-containing staphylococci: relationship to subclasses. Scand J Immunol 1976; 5:1103-08.
43. Grov A. Human colostral IgA interacting with staphylococcal protein A. Acta Pathol Microbiol Immunol Scand (C) 1976; 84:71-72.
44. Biguzzi S. Fc gamma-like deteminants on immunoglobulin variable regions: identification by staphylococcal protein A. Scand J Immunol 1982; 15:605-18.
45. Bruin G, Faber A, Biewenga J. Binding of human IgA fragments to protein A-sepharose studied with ELISA method. Scand J Immunol 1985; 21:49-54.
46. Sasso EH, Silverman GJ, Mannik M. Human IgA and IgG $F(ab')_2$ molecules that bind to Staphylococcal protein A belong to the V_HIII subgroup. J Immunol 1991; 142:1877-83.
47. Ibrahim S, Seppälä I, Mäkelä O. V-region mediated binding of human Ig by protein A. J Immunol 1993; 151:1-7.

48. Herman A, Kappler JW, Marrack et al. Superantigens: Mechanism of T cell stimulation and role in immune responses. Annu Rev Immunol 1991; 9:745-77.

49. Choi Y, Herman A, DiGiusto D et al. Residues of the variable region β chain that interact with S. aureus toxin superantigens. Nature 1990; 346:471-73.

50. Shokri F, Mageed RA, Maziak BR et al. Expression of V_HIII-associated cross-reactive idiotype on human B lymphocytes. Association with staphylococcal protein A binding and Staphylococcus aureus Cowan II stimulation. J Immunol 1991; 146:936-40.

51. Koslowski LM, Kunning SR, Zheng Y et al. Staphylococcus aureus Cowan II -induced human immunoglobulin responses: preferential IgM rheumatoid factor production and VH3 mRNA expression by protein A-binding B cells. J Clin Immunol 1995; 15: 145-51.

52. Zouali M, Thèze J. Probing V_H gene family utilization in human peripheral B cells by in situ hybridization. J Immunol 146: 2885-64.

53. Levinson AI, Tar L, Carafa C et al. *Staphylococcus aureus* Cowan I. Potent stimulus of immunoglobulin M rheumatoid factor production. J Clin Invest 1986; 78:612-17.

54. Rechavi G, Ram D, Glazer L et al. Evolutionary aspects of immunoglobulin heavy chain variable region (V_H) gene subgroups. Proc Natl Acad Sci USA 1983; 80:855-59.

55. Seppala IM, Kaaritinen S, Ibrahim S et al. Mouse Ig encoded by V_H families S107 or J606 bind to protein A. J Immunol 1990; 145:2989-93.

56. Ey PL, Prowse SJ, Jenkin CR. Isolation of pure IgG_1, IgG_{2a}, and IgG_{2b} immunoglobulins from mouse serum using protein A-sepharose. Immunochemistry 1978; 15: 429-36.

57. Chalon MP, Milne RW, Vierman, J-P. Interactions between mouse immunoglobulins and staphylcoccal protein A. Scand J Immunol 1979; 9:359-64.

58. Ternynck T, Avrameas S. Murine natural monoclonal antibodies: a study of their polyspecificities and their affinities. Immunol Rev 1986; 94:99-12.

59. Nakamura M, Burastero SE, Ueki Y et al. Probing the normal and autoimmune B cell repertoire with Ebstein-Barr virus. Frequency of B cells producing monoreactive high affinity autoantobodies in patients with Hashimoto's disease and Systemic Lupus Erythematosus. J Immunol 1988; 141: 4165-72.

60. Casali P, Notkins AL. Probing the human B cell repertoire with EBV: polyreactive antibodies and $CD5^+$ B lymphocytes. Annu Rev Immunol 1989; 7:513-35.

61. Manser T. Evolution of antibody structure during the immune response. The differentiative potential of a single B lymphocyte. J Exp Med 1989; 170:1211-30.

62. Ueki Y, Goldfarb IS, Harindranath N et al. Clonal analysis of a human antibody response. Quantitation of precursors of antibody-producing cells and generation and characteization of monoclonal IgM, IgG, and IgA to rabies virus. J Exp Med 1990; 171:19-34.

63. Kocks C, Rajewsky K. Stable expression and somatic hypermutation of antibody V regions in B cell developmental pathways. Ann Rev Immunol 1989; 7:537-59.

64. Randen I, Potter KN, Li Y et al. Complementarity-determining region 2 is implicated in the binding of staphylococcal protein A to human immunoglobulin V_HIII variable regions. Eur J Immunol 1993; 23:2682-86.

65. Kabat EA, Wu TT, Reid-Miller M et al. Sequences of proteins of immunological interest. xi. Bethesda: U.S. Department of Health and Human Services, United States Government Printing Office, 1987; 167-75, 656-58.

66. Pascual V, Randen I, Thompson K et al. The complete nucleotide sequences of the heavy chain variable regions of six monospecific rheumatoid factors derived from Epstein-Barr virus-transformed B cells isolated from the synovial tissue of patients with rheumatoid arthritis. Further evidence that some autoantibodies are unmutated copies of germline genes. J Clin Invest 1990; 86:1320-28.

67. Thompson KM, Randen I, Natvig JB et al. Human monoclonal rheumatoid factors derived from the polyclonal repertoire of rheumatoid synovial tissue: incidence of cross-

reactive idiotopes and expression of V_H and V_K subgroups. Eur J Immunol 1990; 20:863-68.

68. Ibrahim SM, Kaartinen M, Seppälä et al. The alternative binding site for protein A in the Fab fragment of immunoglobulins. Scand J Immunol 1993; 37:257-64.
69. Silverman GJ. Superantigens and the spectrum of unconventional B cell antigens. The Immunologist 1994; 2:51-57.
70. Goodnow CC, Cyster JG, Hartley SB et al. Self-tolerance checkpoints in B lymphocyte development. Adv Immunol 1995; 59: 279-368.
71. Sasso EH, Willems van Dijk K, Milner, ECB. Prevalence and polymorphism of human V_H3 genes. J Immunol 1990; 145 :2751-57.
72. Willems van Dijk K, Schroeder HW Jr, Perlmutter RW et al. Heterogeneity in the human immunoglobulin V_H locus. J Immunol 1989; 142:2547-54.
73. Sasso EH, Willems van Dijk K, Bull A. V_H genes in tandem array comprise a repeated germline motif. J Immunol 1992; 149: 1230-36.
74. Willems van Dijk K, Sasso EH, Milner, ECB. Polymorphism of the human immunoglobulin V_H4 gene family. J Immunol 1991; 146:3646-51.
75. Sasso EH, Willems van Dijk K, Bull A et al. A fetally expressed immunoglobulin V_H1 gene belongs to a complex set of alleles. J Clin Invest 1993; 91:2358-67.
76. Sasso EH, Suzuki LA, Buckner JH. Ethnic differences in polymorphism of an immunoglobulin V_H3 gene. J Clin Invest 1995; 96:1591-00.
77. Braun J., Berberian L, King L et al. Restricted use of fetal VH3 immunoglobulin genes by unselected B cells in the adult. Predominance of 56p1-like VH genes in common variable immunodeficiency. J Clin Invest 1992; 89:1395-02.
78. Yang, P-M, Olsen NJ, Siminovitch KA et al. Possible deletion of a developmentally regulated Vh gene in autoimmune disease. Proc Natl Acad Sci 1990; 87:7907-11.
79. Sasso EH, Suzuki LA, Petri MA. Polymorphism of an Ig V_H3 gene is associated with SLE in blacks but not Caucasians. Arthritis Rheum 1995; 38:S213.
80. Walter GI, Tomlinson IM, Cook GP et al. HAPPY mapping of a YAC reveals alternative haplotypes in the human immunoglobulin V_H locus. Nucleic Acids Res 1993; 21:4524-29.
81. Suzuki I, Pfister L, Glas A et al. Representation of rearranged V_H gene segments in the human adult antibody repertoire. J Immunol 1995; 154:3902-11.
82. Brezinschek HP, Brezinschek RI, Lipsky PE. Analysis of the heavy chain repertoire of human peripheral B cells using single cell polymerase chain reaction. J Immunol 1995; 155:190-02.
83. Dersimonian H, Schwartz RS, Barrett KJ et al. Relationship of human variable region germline genes to genes encoding anti-DNA antibodies. J Immunol 1987; 139: 2496-01.
84. Tomlinson IM, Walter G, Marks JD et al. The repertoire of human germline V_H sequences reveals about fifty groups of V_H segments with different hypervariable loops. J Mol Biol 1992; 227:776-98.
85. Matthyssens G, Rabbitts T. Structure and multiplicity of genes from the human immunoglobulin heavy chain variable region. Proc Natl Acad Sci 1980; 77:6561-65.
86. Chen PP, Liu, M-F, Sinha S et al. A 16/6 idiotype-positive anti-DNA antibody is encoded by a conserved V_H gene with no somatic mutations. Arthritis Rheum 1989. 31:1429-31.
87. Barbas SM, Ditzel HJ, Salonen EM et al. Human autoantibody recognition of DNA. Proc Natl Acad Sci USA 195; 92:2529-33.
88. Adderson EE, Schackelford PG, Quinn A et al. Restricted Ig H chain V gene usage in the human antibody response to *Haemophilus influenzae* type b capsular polysaccharide. J Immunol 1991; 147:1667-74.
89. Silverman GJ, Lucas AH. Variable region diversity in human circulating antibodies specific for the capsular polysaccharide of *Haemophilus influenzae* type b. Preferential usage of two types of V_H3 heavy chains. J Clin Invest 1991; 88:911-20.
90. Berberian L, Goodlick L, Kipps TJ et al. Immunoglobulin V_H3 gene products: natural ligands for HIV gp120. Science (Wash DC) 1993; 261:1588-91.

91. Isenberg DA, Schoenfeld T, Madaio MP et al. Anti-DNA antibody idiotypes in systemic lupus erythematosus. Lancet 1984; 2:417-22.
92. Young F, Tucker L, Rubenstein D et al. Molecular analysis of a germ line-encoded idiotypic marker of pathogenic human lupus autoantibodies. J Immunol 1990; 145: 2545-53.
93. Willems van Dijk K, Milner LA, Sasso EH et al. Chromosomal organization of the heavy chain variable region gene segments comprising the human fetal antibody repertoire. Proc Natl Acad Sci 1992; 89: 10430-34.
94. Rubenstein DB, Symann M, Stewart AK. Restriction fragment length polymorphisms and single germline coding region sequence in VH18/2, a duplicated gene encoding autoantibody. Mol Immunol 1993; 30: 403-12.
95. Chothia C, Lest A, Gherardi E et al. Structural repertoire of human V_H segments. J Mol Bio 1992; 227:799-17.
96. Kipps TJ, Tomhave E, Pratt LF et al. Developmentally restricted immunoglobulin heavy chain region expressed at high frequency in chronic lymphocytic leukemia. Proc Natl Acad Sci USA 1989. 6:5913-17.
97. Crowley JJ, Goldfein RJ, Schrohenloher RE et al. Incidence of three cross-reactive idiotypes on human rheumatoid factor paraproteins. J Immunol 1988; 140: 3411-18.
98. Kipps TJ, Duffy SF. Relationship of the CD5 B cell to human tonsillar lymphocytes that express autoantibody-associated cross reactive itiotypes. J Clin Invest 1991; 87:2087-96.
99. Sasso EH, Johnson T, Kipps TJ. Expression of the Ig V_H gene 51p1 is proportional to its germline gene copy number. J Clin Invest, 1996; 97:2074-80.
100. Pascual V, Liu, Y-J, Magalski A et al. Analysis of somatic mutation in five B cell subsets of human tonsil. J Exp Med 1994; 180:329-39.

CHAPTER 4

Molecular Characterization of the Interaction of Immunoglobulin Variable Region with Staphylococcal Protein A

Saleh M. Ibrahim

INTRODUCTION

Although in the early sixties there was some evidence already suggesting the existence of a reaction between staphylococcal protein A (SpA) and nonimmune immunoglobulins (Ig), it was Forsgren and Sjöquist who first described the unique "pseudo-immune" reaction between SpA and IgG.[1-3] They concluded that the structure which bound SpA resided in the Fc part of IgG. This opened the way for systematic and detailed analysis of the SpA-IgG "classical binding" and to the discovery of other bacterial Ig-binding proteins.[4-8] These studies showed that almost all mammalian species sera are reactive with SpA.[9-11] However, it was not until 1974 that Harboe and Fölling demonstrated the binding of Ig isotypes other than IgG to SpA.[12] A group of human monoclonal IgM and IgA were shown to bind the Cowan II strain of *S. aureus* while another group failed to bind. Johansson and Inganäs reported that certain IgG, IgM and IgA myeloma proteins inhibited the binding of IgE to SpA.[13] This inhibitory effect was retained in the respective $F(ab')_2$ fragments, indicating the existence of two separate interactions: one compatible with the well known (classical) Fc-binding and the other named the 'alternative Fab interaction'. Other studies soon confirmed these findings.[14-17] Endresen was the first to suggest that the epitope for SpA resides on the Fab and

Human B Cell Superantigens, edited by Moncef Zouali. © 1996 R.G. Landes Company.

that it is distinct from the Ag binding site,[18] a finding that was confirmed by others.[19-20] The Fab binding was defined further by Sasso et al who studied the binding of human monoclonal IgM proteins to SpA and determined their V_H and V_K subgroups.[21] Binding to SpA was observed with most V_H3 IgM proteins but not with Igs belonging to other subgroups. The same phenomenon was observed with human polyclonal IgM, IgA and with $F(ab')_2$ fragments of IgG.[22] Regardless of the Ig subclass a restricted binding of V_H3 molecules was demonstrated.

The Fab mediated SpA reactivity was shown to exist in many mammalian Ig such as mouse, guinea pig, dog and chimpanzee. However, most avian Ig and some mammals such as the rabbit lacked the alternative binding.[11,23] The conservation of this interaction among different species suggests that it is a biologically important phenomenon. This chapter will review studies aimed at further characterization of the molecular basis of SpA-V_H interaction and its possible biological significance.

KEY IMMUNOGLOBULIN GENE SEGMENTS DETERMINING THE FAB-SPA BINDING

The binding of only a subset of monoclonal IgM and IgA antibodies (mAb) and IgG fab fragments to SpA suggested a role for the variable region of Ig in this interaction. To determine what gene segments are involved we tested 51 mouse and human monoclonal IgM, IgA, and IgG1 of known V-region sequences for SpA binding. They were tested by allowing them to bind to a SpA-Sepharose column and were then eluted with a pH gradient (Fig. 4.1). Only isotypes that do not bind to SpA via the Fc fragment were tested and representatives of as many V_H and V_K families as possible were included (see Table 4.1 for details).[24-25] When antibodies required a pH 5 or lower for elution they were considered binders, half of the monoclonal antibodies tested bound to SpA (Table 4.1). When a correlation between the binding characteristics and the V region sequence was sought (Table 4.1, Fig. 4.2), a striking difference in gene usage between SpA binders and non binders was apparent. All binders were encoded by mouse V_H genes from the S107 or J606 families and from the human V_H3 gene family. Non-binders were encoded by genes from a diverse set of V_H families.

The relationship between SpA binding status and Ig amino acid sequence indicated that the encoded V_H gene segment was not only a major determinant but the only one which matters for binding. The V_L domains of Ig binders varied greatly, with examples of Ig having less than 50% homology both in the V_L gene and in J_L gene segments. For other Ig, a binder and a nonbinder have almost identical V_L and J_L sequences. For example, 4B8 Ig (a SpA binder) and 15E7 Ig (a SpA nonbinder) have only one amino acid difference in their V_L-J_L region (data are not shown). Within the V_H it is fairly safe to rule out a role of the D_H and J_H in SpA-binding. Only limited heterogeneity is observed in the J_H region of SpA binders and nonbinders, they often have identical FR4 sequences. In contrast to the V_H-CDR3 (D_H) sequences which exhibit a great deal of length and sequence heterogeneity within binders (Fig. 4.2).

Comparative analysis of the remaining regions of the V_H domain in SpA-binders and nonbinders suggested a role for two FR stretches in binding. Large portions of the FR1 region of all V_H-binders were highly homologous. Apart from the low-affinity binders 10F7 and 13G7, no Ig binder deviated from the consensus sequence by more than three residues (87% homology). This peptide motif is also solvent-exposed, and a portion of it (6-24) is conserved in evolution.[26-29] Although this suggests a role of this peptide in SpA binding, there is also evidence against this conclusion. Two Ig nonbinders (MOPC-21 and RPC44) had sequences at positions 6-29 homologous to binders. Another stretch in

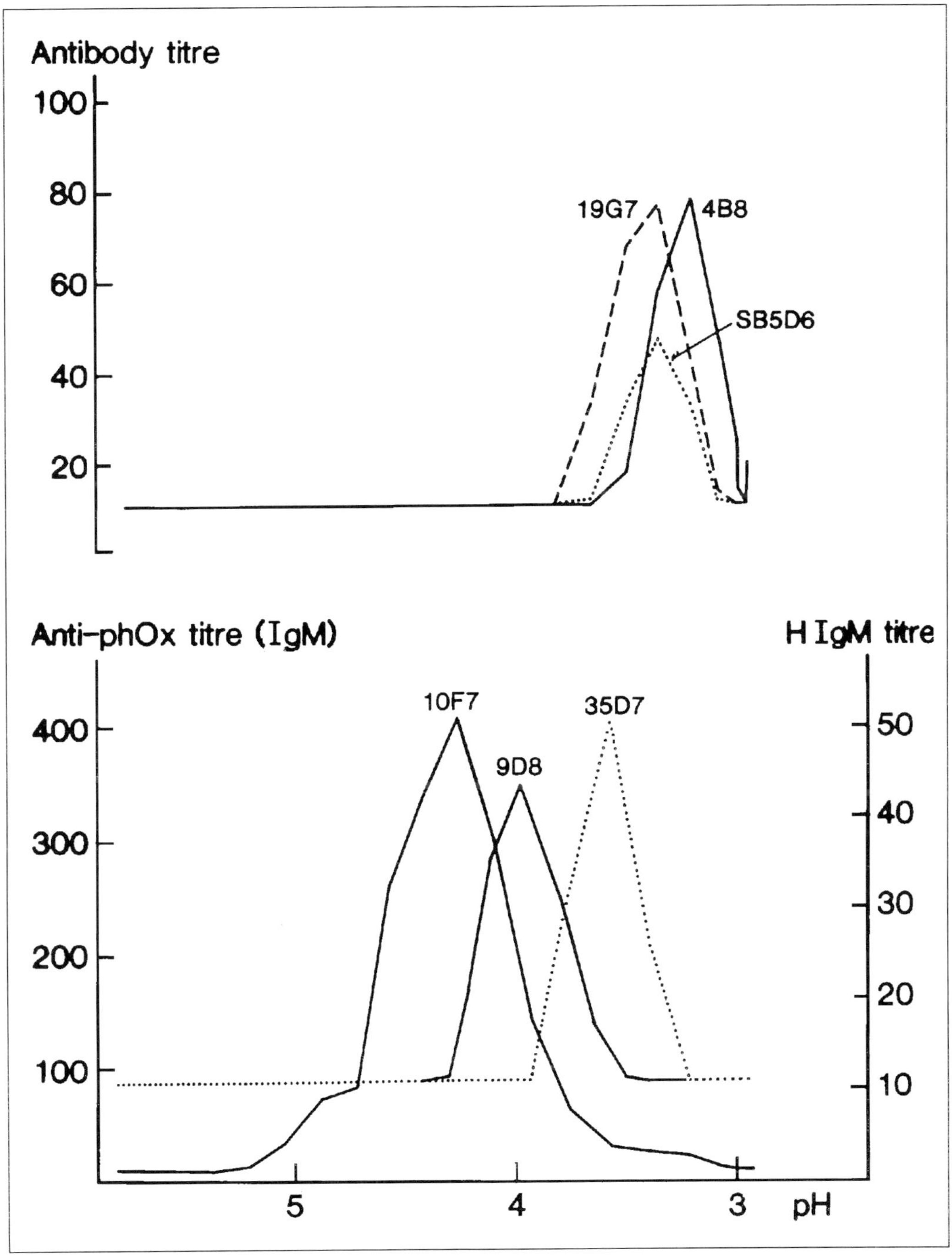

Fig. 4.1. Elution patterns of a group of mAb from SpA-Sepharose columns. The elution was carried out with a pH gradient, and the pH and Ig concentration or antibody titer in each fraction were determined. The scale of human IgM titer on the right of the bottom part refers to 35D7 Ig. The elution pattern of the three antibodies in the top section was determined in one experiment whereas in the bottom part this was the result of two experiments. phOx: 2-phenyl-4-ethoxymethylene-5-oxazolone. (Reprinted with permission from: Ibrahim S et al. Scand J Immunol; 37:257-64, ©1993.)

the FR3 encompassing residues 67-85 is conserved in evolution as well and is also solvent-exposed.[26-29] However, the homology among binders is lower than in the FR1 area (some high-affinity binders had only 58% homology with the majority). Based on sequence homology alone it is rather difficult to localize the Ig ligand for SpA. Nevertheless, this analysis, the ability of mAb to sustain both SpA and Ag binding simultaneously (see below), and in vitro mutagenesis studies by others suggest that SpA binds to a conformational epitope in the V_H-FR1, FR3 and possibly CDR2.[30,31]

V_H-Binding is Distinct from the Classical Fc-Binding and is Mediated by a Limited Number of SpA-Domains

SpA has five domains, each is approximately 58 amino acids long. Comparison of the amino acid sequences of these domains suggests that SpA evolved by tandem duplication events followed by genetic drift. This results in a homology gradient between the domains, with the first three domains (C, B of A, those closer to the C-terminal cell wall binding region) being more homologous to each other than to the last two domains (D and E). All domains bind IgG through the Fc region.[32] However,

Table 4.1. Characteristics of monoclonal immunoglobulins tested for SPA-binding

	pH of elution	Source	Antibody specificity	Isotype	V_H gene family	J_H	V_L gene family	J_L
VH-Binders								
19E11	3.51	BALB/c	phOx	IgMK	S107	J_H3	K-1	J_K4
4B8	3.2	SJL	phOx	IgMK	S107	J_H3	K-1	J_K2
15F7	3	AKR	phOx	IgMK	S107	J_H3	K-1	J_K2
20D4	3.33	AKR	phOx	IgG1K	S107	J_H3	K-1	J_K1
17E4	3.7	CE	phOx	IgG1K	S107	J_H3	K-1	J_K2
18D7	3.5	CE	phOx	IgMK	S107	J_H3	K-1	J_K2
19G7	3.44	CE	phOx	IgG1K	S107	J_H3	K-1	J_K2
3B5	3.21	CBA	phOx	IgG1K	S107	J_H3	K-1	J_K4
4D6	3.42	CBA	phOx	IgMK	S107	J_H3	K-1	J_K4
10H10	3	NZB	phOx	IgMK	S107	J_H3	K-1	J_K4
9D8	3.98	RF	phOx	IgMK	S107	J_H3	K-1	J_K2
35D7	3.56	Human	TT	IgMλ	V_H3	J_H4	λIII	$J_\lambda 2$
ED8.4	3	Human	PRP	IgMK	V_H3	J_H6	?	?
RAY4	3	Human	PRP	IgA2λ	V_H3	J_H4	λII	$J_\lambda 2/3$
SB5D6	3.36	Human	PRP	IgA1λ	V_H3	J_H4	λII	$J_\lambda 2/3$
TEPC15	4.3	BALB/c	PC	IgAK	S107	J_H1	K22	J_K5
M167	3.7	BALB/c	PC	IgAK	S107	J_H1	K24	J_K5
M511	4.1	BALB/c	PC	IgAK	S107	J_H1	K24	J_K5
4D4	3.8	BALB/c	phOx	IgG1K	S107	J_H3	K-1	J_K4
6F8	3.7	C57BL/10	phOx	IgMK	S107	J_H3	K-1	J_K2
8F11	3.5	C57BL/10	phOx	IgMK	S107	J_H3	K-1	J_K2
17G5	3.6	C57BL/10	phOx	IgG1K	S107	J_H3	K-1	J_K2
16C10	5	RII	phOx	IgG1K	J606	J_H3	K-1	J_K1
13G7	4.6	BALB/c	phOx	IgMK	J606	J_H2	K-1	J_K2
10F7	4.6	BALB/c	phOx	IgMK	J606	J_H3	K-1	J_K1

it is not yet known whether they all contribute to the V_H-binding or whether it is the function of a specialized domain(s).

To distinguish between the two possibilities a series of competition experiments were conducted between an IgM V_H-binder and various monoclonal IgG Fc-binders that do not bind SpA through the V_H region (Fig. 4.3).[33] Another experiment tested the ability of one SpA domain (B) to bind monoclonal Ig of different isotypes through the Fc and/or the V_H region (Fig. 4.4). No competition was seen between the V_H-binder and the Fc-binders for binding to SpA. On the contrary, enhancement of binding was often observed and Fc-binders inhibited the binding of SpA to the Fc-binder FLOPC 21 (a mouse IgG3 monoclonal Ig). If different domains are responsible for the two bindings, a V_H binder and a Fc binder can exhibit enhancement because the solid-phase SpA is capable of binding another Ig molecule which again can bind a new SpA molecule. The results provide evidence supporting the second alternative. A conclusion which is supported by the finding that Ig bind to domain B of SpA only through the Fc region and not through the V_H region. Taken together these data suggest that V_H-binding is localized to one or more specialized SpA domain(s). Having excluded domain B as a V_H-binding domain it is

Table 4.1. (continued)

	pH of elution	Source	Antibody specificity	Isotype	V_H gene family	J_H	V_L gene family	J_L
Non-binders								
10C5	6	BALB/c	ABA-HOP	IgG1K	7183	J_H2	KVI	J_K1
7F2	6	BALB/c	ABA-HOP	IgG1K	7183	J_H3	K-21E	J_K2
16B8	6	BALB/c	ABA-HOP	IgG1K	Q52	J_H3	KVI	J_K5
1G5	6	RF	phOx	IgG1K	J558	J_H3	KVI	J_K4
94.3	8	BALB/c	phOx	IgMK	7183	J_H4	K23	J_K2
XRPC44	8	BALB/c	?	IgAK	441-4	J_H3	K-4	J_K2
ABE48	8	BALB/c	?	IgAK	441-4	J_H3	?	?
MOPC467	8	BALB/c	?	IgAK	J558	J_H2	K-1	J_K1
J558	8	BALB/c	dex	IgAλ	J558	J_H1	λ1	$J_\lambda 3$
7SA11	8	Human	?	IgG3λ	V_H2	J_H3	λI	$J_\lambda 2$
LSF2T	8	Human	PRP	IgA1λ	V_H3	J_H4	λII	$J_\lambda 2/3$
9B7	5.7	C57BL/10	phOx	IgG1K	Gam 3-8	J_H3	K-1	J_K1
MOPC21	6.2	BALB/c	?	IgG1K	7183	J_H4	K19	J_K2
17B6	6	BALB/c	phOx	IgG1K	7183	J_H1	?	J_K4
M406	8	BALB/c	phOx	IgAK	X24	?	?	?
M315	8	BALB/c	DNP	IgAλ	36-60	?	?	
5G11	5.9	A/J	phOx	IgG1K	Q52	J_H4	K31	J_K5
H12	5.8	BALB/c	phOx	IgG1K	Q52	J_H2	K10	J_K2
7F11	5.8	C57BL/10	phOx	IgG1K	J558	J_H2	K10	J_K1
M104E	8	BALB/c	dex	IgMK	J558	J_H1	?	?
NQ2.6.1	5.8	BALB/c	phOx	IgG1K	J558	J_H4	K31	J_K5
NQ2.45.1	5.8	BALB/c	phOx	IgG1K	J558	J_H3	K-1	J_K5
5D3	8	C57BL/10	phOx	IgMK	J558	J_H2	K5	J_K5
18C10	8	BALB/c	phOx	IgMK	J558	J_H2	K10	J_K2
8D5	5.9	BALB/c	phOx	IgG1K	J558	J_H3	K5	J_K1
15E7	5.8	BALB/c	phOx	IgG1K	J558	J_H3	K-1	J_K1

. phOx: 2-phenyl-4-ethoxymethylene-5-oxazolone; TT: Tetanus Toxoid; PRP: polyribosylribitol phosphate; PC: phosphorylcholine; ABA-HOP: p-azobenzenearsonate coupled to hydroxyphenylacetic acid; dex: dextran; DNP: dinitrophenyl.

```
Binders                     10         20          30  CDR1   36                  50      CDR2
                             .          .           .          .                   .  abc
4B8            EVKLMESGGGLVQPGASLRLSCAASGFTFT  DYYMS  WVRQPPGKAPEWLG  LIRNKANGYTTEYTASVKG
4D6            ----V----------G--S-----------  -----  ----------L---A  -------------S-----
SB5D6*         --Q-V-------K--G--------------S  NAW-N  ---------GL--V-  R-KT-TD-G--D-A-P---
ED8.4*         --Q-L-------Q--G--------------S  S-A--  --L-----GL--VS  A-SG..SGGR-Y-AD----
19E11          ----V----------G-------T------  -----  ----------L----  F------------S-----
4D4            ----V----------G--S----T------  -----  ----------L---    ------------S-----
19G7           ----V------------------T------  -----  - --------L---  F------------S-----
MOPC167        ---VV----------G-------T-----S  -F--E  ----T---RL--IA  AS-S--HD-R---S-----
9D8            -- -    --  A---G-------T----L-  ----T  ----------L---    ------------S-----
16C10               ----A-----G-MK---V------N  Y-W-N  -SARS-A-GL--VA  E--L-S-  --H-AE----

Non-binders
M21            D-Q-V----------G-RK----------S  SFG-H  ----A-E-GL--VA  Y-SS..-SS-LD-AHT---
10C5                                         S  T-D -  ----T-E-GL--VA  Y-TS..G-VS-Y-SDT---
7F2                                     --I-L-  SLE-H  ---KA-E-GL--VA  Y-SG..DSC-IY-ADTL--
XRPC44         ----L----------G--K---------D-S  R-W--  ----A---GL--I-  E--P..DSC-IN--P-L-D
ABE48                                            -W--  ----A--RGL--I-  E--P..DSC-IN--P-LRD
LSF2*          --Q-V------IK--G--T--------I--S  NAW-N  ----A---GL--V-  R-KK-TD-G--D-A-P---
H12            Q-Q-K---P---A-SQ--SIT-TV---SL-  S-GVH  ---------GL----  V-W...A-GS-N-N--LMS
8D5            Q-Q-QQP- E--K-- -VK---K---Y---  S-W H  --K-R--Q L--I-  N--P..SNGG-N-NEKF-S
7F11           --Q-QQ-  E--K----VKM--K---Y---  E-N-H  --K-SH--SL- I-  Y--P..-NGG-S-NKKF--
M315            -Q-Q---P---K-SQ--S-T-SV--YSI-  SG-FW  -I--F--NKL--L-  K-K...YDGS-YGAP-L-N
7SA11*             -H---P- -K-SHT-S-T--V--YSIS  SSNWW  G -- - -GL--I-  YF-...-RWS-Y-NL-L-S

                   70          80                 94   CDR3  103
                   .           .  abc              .        abcde  .
4B8             FTISRDDSQ ILYLQMNTLRAEDSATYYCVK  AVMG.......AY W  J3
4D6            R---------S-------A-----------AR  GYYDGAWF...-- -  J3
SB5D6*         A-----N--KNT------S-KT--T-V---TT  GGGV-........ -  J4hum
ED8.4*         R-----EN-KNT--V---S--V--T-V---T-  GYGMDV....... -  J6hum
19E11          R---------S-------------------AR  GAAT-AWF...-- -  J3
4D4            R---------S-------A-----------AR  GKYY-T--...-- -  J3
19G7           R---------S-------------------AR   SGY- - ...-- -  J3
MOPC167        R---------SV------A----------TAR  DADY-DSY...FG -  J1
9D8            R---------S--------------------R  -NWT----...-- -  J3
16C10          R -------KSSV-----NF-S--TGI---TR  DAGPYVSPTFF-H -  J3

M21            R-------PKNT-F----S--S--T-M---AR  HGNYPWAM...D- -  J4
10C5            -------AKNT-F---S--KS--T-M---AR  HWY-NRYS...-- -  J2
7F2             -------PKNTNE-LLH-DQS--T-I---ER  SGY-NYGLG..-- -  J3
XRPC44         K-I-----AKNT-----SKV-S--T-L---AR  LHYY-YA....-- -  J3
ABE48          K-I-----GKNT-----SKV-SD-T-L--YAA  NWDR-F.....-- -  J3
LSF2*          R--V----N-STV----SS--T--T-V---GT  RDY.......... -  J4hum
H12            RLS--K---KSQVF-K--S-QT--T-M---AR  DGG........Y- -  J2
8D5            KA-LTV-K-SSTA-M-LSS-TS----V---AR   IYY-S.....DW -  J3
7F11           KA-LTV-K-SSTA- GLRS-TS----V---AR  R-V-N......DY -  J2
M315           RVS-T--T-ENQFF-KLDSVT   T-----AG  DNDHLYF....DY -  J2
7SA11*         RVT--L-T-ENQSS-TL-S-T-A---V---AT  TGDFWSGPTALNI -  J3hum
```

Fig. 4.2. Amino acid sequences of the V_H regions of binder Ig (top portion) and non-binders (bottom portion). All V_H segment sequences have been published.[24-25] Residue numbering is according to Kabat et al.[26] Dashes indicate a residue identical to that in the top row and empty spaces an undetermined residue. Deletions are indicated by dots. These Ig have been selected to represent different sequence types. They are ordered according to their affinity to SpA with the highest affinity Ab at the top. Human Ig are indicated by asterisks, the rest are mouse Ig. (Reprinted with permission from: Ibrahim S et al. Scand J Immunol; 37:257-64, ©1993.)

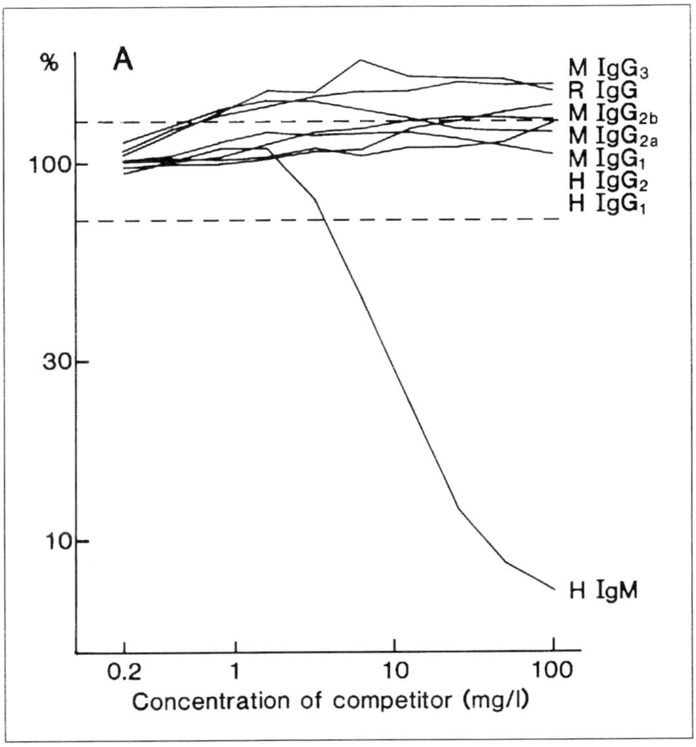

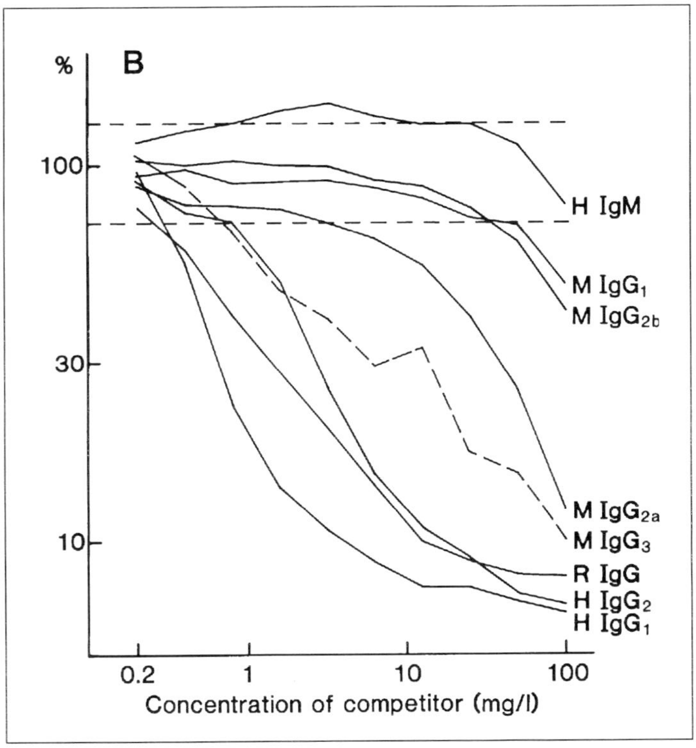

Fig. 4.3. Effect of various competing mAb on binding of biotin labelled SpA to wells coated with human IgM V_H-binder WEC (panel A) or mouse IgG3 Fc-binder FLOPC21 (panel B). The competing Ig were preincubated, at different concentration, with a constant amount of SpA and then transferred to the coated wells. One hundred percent binding was determined by adding SpA only. The vertical axis shows inhibition as a percentage of maximal binding and the horizontal axis the concentration of the competing mAb (µg/ml). M: mouse, H: human and R: rabbit. (Reprinted with permission from: Ibrahim S. Scand J Immunol; 38: 368-74, ©1993.)

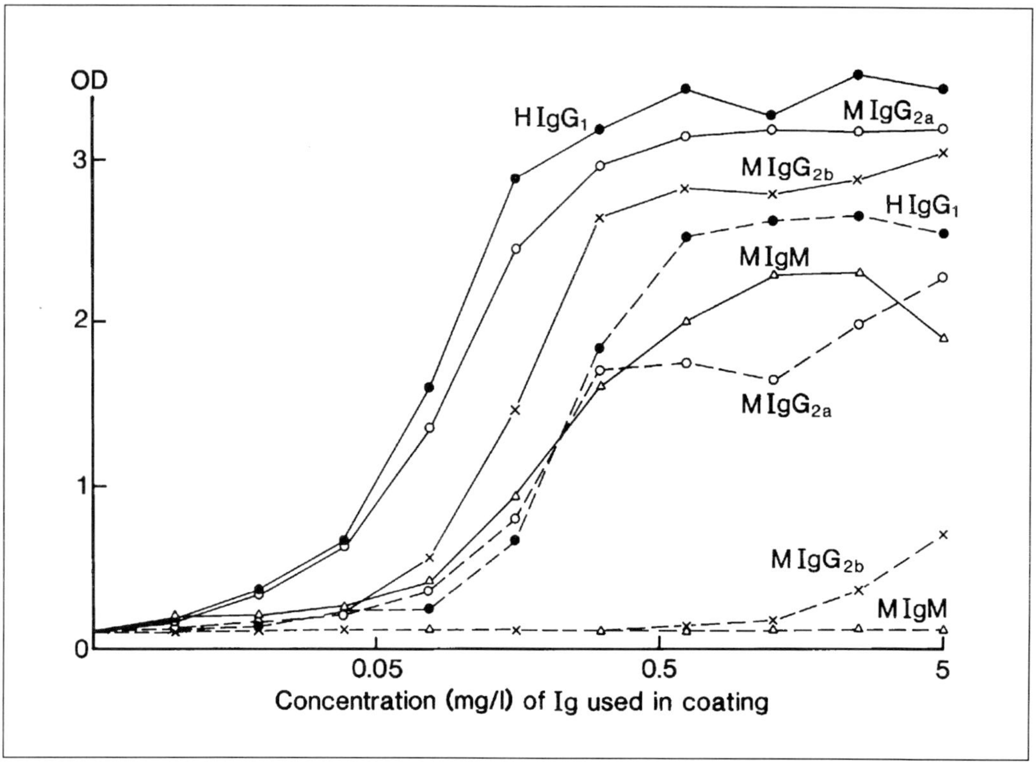

Fig. 4.4. Binding of labeled SpA (solid lines) or domain B (broken lines) to Ig coated plates. Four mAb were tested: 4D6 (MIgM, V_H-binder), and the Fc-binders, H11 (MIgG2a), DKE9 (MIgG2b) and KAR (HIgG1). M: mouse and H: human. The vertical axis gives the optical density (OD) and the horizontal axis the coating concentration of the mAb (µg/ml). (Reprinted with permission from: Ibrahim S. Scand J Immunol; 38: 368-74, ©1993.)

likely that the binding domain(s) are either E, D or both. A recent published report suggests that this is the case.[34] However, further experiments need to be done to address this question.

SpA-Binding Site is Distinct from the Conventional Ag-Binding Site

To see whether a mAb can sustain V_H-binding of SpA and Ag binding at the same time a series of experiments were carried out. The Ag (hapten-bovine serum albumin) was coated on plastic wells. Various mAb (IgM, V_H-binders) were then let to bind onto the antigen and, after washing, labeled SpA was added. To monitor the amount of the mAb bound, anti-kappa chain antibody was added as a reference to a replica row of wells (Fig. 4.5).

Different mAbs gave different results in these experiments. On one hand Ag-bound 4B8 mediated subsequent SpA binding efficiently. On the other hand, 10F7 and 13G7 failed to mediate SpA binding. The other mAbs gave intermediate results. while all mAbs bound anti-kappa chain antibody with the same magnitude (OD 2.0 was obtained with concentrations ranging from 0.3 to 0.6 µg/ml), they exhibited a gradient of SpA binding capacities. The concentrations of the mAbs which led to OD 2.0 in the SpA binding varied from 0.03 µg/ml in the case of 4B8 to 8 µg/ml in the case of 9D8 and > 10 µg/ml in the case of 10F7 and 13G7. The capacity of Ag-bound mAb to bind SpA correlated with its affinity for SpA as defined by the pH of elution from a SpA column (Table 4.1).[24-25] In two further experiments separate plates were directly coated with varying

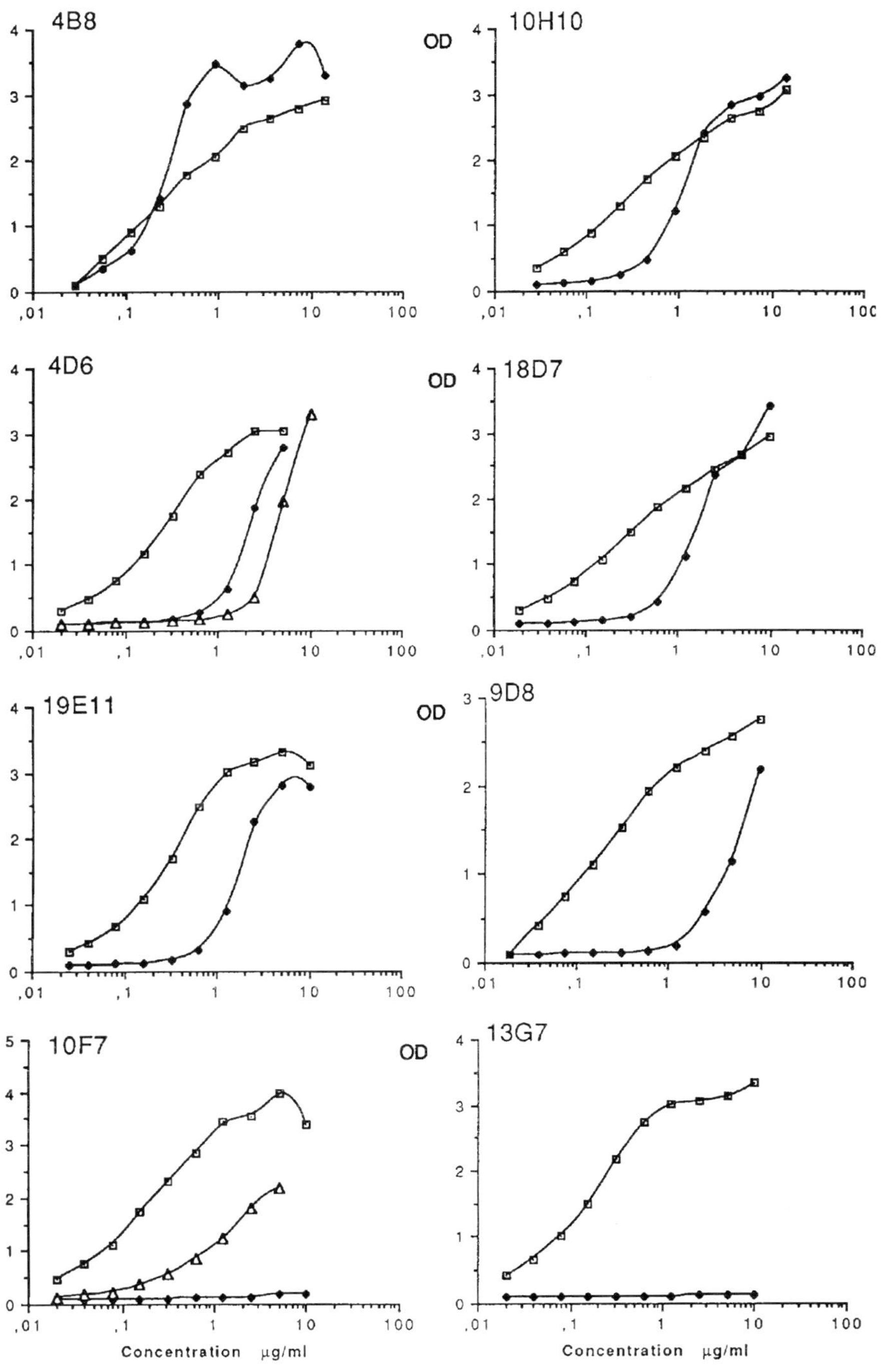

Fig. 4.5. Binding of SpA to Ag-bound monoclonal IgM antibodies (V_H-binders). Wells of microtiter plates were coated with Ag (phOx-BSA) and varying concentrations of mAbs were added. Binding was revealed by adding biotinylated SpA (solid squares) or biotinylated anti-kappa chain (open squares). The vertical axis gives the optical density (OD) and the horizontal axis the concentration of the mAb (µg/ml). An additional experiment was performed with two purified antibodies 4D6 and 10F7. The mAbs were directly coated on the plate and SpA was applied as in the main experiment (triangles).

Table 4.2. Proportions of SpA-binders among human Ig of various origins

Immunoglobulins tested	Isotype				
	IgM	IgA	IgA1	IgA2	IgG3
Myeloma proteins	35%		11%	25%	13%
Polyclonal Ig (adults)	32%		13%	24%	14%
Polyclonal Ig (4 m)	47%		35%	39%	38%
Polyclonal Ig (14 m)	44%		29%	37%	29%
Antibodies to Tetanus toxoid	43%	13%			
Antibodies to Diphtheria toxoid	38%	14%			
Antibodies to *Haemophilus influenza* type b polysaccharide	65%	36%			
Antibodies to Pneumococcal polysaccharide					
type 3	40%	29%			
type 18C	45%	33%			
type 14	52%	45%			
CPS	46%	24%			

Myeloma proteins of different H chain isotypes, polyclonal Ig from adults, 4 month old and 14 month-old infants and anti-microbial antibodies are considered. CPS: capsular polysaccharide.

concentrations of purified mAb. In the case of 4D6 the electrostatically bound mAb was inferior to the Ag-bound mAb regarding the binding of SpA but the reverse was true of 10F7. Plates directly coated with 10F7 mediated binding of SpA, those coated with 10F7 via the antigen failed to do so (Fig. 4.5).

These data as well as earlier studies suggest that an Ig can bind antigen and SpA at the same time, and that some degree of steric hindrance between the two "ligands" of a mAb exists.[18-19,25] SpA can bind to an Ag-bound Ig when the affinity is high for the Ig, but it does not bind when the affinity is low. Taken together, these data suggest that the SpA epitope is close but separate from the Ag-binding site.

SpA-BINDING AS A MARKER OF A HUMAN IMMUNOGLOBULIN SUBSET

By 1993 a total of 30 human mAbs with a known V_H family have been typed for SpA-binding.[21,25,35] Fourteen (V_H3^{+}) were binders and sixteen were nonbinders, two of which belonged to the V_H3 family. These two V_H3^+ Ig that do not bind SpA could be the product of a nonbinding germline gene or of somatic mutations converting a binder to a nonbinder Ig. However, eight replacement mutations in the V_H segment of one monoclonal Ig (MOPC 167, a product of a binder-encoding gene) have not changed its binding status (Table 4.2) suggesting that, at least for this antibody, somatic mutations does not greatly influence binding to SpA. Based on this observation it can be concluded that V_H-binding is a fairly good but incomplete marker of V_H3^+ Ig. Taking advantage of this phenomenon a series of experiments in which V_H-binding to SpA was used as the marker of this subset of human V_H3 immunoglobulins were conducted. The proportion of human Ig molecules which bind to SpA (V_H3 encoded Ig) were determined in different isotypes, age groups and specific antibodies.[36-37] Only IgM, IgA1, IgA2, and IgG3 were tested as the structure of the constant domains of these isotypes is such that binding must be mediated by the V domains and two approaches were taken. First, 115 monoclonal Ig of these isotypes were typed as binders or nonbinders. Second, an independent estimate of the bound fraction in a particular isotype was obtained from the polyclonal Ig of ten adults and ten 4- of 14-month-old children. The proportion of alternative binders in polyclonal and monoclonal Ig was determined by absorbing aliquots of normal serum with SpA-Sepharose and BSA-Sepharose (nonspecific binding), and determining IgM, IgA, IgA2, and IgG3 in the two supernatants using isotype or antibody-specific ELISA.[36-37] We assumed that the differences between the two was due to specific binding to SpA. Samples were tested more than once, and values in Table 4.2 are means of 4 or 5 tests.

FREQUENCY OF SPA-BINDERS IN IMMUNOGLOBULIN ISOTYPES

Since the VDJ rearrangement and Ig class switch are independent events the simple prediction is that the proportion of V_H-binders is approximately the same in all Ig classes of a species. Apparently this is not the case; the proportion of V_H-binders varies considerably from one heavy chain isotype to another (Table 4.2). The proportion of V_H-binders was considerably lower among IgA1 or IgG3 than among IgM paraproteins. A corresponding difference was observed in normal polyclonal Ig isotypes of adults. The average proportion was only 13-14% in IgA or IgG3 whereas it was approximately one-third in IgM ($p = 0.0029$). The curious additional finding was that a significantly higher proportion of IgA2 than IgA1 were V_H-binders (24 vs 13%, $p = 0.00035$).

FREQUENCY OF SPA BINDING AS A FUNCTION OF AGE

Ig of infants aged 4 months were richer in SpA-binders than adult Ig (Table 4.2). The mean for each Ig was significantly higher than the corresponding mean in adults ($p < 0.0001$). Children aged 14 months had slightly lower IgA and IgM SpA-binders than the 4-month-old infants. Smaller inter-isotypic differences, similar to those observed in adults, were seen in young infants. In adults, the difference between IgM and IgA1 and IgG3 was 2.5-fold; at the age of 4 months it was only 1.3-fold. The small size of the difference was due to the high proportion of alternative binders in infant IgA1 and IgG3 (more than 30%). Children aged 14 months took an intermediate position but were closer to infants than adults.

FREQUENCY OF SPA-BINDERS IN AG-SPECIFIC ANTIBODY POPULATIONS

Several antibody responses have been shown to use a limited number of V_H or V_L genes. Early experiments were carried out in mice. Adderson et al were the first to demonstrate the phenomenon in man in a study of the antibody response to type b polysaccharide of *Haemophilus influenzae*, where the V_H3 gene family is predominantly used.[38] V_H-binding to SpA can also be used for a search of antibody responses with a restricted V_{H3} gene usage. The results will be less informative than traditional methods such as generation of hybridomas and sequencing of Ag-specific mAbs but they are easier to obtain. Therefore a number of antibody responses, each in several individuals, can be studied.

The IgM and IgA antibody responses to seven bacterial antigens were studied. In responses to two protein antigens (tetanus toxoid and diphtheria toxoid) no evidence was found for a restricted V_H gene usage (Table 4.2). Both in IgM and in IgA antibodies the mean proportion of V_H-binders was approximately the same as in total IgM or IgA. This is probably because antibody responses to the two toxoids may be directed to several epitopes. It is possible that the response to one epitope of tetanus toxoid has a bias towards the use of V_H3 family but the response to other epitopes is derived from other gene families; the total response studied may then exhibit no bias.

Antibodies to polysaccharides had significantly higher proportions of SpA-binders compared with the total serum Ig (Table 4.2).[37] The excess was 1.3- to 2-fold in IgM and 1.7- to 2.5-fold in IgA. This suggests that the five anti-polysaccharide responses studied use a restricted set of V_H genes with a bias for the V_H3 family. Inter-individual variation was considerable especially in anti-Hib antibodies of IgA isotype (data are not shown).

DISCUSSION

SpA is considered a virulence factor.[39] Infection experiments, subcutaneous abscess and perotinitis in mice with a SpA-deficient strain showed that it is less virulent than the wild type strain.[40] SpA has also been shown to block opsonization in vitro.[39] The uptake of the wild type bacteria in the presence of normal human serum was significantly lower than with the SpA-mutant strain. Whether the classical Fc binding or the V_H-interaction is the cause for this effect is still unknown. The effect of Fc-binding on opsonization and phagocytosis is easily explained by interference with the recognition by the Fc receptors on leukocytes. Another possible explanation is that covering the bacterial surface with the host's IgG molecules helps the bacterium evade the immune system by masking the binding sites for opsonins present in normal serum.[39] However, IgG bound to SpA through the Fc can still activate complement.[41] Although these early experiments did not take into account the existence of the V_H-interaction, complement activation can be of advantage to the bacterium. Bacteria can deplete complement components, especially in the case of localized infections like those of *Staphylococcus aureus*, by activating complement at a distance from the cell wall. A strategy that is adopted by other bacterial strains as well.[42-44]

The distinction between V_H-binding and Fc-binding domains suggests that V_H binding has evolved recently as an independent function, and it must be beneficial for the bacterium. It is tempting to speculate that pathogens have evolved an elaborate mechanism to evade the immune system by activating and deleting B cells expressing families of V genes that are most likely to be used in anti-bacterial responses. Indeed, the antibody responses to several bacterial antigens, notably polysaccharides, are dominated by V_H genes that belongs to the V_H3 clan (V_H3 gene family in man, J606, S107, X24, and 7183 in mouse).[26] However, more evidence is needed to support this intriguing possibility.

The decrease of V_H-binders with age and their lower proportion in IgA1 and IgG3 than in IgM is another interesting phenomenon. It can be explained by postulating that the ontogenically early B cell population has a high proportion of cells producing V_H3^+ Ig with antigens in our environment stimulating preferentially B cells producing Ig encoded by other V_H gene families. The experiments with specific antibodies provide some tentative explanation for the preferential use of these early V_H genes. The same V_H genes encoding binder-Ig are responsible for a high proportion of human anti-polysaccharide antibodies. In the mouse, too, they seem to be responsible for a great number of anti-carbohydrate antibodies. According to Kabat et al 72% of mAbs of the J606 and S107families were anti-polysaccharide antibodies.[26] Only 18% of mAbs of other families were anti-polysaccharide antibodies. This suggests that evolution has selected for those V_H genes that encode antibodies recognizing important microbial structures to facilitate an early strong primary response to those common pathogens.

ACKNOWLEDGMENTS

This work was performed in the laboratories of Professor Olli Mäkela and Dr. Ilkka Seppälä, both of whom I thank for continuous support, encouragement and intellectual contributions. This study was supported by the University of Helsinki, the Paulo Foundation and the Centre for International Mobility (CIMO).

References

1. Löfkvist T, Sjöquist J. Chemical and serological analysis of antigen preparations from *Staphylococcus aureus*. A comparison between the products obtained by Verwey's and Jensen's techniques. Acta Path Microbiol Scand 1962; 56:295-304.
2. Grov A, Myklestad B, Oeding P. Immunochemical studies on antigen preparations from *Staphylococcus aureus*. 1. Isolation and chemical characterization of antigen A. Acta Path Microbiol Scand 1964; 61:588-96.
3. Forsgren A, Sjöquist J. "Protein A" from *S. aureus*. I. Pseudo-immune reaction with human γ-globulin. J Immunol 1966; 97:822-27.
4. Björck L, Kronvall G. Purification and some properties of streptococcal protein G, a novel IgG-binding reagent. J Immunol 1984; 133:969-74.
5. Reis KJ, Hansen HF Björck L. Extraction and characterization of IgG Fc receptors from group C and group G streptococci. Mol Immunol 1986; 23:425-31.
6. Forsgren A, Grubb A. Many bacterial species bind IgD. J Immunol 1979; 122: 1468-72.
7. Frithz E, Hedén L-O, Lindahl G. Extensive sequence homology between IgA receptor and M proteins in *Streptococcus pyogenes*. Mol Microbiol 1989; 3:1111-19.
8. Gomi H, Hozumi T, Hattori S et al. The gene sequence and some properties of protein H. A novel IgG-binding protein. J Immunol 1990; 144:4046-52.
9. Kronvall G, Seal US, Finstad J et al. Phylogenetic insight into evolution of mammalian Fc fragment of γG globulin using staphylococcal protein A. J Immunol 1970; 104:140-47.
10. Grov A, Oeding P, Myklestad B et al. Reactions of staphylococcal antigens with normal sera, γG-globulins, and γG-globulin fragments of various species origin. Acta path microbiol scand Sect B 1970; 78: 106-11.
11. Kronvall G, Seal US, Svensson S et al. Phylogenetic aspects of staphylococcal protein A-reactive serum globulins in birds and mammals. Acta Path Microbiol Scand Sect B 1974; 82:12-18.
12. Harboe M, Fölling I. Recognition of two distinct groups of human IgM and IgA based on different binding to staphylococci. Scand J Immunol 1974; 3:471-82.
13. Johansson SGO, Inganäs M. Interaction of polyclonal human IgE with protein-A from *Staphylococcus aureus*. Immunol Rev 1978; 41:248-60.
14. Biguzzi S. Fcγ-like determinants on immunoglobulin variable regions: identification by staphylococcal protein A. Scand J Immunol 1982; 15:605-18.
15. Erntell M, Myhre EB, Kronvall G. Non-immune $F(ab')_2$- and Fc-mediated interactions of mammalian immunoglobulins with *S. aureus* and group C and G streptococci. Acta Path Microbiol Immunol Scand Sect B 1986. 94:377-85.
16. Erntell M, Sjöbring U, Myhre EB et al. Non-immune Fab- and Fc- mediated interactions of avian Ig with *S. aureus* and group C and G streptococci. Acta Path Microbiol Immunol Scand 1988; 96:239-49.
17. Inganäs M, Johansson SGO, Bennich HH. Interaction of human polyclonal IgE and IgG from different species with protein A from *Staphylococcus aureus:* Demonstration of protein-A-reactive sites located in the Fab_2 fragment of human IgG. Scand. J Immunol 1980; 12:23-31.
18. Endresen C. The binding to protein A of immunoglobulin G and of Fab and Fc fragments. Acta Path Microbiol Scand Sect C 1979. 87:185-89.
19. Young WW JR, Tamura Y, Wolock DM, Fox JW. Staphylococcal protein A binding to the Fab fragments of mouse monoclonal antibodies. J Immunol 1984; 133:3163-66.
20. Vidal MA, Conde FP. Alternative mechanism of protein A-immunoglobulin interaction: the V_H-associated reactivity of a monoclonal human IgM. J Immunol 1985; 135:1232-38.
21. Sasso EH, Silverman GJ, Mannik M. Human IgM molecules that bind staphylococcal protein A contain V_HIII H chains. J Immunol 1989; 142:2778-83.
22. Sasso EH, Silverman GJ, Mannik M. Human IgA and IgG $(F(ab')_2$ that bind to staphylococcal protein A belong to the V_HIII subgroup. J Immunol 1991; 147:1877-83.

23. Endresen C. Protein A reactivity of whole rabbit IgG and of fragments of rabbit IgG. Acta Path Microbiol Scand Sect C 1978. 86:211-14.
24. Seppälä I, Kaartinen M, Ibrahim S et al. Mouse Ig coded by V_H families S107 or J606 bind to protein A. J Immunol 1990; 145:2989-93.
25. Ibrahim S, Kaartinen M, Matoso-Ferreira A et al. The alternative binding site for protein A in the Fab fragment of immunoglobulins. Scand J Immunol 1993; 37:257-64.
26. Kabat EA, Wu TT, Perry HM et al. Sequences of proteins of immunological interest, 5th edition NIH Publication 91-3242. 1991.
27. Schroeder HW JR, Hillson JL, Perlmutter RM. Structure and evolution of mammalian V_H families. Int Immunol 1990; 2:41-49.
28. Kirkham PM, Mortari F, Newton JA et al. Immunoglobulin V_H clan and family identity predicts variable domain structure and may influence antigen binding. EMBO J 1992; 11:603-9.
29. Padlan EA. Anatomy of the antibody molecule. Mol Immunol 1994; 31:169-217.
30. Randen I, Potter KN, Thompson KM et al. Complementary-determining region 2 is implicated in the binding of staphylococcal protein A to human immunoglobulin V_HIII variable regions. Eur J Immunol 1993; 23: 2682-86.
31. Hillson JL, Karr NS, Oppliger IR et al. The structural basis of germline-encoded V_H3 immunoglobulin binding to staphylococcal protein A. J Exp Med 1993; 178:331-36.
32. Moks T, Abrahamsén L, Nilsson B et al. Staphylococcal protein A consists of five IgG-binding domains. Eur J Biochem 1986; 156:637-43.
33. Ibrahim S. Immunoglobulin binding specificities of the homology regions (domains) of protein A. Scand J Immunol 1993; 38:368-74
34. Robin PW, Salem AN, Silverman GJ. V_H3 family antibodies bind domain D of staphylococcal protein A. J Immunol 1995; 154:6437-45.
35. Silverman GJ. Human antibody responses to bacterial antigens: studies of a model conventional antigen and a proposed model B cell superantigen. Int. Rev. Immunol 1992; 9:57-78.
36. Ibrahim S, Seppälä I, Mäkelä O. The V-region mediated binding of human Ig by protein A. J Immunol 1993; 151:3597-603.
37. Ibrahim S, Seppälä IJT, Sarvas H et al. Proportion of protein A bindable molecules in human IgM and IgA antibodies to seven antigens. Microbial Pathogenesis 1993; 15:159-68.
38. Adderson EE, Shackelford PG, Quinn A et al. Restricted IgH chain V gene usage in the human antibody response to *Haemophilus influenzae* type b capsular polysaccharide. J Immunol 1991; 147:1667-74
39. Foster TJ, McDevitt D. Surface-associated proteins of staphylococcus aureus: their possible roles in virulence. FEMS Microbiol Letters 1994; 118:199-206.
40. Patel AH, Nowlan P, weavers ED et al. Virulence of protein a-deficient and alpha-toxin-deficient mutants of *Staphylococcus aureus* isolated by allele replacement. Infect Immun 1987; 55:3103-10.
41. Sjöquist J, Stålenheim G. Protein A from *Staphylococcus aureus*. IX. complement-fixing activity of protein A-IgG complexes. J Immunol 1969; 103:467-73.
42. Brown EJ. Interaction of gram-positive microorganisms with complement. In: Loos M, ed. Current Topics in Microbiology and Immunology. Bacteria and Complement. Heidelberg: Springer-Verlag 1985; 159-82.
43. Joiner KA. Complement evasion by bacteria and parasites. Ann Rev Microbiol 1988; 42:201-30.
44. Jones KF, Fischetti VA. The importance of the location of the antibody binding on M6 protein for opsonization and phagocytosis of group A M6 streptococci. J Exp Med 1988; 167:1114-23.

CHAPTER 5

B Cell Superantigens and the Somatic Diversification of Immune Repertoires: Molecular and Cellular Implications

Gregg J. Silverman

INTRODUCTION

Superantigens (SAg) have received considerable attention due to their ability to induce global changes in the overall composition of the immune repertoire. Unlike a conventional peptide antigen (Ag) that can generally stimulate less than 0.01% of naive lymphocytes, a superantigen can stimulate greater than 5% of the lymphocyte pool,[1] which represents a 500-fold enhanced lymphocyte mitogenic potential. In several different cases, this broad reactivity has been documented to occur largely because the T cell SAg is recognized by most (or all) lymphocytes that express T cell receptors (TcR) that derive from a particular β chain variable region ($V_β$) family, and reactivity in many cases did not appear to be significantly affected by differences in $V_β$ junctional sequences or by the α chains that are coexpressed. Studies of a virally encoded T cell SAg indicate that binding is mediated through contact residues in the first and third framework regions (FR) of the $V_β$ chains shared by all members of a $V_β$ gene family. These framework region residues are spatially distinct from the putative TcR Ag combining site.[2]

The potent in vivo immunomodulatory abilities of T cell SAgs have been extensively investigated.[3] T cell SAg exposure can result in large scale lymphocyte clonal expansions and/or deletions. In a susceptible animal strain, SAg exposure can have different outcomes; costimulation can augment the response to a conventional peptide Ag,[4] induce immunosuppression[3] or result in the production of auto-antibodies (Abs).[5] T cell SAgs have also been implicated in the pathogenesis of human diseases, such as toxic shock syndrome[6] and Kawasaki's disease.[7] A possible role for a T cell SAg in the initiation of autoimmune diseases, such as rheumatoid arthritis has also been proposed.[8] Because T cell superantigens specifically trigger lymphocytes via a TcR-mediated mechanism, and these cells can subsequently be traced with serologic and genetic markers, these SAg studies have also greatly contributed to our current understanding of the fundamental properties of T cells and their in vivo regulation.

Compared to the extensive data on T cell superantigens, much less is known about proteins with comparable interactions with B lymphocytes. Following our first descriptions of a bacterial protein with V gene family-specific binding interactions with immunoglobulins (Igs),[9] we reviewed available T cell SAg data and proposed a series of diagnostic properties that we believe should be documented before a protein can be characterized as a SAg for B lymphocytes:[10,11]

General Properties of B cell Superantigens

i. Superantigens should interact with a large fraction (e.g., > 5%) of the Fab of nonimmune Ig of different isotypes and with surface Ig of B cells.
ii. Abs and B cells that bind conventional Ags can also bind a SAg, and SAg binding should not interfere with the simultaneous binding of a conventional Ag.
iii. Superantigen binding activity should be restricted to Ab from specific V gene families and should involve sites outside of the conventional Ag binding site.
iv. Lymphocyte stimulation should result in shifts in V_H family-restricted B cell populations that are much greater than can occur with a conventional Ag.

We have recently presented a methodological approach to the evaluation of putative B cell superantigens,[11] based on our investigations of the bacterial membrane protein, Staphylococcal protein A (SpA), which is now the best characterized of all known bacterial Ig receptors. SpA has two separate Ig binding specificities. Most attention has focused on the classical Ig binding interaction of SpA that is specific for the Fc fragment of the human IgG1, IgG2, IgG4 heavy (H) chain constant region subclasses.[12] SpA also has an alternate Ig binding site, with specificity for the Fab portion of many Igs. This frequent Fab-mediated reactivity does not require prior exposure to SpA[13] and does not usually interfere with the binding of a conventional Ag.[14] Fab-mediated binding is expressed by 10-40% of human monoclonal and polyclonal Ig irrespective of the isotype of H and light (L) chains,[13] and these binding interactions are now known to involve the V_H domain of the H chain.[9,15] Different antibodies (Abs) compete for Fab-mediated binding to SpA,[16] which indicates that all interactions are mediated by the same unconventional Fab binding site(s). Studies from our group[9,10,15-18] and others[19-24] have documented that SpA has an unconventional human V_H3 gene family-specific Fab-binding activity that imparts properties predicted for a B cell SAg, although the response to in vivo exposure has not been investigated.

Recent studies from our laboratory have also demonstrated that an endogenous human sialoprotein, termed protein Fv (pFv), also has the binding properties of a B cell SAg.[25] pFv is a 175 kDa dimeric sialoprotein that was originally discovered by Bouvet and co-workers in the enteric contents of patients suffering from viral liver diseases.[26] pFv has six separate functional sites for interacting with the Fab of a large proportion (>20%) of human adult IgM, IgA, IgG and IgE.[27] Among the in vitro properties characterized, binding of pFv has been shown to trigger complement activation by IgG or IgM Abs[28] and it can induce the activation of IgE-sensitized basophils.[29] In addition, pFv can augment pathogen agglutination by anti-virus and anti-bacterial Abs.[30] It has been proposed that through these properties pFv contributes to the humoral immune defenses in the gut.[30] We have recently demonstrated that pFv binding is primarily restricted to the products of the V_H3 and V_H6 gene families and that the properties of SpA and pFv display many similarities.[25]

In the current review, we present our observations from studies that have sought to elucidate the molecular and cellular correlates for the unconventional Ag-Ab interactions of SpA and pFv. Our observations suggest that the molecular bases for the binding properties of the T cell SAgs and B cell SAgs are highly analogous. We have also determined that the microbial and endogenous proteins, SpA and pFv, generally recognize related and overlapping unconventional sites in V_H regions. The possible implications of these findings for the development of B cell repertoires and the (dys)regulation of immune responses are discussed.

SPECIFICITY AND AFFINITY OF AB BINDING TO SPA

Unlike studies of T cell SAgs, which initially focused on cellular and in vivo responses and only much more recently have made use of isolated TcR, our first molecular studies were greatly simplified by the availability of soluble monoclonal and polyclonal Ig that include the Fab (Ag binding) structures that also act as the membrane receptors of B cells. Thus, our initial studies evaluated the structural bases for Fab-mediated binding of SpA by correlating the binding capacity for SpA with Ab V region usage.[9,15] These studies were facilitated by the application of a novel panel of V family-specific serologic reagents that can identify the V family origins of Ig samples.[9,15,31,32] We found that Fab-mediated SpA binding is common amongst monoclonal V_H3 Abs, but absent in a large panel of monoclonal IgM and IgG from the other V_H families. These primary sequence-specific reagents also enabled the observation that the subsets of polyclonal IgM, IgA and IgG $F(ab')_2$ that bind to an SpA-affinity column are highly enriched in the products of the V_H3 family.[9,15]

To further investigate the molecular and genetic correlates of SpA binding interactions, we created combinatorial Ig expression libraries in the phagemid vector, pComb3 (the gift of Dr. Carlos Barbas III, The Scripps Research Institute) that enables the efficient cloning and in vitro expression of human Ig H and L chains, either separately or in combination. This combinatorial library approach offers many unique advantages. Large libraries with greater than 10^7 H chains and 10^7 L chains are created with mRNA from lymphocytes. V_H-C_H1 rearrangements, and rearranged L chain genes are amplified with a large series of sequence-specific primers that enable directional cloning into pComb3. Bacteria transformed with a library of these constructs are "rescued" with helper filamentous phage, resulting in the creation of a library of phage that contain the DNA construct and which express the encoded H-L chain Fab dimer on their surface. From these libraries, we can evaluate unconventional SAg binding interactions with the Ag receptors of B cells from any lymphoid compartment or from any point of immune development. Compared to the inefficiency of studying Abs from B cell lines, this represents a more efficient "high throughput" system to evaluate a virtually unlimited number of Abs. In addition, sequence determination of the Ab genes cloned into the expression vector is technically simplified, and the cloned genes are also easily manipulated for H-L chain pairing and mutagenesis studies. This expression vector does not include the C_H2 and C_H3 domains, so the Fc binding activity of SpA is irrelevant.

Our first combinatorial Ab library, subsequently designated JG, was created from the peripheral blood cells of a healthy adult donor.[16] This library was constructed with diverse κ and λ L chain genes paired with rearranged γ H chain genes to study the effect of the hypermutation on SpA binding. With the phage-display form of the library, Abs were selected by biopanning on microtiter wells coated with

SpA. During subsequent rounds of panning, we documented a competition for selection based on superior SpA binding affinities.[16] Thus, Abs from these libraries can be used for sequence correlations of SpA binders and nonbinders to evaluate the minimal structural and genetic requirements for binding, and for a possible effect of somatic hypermutation on binding. By using Ab from SpA selected libraries, the determinants associated with optimal SpA binding capacity can be identified. The central findings regarding V_H gene expression and SpA binding include:

i. While this IgG Fab phage-display library contained a V_H family usage roughly representative of the in vivo distribution, we found that about 17% of Ab-expressing clones in the library bound SpA.
ii. About 60% of V_H3 Fab in the unselected IgG library had SpA binding capacity.
iii. Biopanning with SpA resulted in selection based on relative SpA binding affinities.
iv. SpA binding was completely restricted to Fab with V_H3 H chains.
v. All Abs competed for binding at the same (or adjacent) site(s) on SpA.
vi. From V region sequence analyses of over 40 SpA-binding Abs, SpA binding activity was shown to be common to Ab with highly diverse complementarity-determining regions (CDR1 and 2) subdomain sequences, and Fab that bind SpA do not display conserved V_H CDR3 sequence or J_H usage.
vii. Both mutated and germline V_H3 sequences can bind SpA, and the proportion of B cells with SpA binding activity remains high even following somatic hypermutation (although some SpA binding activity is lost) (Fig. 5.1).

Because these studies included affinity measurements of diverse Fab, we were able to demonstrate that V_H3 Abs display a hierarchy of binding affinities for SpA, based on V region usage (discussed further below). These data, taken together with sequence correlations from other groups,[19,21,22,24] indicate that at least 15 (and perhaps all) of the 26-32 known potentially functional germline V_H3 gene segments can encode for an SpA binding site (Fig. 5.1).[10,16,33] It is also evident that SpA binding capacity is not limited to only certain V_H3 gene products with particular CDR sequences or with certain canonical CDR structures.

To further evaluate the structural requirements for SpA binding, H-L chain

Legend for Fig. 5.1 (opposite page):

[a] V_H regions with a V_H3 gene segment in germline configuration are indicated below "Germline". Certain H chains were obtained from fetal tissues and are presumed to contain V_H segments in germline configuration,[19] although the germline source has not been independently isolated.

[b] SpA binding activity is frequently expressed by V_H3 antibodies that also have a conventional antigen binding activity, which is indicated below "Ag".

[c] The immunoglobulin isotype is indicated below "Isotype". The IgG Fab were derived from a combinatorial antibody expression library (20), all others were derived via conventional cellular approaches.

Sequences are compiled from previous reports by Silverman[10] designated[d], by Sasano et al[16] designated[e], by Ibrahim et al[21] designated[f], by Randen et al[24] designated[g], by Hillson et al[19] designated[h], and by Sasso et al[9] designated[i]. The V_H sequence for CA4/PRP12 is previously unreported[10,19] (AH Lucas, personal communication). Amino acid residues are indicated by the single letter code. X is an indeterminate residue. "-" indicates identity with the amino acid in the same position in the 18/2 sequence.

* marks the amino acid positions in V_H3 FR3[16] and CDR2[24] that have been implicated as critical to expression of SpA binding activity. From mutagenesis experiments with a V_H3-encoded IgM RF, Randen et al[24] have reported that at the indicated position in CDR2, K endows SpA binding capacity, while E abolishes SpA binding. However, the absence of SpA binding by PRSJ1 and SpA1-17 indicates that this is not a universal rule. The role of the loop (HV4) in the FR3 subdomain is suggested by antibody 0-19, which has very weaked SpA binding activity.[16] Adapted from Silverman.[38]

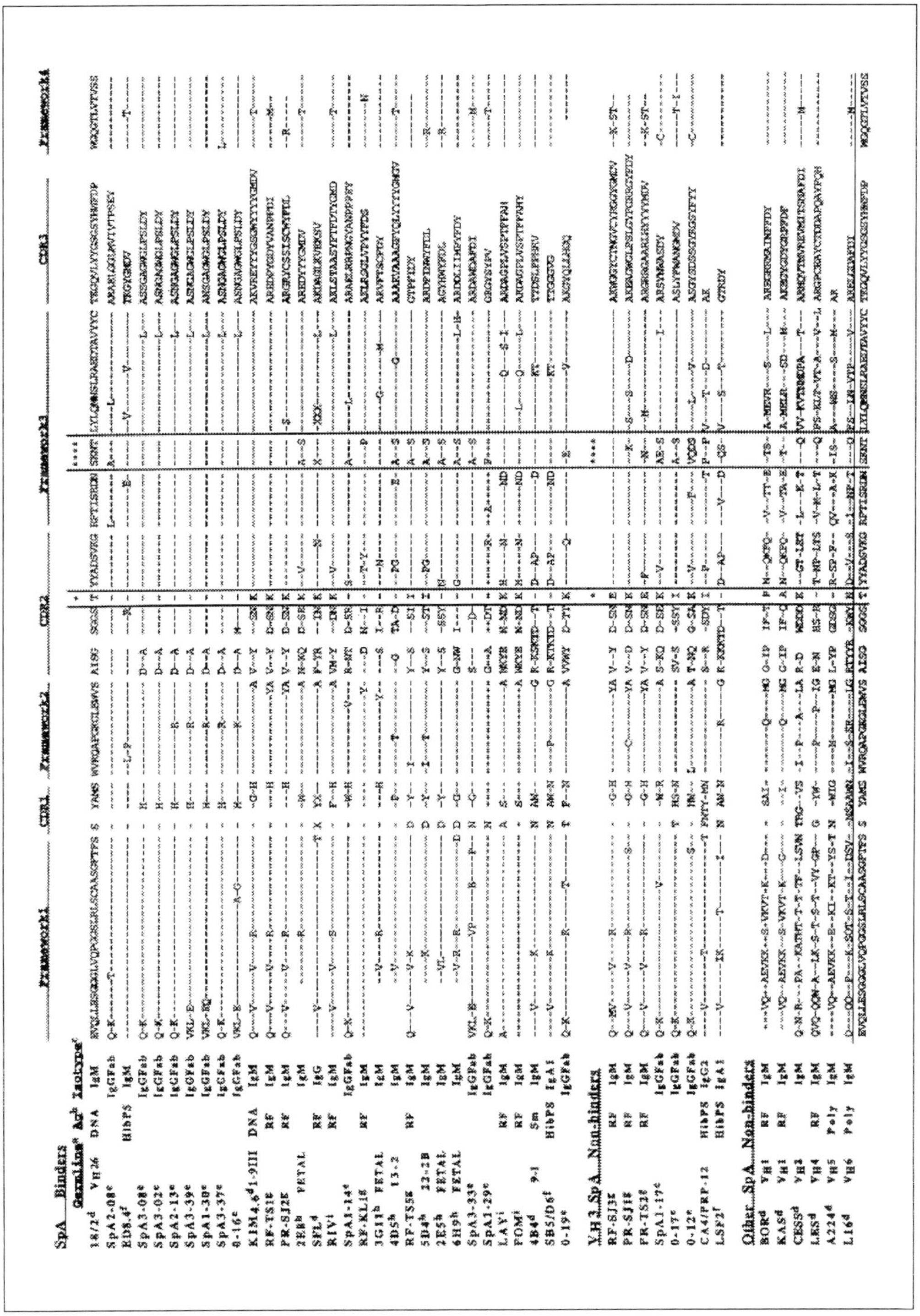

Fig. 5.1. SpA binding and VH utilization. Antibody sequences and relative reactivity with the Fab-mediated binding site of SpA are compiled. VH regions are grouped by VH gene segment family and SpA reactivity. (Legend for Fig. 5.1 on opposite page).

recombination experiments were also performed. The same L chain gene was grafted into a series of the JG phagemid constructs with different V_H gene rearrangements. These studies demonstrated that the global capacity to bind (or not bind) SpA is dictated by the specific V_H3 gene usage—a V_H3 H chain from an antibody without SpA binding activity did not acquire SpA binding activity when it was associated with a L chain from a high affinity SpA binder. We looked for evidence of an effect of V_H3 gene hypermutation on SpA binding activities, using phagemids with the same L chain gene and a limited series of related V_H gene rearrangements that differed by up to three replacement mutations. In Fab with the JGSpA3-37 and JGSpA2-13 H chains, we found that a somatic replacement mutation that changed a tryptophan to a leucine in the FR4 portion contributed by the J_H gene segment resulted in significant, but minor (2-fold), decrease in relative SpA binding affinity.

These differential H-L chain pairing studies also enabled the first direct evaluations of the contribution of L chains to SpA binding activity. Significantly, in certain cases changing only the L chain usage caused up to a 4-fold change in SpA binding affinity. We believe that this does not necessarily indicate that L chains are directly involved in SpA binding. It seems more likely that certain L chains better facilitate the stabilization of desirable V_H region conformations or improve the accessibility to V_H region contact sites.

THE GERMLINE GENE V_H3-23 APPEARS TO ENCODE FOR OPTIMAL SPA BINDING ACTIVITY

Following three rounds of SpA panning of the IgG Fab library, individual Fab-producing clones were isolated, and their high affinity for SpA confirmed.[16] The complete sequences of the V_H genes encoding nine of these highly selected SpA binders were determined.[16] As mentioned above, ELISA-based affinity measurements confirmed that throughout this process Fab clones were selected based on relative SpA binding affinity. Interestingly, sequence analysis of the SpA binders obtained after three rounds of panning demonstrated that the H chains derived from only two unique V-D-J rearrangements. The dominant clone from the JG library, representing seven of these nine sequences, was most homologous to the V_H26c/V3-23 germline gene, with only four replacement mutations.[16] To further evaluate the germline origin of these rearrangements, the V_H3 genes in the genomic DNA of the donor were amplified by the polymerase chain reaction, and then blotted and probed with an oligonucleotide with the exact CDR2 sequence unique to the representative clone, JGSpA3-08 (GJS, unpublished). A replicate blot was hybridized with an equivalent oligonucleotide probe from the V_H26c/V3-23 sequence. While the donor was shown to have inherited genes akin to the V_H26c/V3-23 gene, we did not detect a germline gene segment closer to the highly selected sequences of the JGSpA3-08 related Fabs. These studies further suggested that the Fab with optimal SpA binding activity in the JG library are most likely derived from the V_H26c/V3-23 gene segment.

To extend our observations, we then created an IgM Fab library, designated JM, beginning with the same L chain library and using V_H-mu rearrangements amplified from the same peripheral blood sample of the donor of the JG library. After three rounds of panning of this IgM Fab library on SpA, seven V_H sequences of these highly selected SpA binders were determined (GJS, unpublished). Five of these highly selected rearrangements were found to contain the exact germline configuration of the V_H26/V3-23 gene. These rearrangements, which include the phagemid clone termed JMSpA3-15, have different V_H CDR3 than the JGSpA3-08 related Fab, and they do not appear to derive from the same lymphocyte source (Fig. 5.1).

In a recent report, we described studies of the binding of Abs to SpA with the BIAcore™ surface plasmon resonance device (Pharmacia) that enables real-time measurements of the kinetics of macromolecular binding interactions.[18] We evaluated the binding of Fab because these Abs are capable of only monovalent SpA binding interactions. The highly selected IgG Fab, JGSpA3-08, and IgM Fab, JMSpA3-15, were of particular interest because they share near identical V_H gene segment contributions but have completely different V_H CDR3, heavy chain constant regions and L chains (Vλ1 and Vκ2, respectively). These measurements demonstrated apparent K_D of 1.6×10^{-7} M and 2.1×10^{-7} M for the JGSpA3-08 and JMSpA3-15 Fab, respectively [18] (Table 5.1). These data independently confirmed the dominant contribution of the V_H gene segment in determining SpA binding capacity. Native V_H3 IgM had significantly stronger binding (>100-fold stronger), presumably due to multivalent binding interactions (Table 5.1).

The observation that rearrangements of the V_H26c/V3-23 gene in human repertoires express the strongest affinity for SpA is potentially important for several reasons. Within the human genome, V_H26c/V3-23 encoded H chains contain one of the most highly conserved V_H FR1/FR3 surfaces,[34] and this gene is also closest to the consensus sequence of germline human V_H3 gene segments.[35] While the repertoires of many other mammalian species also commonly express Fab-mediated SpA-binding activity,[36] their Ab genes also share great(est) homology with the human V_H26c/V3-23 gene.[37]

LOCALIZATION OF THE V_H REGION BINDING SITE FOR *STAPHYLOCOCCAL* PROTEIN A

As described above, extensive data clearly indicate that SpA binding activity correlates with V_H region usage but not with CDR sequences. These sequence data and the finding that SpA binding does not interfere with the binding of conventional Ags binding (that generally involve CDR sites) all suggest that V_H framework region (FR) contact sites are responsible for SpA binding. We have recently discussed this topic in detail.[38] The FR1 and FR3 subdomains together create a large solvent exposed Fab surface that is not directly in contact with the L chain and which is separate from the classical Ag binding site.[34,39] While we believe that the V_H FR portions are involved in SpA binding, the localization of the SpA binding site has been complicated by the fact that all of the members of a V_H family have limited variation in their FR1 and the FR3 subdomains,[34] and many of these residues are required to maintain the overall "immunoglobulin fold".[39] Therefore, it is not possible to rigorously examine this question by comparing SpA binding in Abs that have all potential FR mutations in the V_H region, because many mutations are not structurally allowable. These studies have to consider that single mutations may alter the conformation of the overall Ig fold.

Capra and co-workers have reported that a single nonconservative amino acid change at position 57 (lysine to glutamic acid) in the V_H CDR2 of a V3-30/hv3005-encoded V_H3 rheumatoid factor can destroy SpA binding.[24] However glutamic acid is present at this position in only a minority of the V_H3-encoded SpA nonbinders, and many V_H3 Abs with lysine at position 57 have been described as SpA nonbinders (Fig. 5.1).[33,38]

While far from conclusive, in association with M. Hakoda (Tokyo Women's College) we have recently evaluated the binding of SpA and Mod SpA (see below) to oligopeptides (14-20 amino acids) with sequences from V_H gene segments to look for evidence of possible SpA V_H region contact sites. These studies failed to detect any binding to a previously described series of V_H3 CDR2 derived peptides.[40,41] Thus we doubt that the CDR2 subdomain commonly contributes important SAg contact sites in all V_H3 Ab. These subdomains more likely play an indirect role by affecting remote conformation. By comparison, several peptides with V_H3 FR3 sequences had significant direct SpA binding activity while peptides with comparable sequences from other V_H families were nonreactive[40] (M. Hakoda and GJS, manuscript submitted). These data further support a central role for an unconventional V_H3 FR Ab site in SpA binding interactions.

Table 5.1. The kinetics of B cell superantigen binding interactions

Ig	V_H usage	V_L usage	Isotype		SpA	Protein Fv
Fab fragments (monomeric)						
JMSpA3-15	V_H3	$V_\kappa 3$	IgM Fab	$k_{on}\ (M^{-1}s^{-1})$	4.3×10^3	6.0×10^3
	$V_H26c/V3\text{-}23$			$k_{off}\ (s^{-1})$	8.8×10^{-4}	3.1×10^{-3}
	(100%)			$K_a\ (M^{-1})$	4.8×10^6	1.9×10^6
				$K_D\ (M)$	2.1×10^{-7}	5.3×10^{-7}
JGSpA3-08	V_H3	$V_\lambda 1$	IgG Fab	k_{on}	1.5×10^3	9.8×10^3
	$V_H26c/V3\text{-}23$			k_{off}	2.3×10^{-4}	2.7×10^{-3}
	(94.8%)			K_a	6.2×10^6	3.5×10^6
				K_D	1.6×10^{-7}	2.9×10^{-7}
IgM (polymeric)						
18/2	V_H3	$V_\kappa 1$	IgM	k_{on}	1.3×10^5	3.75×10^4
	$V_H26c/V3\text{-}23$			k_{off}	1.2×10^{-4}	2.5×10^{-4}
	(100%)			K_a	1.1×10^9	1.5×10^8
				K_D	9.1×10^{-10}	6.7×10^{-9}
Kim4.6	V_H3	$V_\lambda 1$	IgM	k_{on}	9.7×10^4	4.3×10^4
	1.9III/V3-30			k_{off}	1.7×10^{-4}	6.4×10^{-5}
	(100%)			K_a	5.7×10^8	6.7×10^8
				K_D	1.8×10^{-9}	1.5×10^{-9}
Hum2-3	V_H3	$V_\lambda 7$	IgM	k_{on}	6.9×10^3	3.4×10^3
	MTGL/V3-73			k_{off}	2.9×10^{-4}	2.4×10^{-4}
	(90%)			K_a	2.1×10^7	1.4×10^7
				K_D	4.8×10^{-8}	7.1×10^{-8}
Hum14-3	V_H3	$V_\kappa 4$	IgM	k_{on}	7.1×10^3	5.0×10^3
	H11			k_{off}	2.2×10^{-4}	4.5×10^{-4}
	(97%)			K_a	3.2×10^7	1.1×10^7
				K_D	3.1×10^{-8}	9.1×10^{-8}
L16	V_H6	V_λ	IgM	k_{on}		1.76×10^4
	6-1R1			k_{off}		2.0×10^{-4}
	(100%)			K_a		8.8×10^7
				K_D	NR	1.1×10^{-8}
$Fc\gamma$				k_{on}	4.1×10^4	
hi				k_{off}	1.8×10^{-4}	
				K_a	2.2×10^8	
				K_D	4.5×10^{-9}	NR
$Fc\gamma$				k_{on}	4.1×10^4	
low				k_{off}	3.6×10^{-3}	
				K_a	1.2×10^7	
				K_D	8.3×10^{-8}	NR

Binding kinetics were measured using the BIAcore[R] apparatus (Pharmacia). k_{on} ($M^{-1}s^{-1}$), k_{off} (s^{-1}), K_a (M^{-1}) K_D (M). The K_a (association constant) is the ratio of the k_{on}/k_{off} kinetic constants and the K_D (dissociation constant) is the ratio of the k_{off}/k_{on} kinetic constants. The closest known V_H gene segments are indicated, and the % DNA sequence homology to the closest known germline gene. All are V_H3 antibodies, except L16 which is encoded by the germline configuration of the V_H6 gene. The V_L family and the isotype are also indicated. Compiled from Silverman et al.[25] and Roben et al.[18]

CHARACTERIZATION OF THE SITE(S) ON SPA THAT BIND ABS

To understand the structural and biologic SAg properties of SpA, we have begun to characterize the site(s) on this bacterial protein that is responsible for SAg activity. The protein and DNA sequences of this 45 kDa bacterial membrane protein indicate that there are 5 extracellular domains in tandem, E, D, A, B, C, and an additional transmembrane domain, X.[42-45] Each of these extra-membrane domains consists of 58-61 amino acids and they are about 80% homologous at a protein level[44] (Fig. 5.2). We know that the Fab and Fcγ binding sites of SpA are structurally and functionally separate because chemical modification of SpA by hyper-iodination can create a molecule termed Mod SpA (see below) that retains Fab binding activity but is devoid of Fc binding activity.[17,46] In addition, earlier reports have suggested that these two distinct Ig binding activities are noncompetitive,[47,48] but these studies are difficult to interpret because multiple domain proteins were studied. A V_H3 Fab-binding site had not previously been localized to a single domain of SpA.

MOLECULAR ANALYSES OF THE PROPERTIES OF SINGLE DOMAIN MOLECULES OF SPA

We selected domain D of SpA for molecular characterization because of a unique structural/genetic feature that distinguishes it from the other extracellular domains.[18] Domain D is the domain of SpA that has a three codon insert that encodes Ala-Gln-Gln (A-Q-Q) between the second and third amino acids of the consensus sequence of the extra-membrane domains (see Fig. 5.2). We cloned and expressed in *Eschericia coli* the 61 codons that compose domain D.[18] Unexpectedly, we discovered that this small protein exhibited both the V_H3 Fab and Fcγ binding specificities.[18] Sandwich ELISA confirmed that domain D can express both activities simultaneously. Competition ELISA suggested that V_H3 Fab binding of this single domain protein does not interfere with Fcγ binding or vice versa.[18]

Multidomain form of SpA			VH3 IgM	Fcγ
Native SpA			9.0×10^{-10} M	4.4×10^{-9} M (hi)
				8.7×10^{-8} M (lo)
Mono- domain forms of SpA				
Domain D		ADAQQNNFNKDQQSAFYEILNMPNLNEAQRNGFIQSLKDDPSQSTNVLGEAKKLNESQAPK	5.0×10^{-9} M	6.7×10^{-8} M
ΔtridomD'	--	---	7.7×10^{-9} M	6.2×10^{-9} M
Domain B	--	-K---E--N------HL-----E----------------A-L-A------DA----	6.3×10^{-9} M	4.0×10^{-9} M

Fig. 5.2. Correlation of SpA domain sequence and binding dissociation constant (K_D). The binding afffinities for Fcγ and the monoclonal V_H3 IgM, 18/2,[71] of native (multidomain) SpA is compared with different single domain SpA proteins. Sequence variations of the single domain proteins ΔtridomD' and Domain B are compared with the amino acid sequence of domain D. Different amino acids in the sequence are indicated by the single letter code, while (-) indicates an identical residue and (*) indicates a deletion. Data are compiled from ref. 18 and previously unreported studies of the kinetics of binding interaction with the BIAcore (Pharmacia).

A domain D monomer displays the same V_H3-restricted Fab binding specificity as the parent SpA molecule. The affinity of this binding interaction also varies with specific V_H3 gene usage,[18] confirming our previous findings.[16] The presumed monovalent binding interaction of the Fab, JMSpA3-15, which is encoded by the V_H26c gene, had an apparent affinity constant (K_D) of 4.3×10^{-7} M for domain D in BIAcore studies.[18] These experiments were designed so that we could evaluate an intact V_H3 IgM in solution for multivalent Fab-mediated binding interactions with the domain D molecule immobilized on the biosensor chip. These studies also employed a native monoclonal IgM, termed 18/2, that is also encoded by the germline configuration of the V_H26c gene. This native IgM was shown to bind domain D about 100-fold stronger (apparent K_D 5.0×10^{-9} M). For the V_H3 Abs evaluated, the V_H26c-derived Ab had the strongest binding interactions with both domain D and native SpA. Significantly, these binding interactions have affinities comparable to those associated with primary Ab responses to conventional Ags.

Deletional Mutagenesis of Domain D of SpA

To assess the functional impact of the three amino acid insert in domain D, we genetically engineered the removal of the three amino acid insert (A-Q-Q) in a variant of domain D that we termed ΔtridomD' (Fig. 5.2).[18] In surface plasmon resonance measurements, this deletion did not significantly alter the V_H3 Fab-mediated SpA binding activity compared to the multidomain SpA. However, kinetic studies of the multidomain SpA demonstrated Fcγ binding sites of two different affinities (hi and lo). The Fcγ binding activity of our recombinant domain D was comparable to the weaker (lo) binding site of native multidomain SpA, while the recombinant domain B of ΔtridomD' displayed a 9-fold improved binding affinity for Fcγ that were similar to the stronger (hi) Fc binding activity of SpA. If domain D also retains the features of a triple alpha helical bundle structure of the highly homologous domain B,[49,50] this three amino acid insertion should be adjacent to a helical zone that contributes Fcγ contact residues in domain B.[49,50] Cumulatively, the data indicate that even though the three amino acid insert that is unique to domain D is not critical for V_H3 Fab binding activity; this insert aids the specialization of the functional capacity of this domain through adverse effects on Fcγ binding.

SPA BINDING AMONGST HUMAN B CELL SUBSETS

Investigations of the molecular correlates for Fab-mediated SpA binding predicted that this specificity would be commonly expressed within the B cell repertoire of healthy individuals. To investigate the representation of this binding specificity in different B cell subsets, direct cellular binding has been evaluated in flow cytometric studies.[17] For these studies, we created a biotinylated form of chemically modified SpA (described above), termed Mod SpA, that retains V_H3 Fab-binding specificity and affinity while the Fcγ binding activity is completely absent. From these ongoing studies, we have begun to identify the B cell subpopulations (or lineages) that preferentially express Fab-mediated SpA binding activity (Fig. 5.3).[17] Our observations in the human immune system include:

Cellular Distribution of Fab-Mediated SpA Binding

i. Mod SpA does not interact with T cells and non-B non-T mononuclear cells, but Mod SpA binding activity is highly prevalent (14-54%) among human B cells.
ii. Mod SpA binding activity is equally prevalent among B cells with κ or λ L chains.
iii. Mod SpA binding activity is much more common among IgM-bearing than IgG-bearing B cells.
iv. Binding of Mod SpA by IgM-bearing B cells is generally stronger than by IgG-bearing B cells.

v. Within the peripheral blood of a healthy donor, Fab-mediated binding specificity for SpA is always associated with a greater proportion of B-1 ($CD5^+$) cells than with B-2 ($CD5^-$) cells (Fig. 5.3).

Anatomic Distribution of B Cells that Bind Mod SpA

i. In tonsilar tissue, Mod SpA is bound by frequent clusters of mononuclear cells in the mantle zone and germinal center of every secondary follicle.
ii. Mod SpA binding is also detected in the interfollicular regions in periarteriolar distributions.

By comparison, staining with the murine monoclonal Ab, B6, that identifies the products of about 10% of all human V_H3 germline genes,[51] detected only very few scattered binding B cells in the tonsil, that are primarily at the interface of the mantle

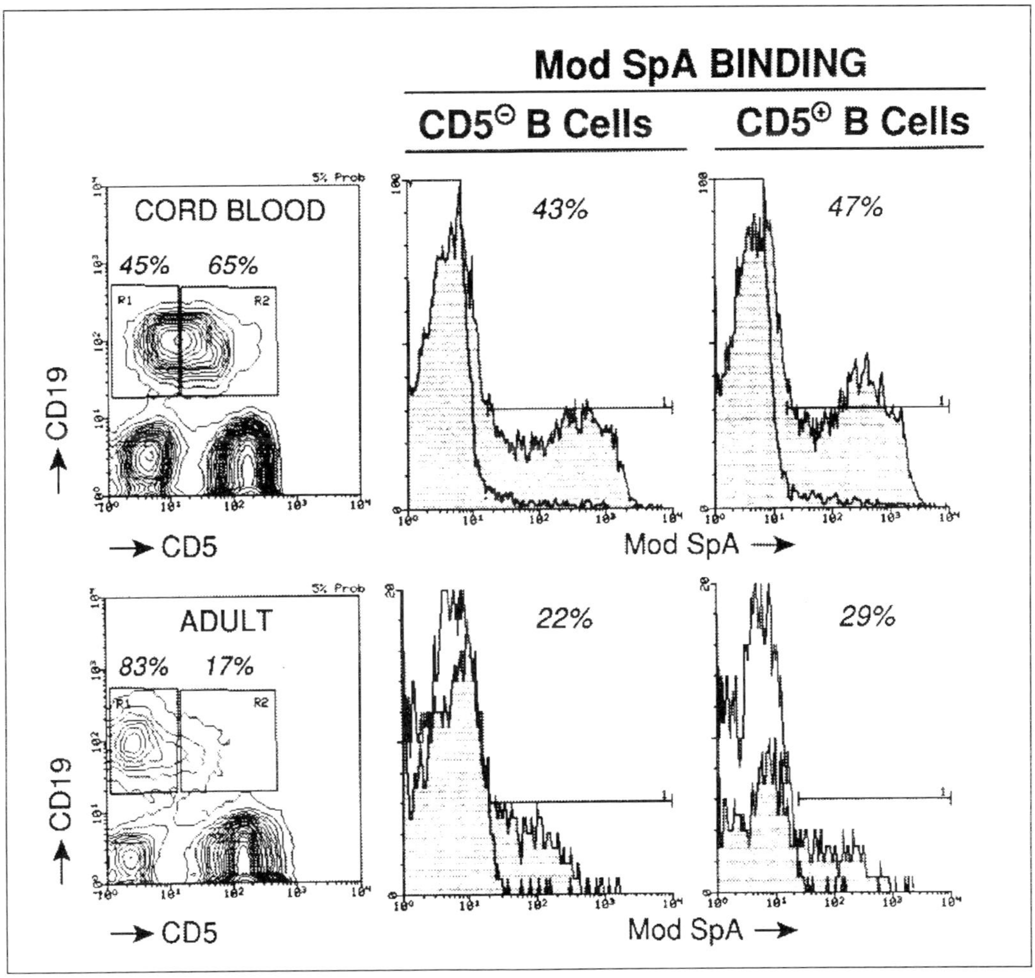

Fig. 5.3. Proportion of CD5-negative and CD5-positive peripheral B lymphocytes that bind Mod SpA. Representative three-color flow cytometric studies of human B lymphocytes that bind Mod SpA (SpA that has been chemically modified to remove Fc binding, but retains V_H3 Fab-mediated binding activity). Mod SpA is bound by both the CD5-negative (R1) and CD5-positive (R2) B cell populations at each age. The proportion of peripheral blood B cells that are CD5-positive decreases with aging, from neonate (cord blood)(65%) to an adult (17%). In both B cell subpopulations, the proportion of B cells that bind Mod SpA is higher in the neonate than in the adult. A greater proportion of CD5-positive B cells bind Mod SpA relative to CD5-negative B cells in both individuals. (Reprinted with permission from Silverman GJ et al. The Journal of Immunology 151(10): 5840-5855. ©1993. The American Association of Immunologists.)

zone and germinal center.[17] These findings are consistent with the notion that Mod SpA interacts with many more V_H3-expressing B cells than are identified with a common V_H3 subfamily-specific cross-reactive idiotype.

Age-Associated Changes in Fab-Mediated SpA Binding

i. There is a dramatic age-associated change in the proportion of peripheral blood B lymphocytes with this V_H3-restricted binding capacity.[17]

ii. In neonates, a large proportion of the peripheral B cells (mean ± SD, 46.0 ± 2.9%) bind this Fab-binding site on SpA, but by 10 months of age this decreases to significantly lower binding levels (30.2 ± 3.3%), which is the same as levels present in adults (Fig. 5.3 & 5.4).

iii. The proportion of Mod SpA binders in both the $CD5^+$ and the $CD5^-$ peripheral blood B cell subsets undergo comparable decreases between 6 and 10 months of age.[17]

Therefore the age-associated decrease in the peripheral blood level of SpA binders is not due to the drop from the high level of human peripheral $CD5^+$ B cells that occurs during the transition from infancy to childhood.

SpA binding is Most Common Among "Naive" B Cells in the Primary (IgM^+IgD^+) Repertoire

In recent studies of adult peripheral blood, we discovered that Fab-mediated

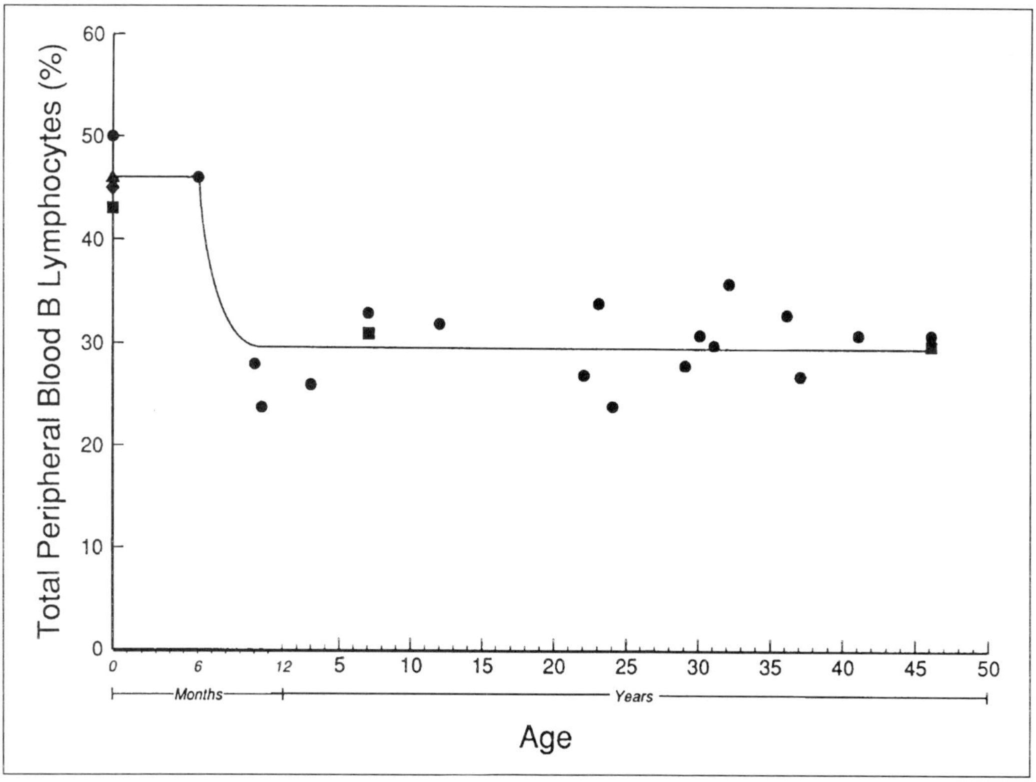

Fig. 5.4. Age-associated changes in binding of Mod SpA by circulating B lymphocytes. Studies of 23 healthy individuals illustrate the correlation of age with the proportion of peripheral B cells that bind Mod SpA. From two and three color flow cytometry experiments, depicted values are the proportion of human peripheral blood B lymphocytes ($CD19^+$) that also bind tagged Mod SpA. The line represents the mean value for the cord blood and 6 month old neonate, and the mean from older individuals. A dramatic decrease in the proportion of B cells that bind Mod SpA is seen between 6 and 10 months of age. (Reprinted with permission from Silverman GJ et al. The Journal of Immunology Vol.151(10):5840-5855. ©1993. The American Association of Immunologists.)

SpA binding is also more common among the sIgM$^+$ B cells that also express surface IgD compared to the minority of sIg$^+$ B cells that are devoid of surface IgD (GJS, manuscript in preparation). Significantly, recent reports indicate that the V genes expressed by sIgM$^+$IgD$^+$ B cells have undergone little or no hypermutation, because they are more likely to be "naive" with regard to exposure to Ag in the periphery. In contrast, V_H rearrangements of sIgM$^+$ IgD$^-$ B cells have generally undergone extensive hypermutation,[52,53] as these likely represent memory or activated B cells. Thus the Ag receptor genes of sIgM$^+$IgD$^+$ B cells appear to more commonly express the germline-encoded binding specificity for SpA.

Taken together, the cumulative data indicate that Fab-mediated SAg binding specificity is very frequent in the primary (preimmune) IgM repertoire and this explains the observed greater prevalence at birth and in the "naive" sIgM$^+$IgD$^+$ B cells of adults. Although also commonly retained (albeit at lower frequencies and generally of lower affinity) in the IgG repertoire, the somatic selection of immune responses to exogenous conventional Ags appears to often result in a loss of B cell SAg binding capacity. It remains to be determined whether a B cell SAg (like protein Fv)(see below) is actively involved in the in vivo selection and expansion of the primary B cell repertoire.

CHARACTERIZATION OF THE AB SITE RESPONSIBLE FOR PROTEIN FV BINDING

In a recent report, several independent approaches were used to evaluate the molecular basis for Fab-mediated binding to protein Fv.[25] These studies have provided significant insights into the structural basis of pFv binding, and aided development of our current hypotheses regarding the physiologic role of pFv. A brief overview includes:

V Region Usage Among Monoclonal Human IgM that Bind pFv

In our first studies of the molecular basis for pFv binding, we studied pFv binding within a large panel of human monoclonal IgM, and correlated pFv binding capacity with V region usage.[25] Central observations in this recent report include:

i. In direct binding ELISA, about 42% of a panel of 52 monoclonal IgM bound pFv, as > 90% of V_H3 IgM and 75% of V_H6 IgM bound pFv. pFv binding capacity did not correlate with V_L region usage (Fig. 5.5).
ii. Few native monoclonal IgM from the V_H1 and V_H4 families had detectable pFv activity, and these IgM have significantly weaker pFv binding activity than displayed by the V_H3 and V_H6 Abs.
iii. From inhibition ELISA, we demonstrated that binding of a monoclonal IgM to pFv could be blocked by the binding of polyclonal IgM or other monoclonal Ig. Thus all Ab binding (even from different V_H families) occurred at the same site(s) on pFv.
iv. Different IgM Ab exhibit a wide range of binding activities with pFv. While Ab that use V_H6 and perhaps all V_H3 gene segments can encode for pFv binding, certain V_H gene segments (e.g., V3-30 and V3-23) especially in germline configuration, may at times endow for optimal pFv binding activity.

Kinetic Measurements of Ab Binding of pFv

As described above in our studies of SpA, we have also used the BIAcore device to measure the strength of the binding interaction between Ab and pFv. The binding strength of the previously described Fabs were evaluated. As discussed, the Fab, JMSpA3-15, is derived from a μ rearrangement paired with a κ L chain (IgM Fab), while the Fab, JGSpA3-08, is a γ rearrangement paired with a λ L chain (IgG

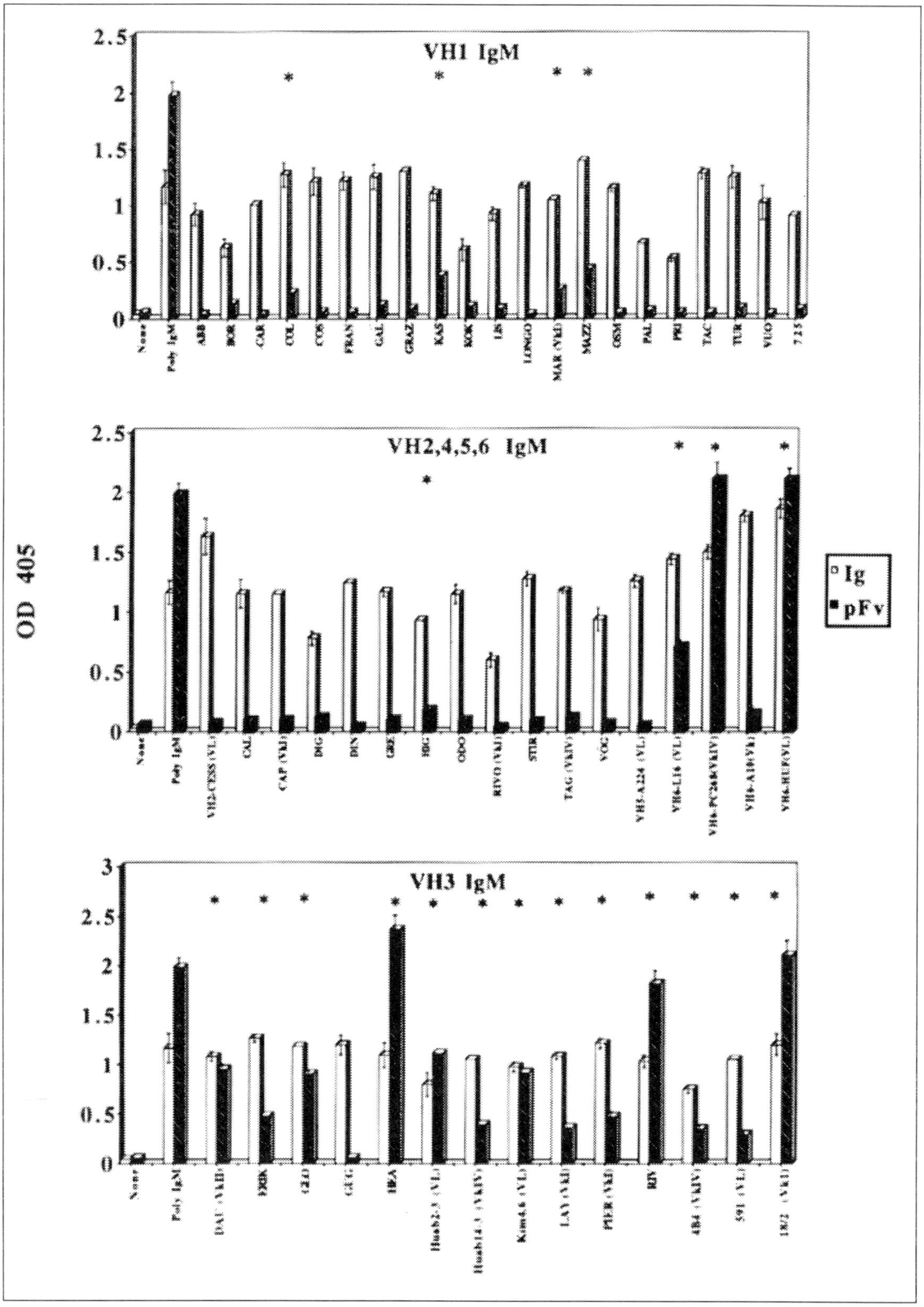
VH1 IgM
VH2,4,5,6 IgM
VH3 IgM
OD 405
Ig
pFv

Fab). These Abs represent different rearrangements of the same V_H gene segment, V_H26c/V3-23. Thus they have V_H CDR3 of very different compositions, but otherwise the V_H regions of these Abs differ by only four amino acids. Significantly, the JMSpA3-15 and JGSpA3-08 bind pFv with apparent association constants (K_a) of 1.9 and 3.5 x 10^6 M^{-1}, respectively (Table 5.1). These data represent strong evidence that L chains are also relatively passive in pFv binding, while pFv binding also appears to be mediated by contact areas in the portion of the Fab that come from the V_H gene segment.

In its native form, pFv has six potential Fab binding sites,[27] and by direct binding and competition ELISA we also demonstrated that native IgM have stronger pFv binding interactions than isolated Fab, presumably due to the capacity of native IgM for multivalent binding.[25] In studies of four purified monoclonal IgM with diverse V_H regions, surface plasmon resonance studies indicated that the V_H6 IgM, L16, binds pFv with an apparent association constant (K_a) of 8.8 x 10^7 M^{-1}, and the four V_H3 IgM bind with K_a of 0.11 to 6.7 x 10^8 M^{-1} (Table 5.1). Two of these IgM, KIM4.6 and 18/2, also have the strongest K_a for binding pFv. Significantly, the intact IgM, 18/2, that uses the same V_H gene segment as the monoclonal Fab described above, has a greater than 75-fold stronger pFv binding interaction than the isolated Fab. The binding affinities for pFv are comparable to SpA-binding interactions. The pFv binding interaction is not generally blocked by binding of an Ab to its conventional Ag,[30,54] which suggests that, similar to SpA, the site on Fab responsible for pFv binding is distinct from the conventional Ag binding pocket.

Phage-Display Ab Expression Libraries and the Investigation of pFv Binding

The above described IgG and IgM phage-display combinatorial Ab libraries were also used to investigate the structural correlates of the binding of pFv.[16,25] The central findings are:

i. In these libraries the V_H family usage was roughly representative of the in vivo usage. We found that about 22% of Fab-expressing clones in the IgM library bound pFv, and about 9.5% of Fab-expressing clones in the IgG library bound pFv.
ii. Antibodies with germline and certain mutated V_H3 and V_H6 sequences can bind pFv strongly.
iii. V_H region sequence analyses of over 40 pFv-binding Abs document that this binding activity is shared by Abs with diverse V_H CDR1 and CDR2 (diverse V_H gene segments).
iv. Fab that bind pFv do not display conserved V_H CDR3 sequences or J_H usage, although we did find that Ab with optimal pFv binding affinity had smaller than normal V_H CDR3 sizes for the adult repertoire (7-11 codons).
v. Panning with pFv resulted in selection for stronger pFv binding affinities. pFv also selected for Abs with identical or clonally related V_H genes associated with different L chains. These data further support the notion that L chains are relatively passive in pFv binding.

These studies supported the evidence from binding assays of native IgM proteins

*Fig. 5.5. (Opposite page) ELISA evaluation of human IgM for pFv binding activity. Direct binding evaluations were performed on a panel of 52 monoclonal human IgM. The proteins are organized according to V_H family, and if known are compiled in ref. 25. V_H region sequences of IgM with strong pFv binding activity are included in Table 5.2. Except where indicated, these IgM use V_κIII L chains, and usage is presented in earlier publications.[6,8,13,14] For comparison, values for Ig content were also obtained. Values were determined in triplicate, and are represented ± SD. * indicates IgM with significant pFv binding capacity, which were greater than 5 S.D. above negative controls. (Reprinted from Silverman et al. J Clin Invest 1995; 96:417-426. ©1995 The American Society of Clinical Investigation.)*

that Abs that bind pFv display preferential V_H3 and V_H6 usage and possess a hierarchy of affinities based on V_H region usage. These studies also provided an unexpected finding (Table 5.2). We also discovered that strong pFv binding was also expressed by certain of these V_H4 IgM Fab that are produced in bacteria, while studies of a large panel of native IgM demonstrated that pFv binding is uncommon among intact V_H4 IgM. Significantly, potential N-linked glycosylation sites are present in most (or all) V_H4 Abs but are generally absent in other families, and in two cases glycosylation of a V_H4 region has been documented.[55,56] However, N-linked glycosylation does not occur in these bacterial products. It has been reported that glycosylation of equivalent sites on a T cell receptor can abolish binding of a T cell SAg.[57] Therefore, we have speculated that V region glycosylation is responsible for the loss in pFv binding activity by V_H4 Abs from mammalian sources.[25] Conformational folding differences may also be contributory.

PROTEIN FV AND SPA BIND TO SIMILAR V_H FAB SITES

In a recently completed series of studies also performed in collaboration with J.-P. Bouvet (Pasteur Institute), we have investigated the molecular relationship between the SpA and pFv binding sites on human Abs. Confirming our previous observations in monoclonal IgM,[9,10,16,25] we found that a greater proportion of polyclonal IgM display pFv binding capacity compared to SpA binding capacity. In studies of IgM fractionated on an SpA-affinity column, virtually all Abs with SpA binding capacity can also bind pFv, but about 20% of the pFv binding activity was associated with the IgM that did not bind SpA. To investigate whether binding of SpA and pFv involves similar V_H region sites, we have also performed a series of competitive inhibition studies. We found that each of the pFv samples from different donors could completely inhibit all SpA binding of a monoclonal V_H3 IgM (Fig. 5.6), and SpA could also inhibit all pFv binding, which suggests that SpA and pFv are bound to a V_H3 Ab at the same (or overlapping) Fab sites. Inhibition was observed at lower molar concentrations of pFv and SpA. Therefore, while pFv and SpA appear to be very different structurally and pFv has generally wider range of V_H region binding interactions, the binding interactions of pFv than SpA can involve the same or similar sites on V_H3 Ab.

DISCUSSION

Our investigations of SpA and pFv have revealed that many of the features of the binding of B cell superantigens are completely analogous to the interactions of T cell superantigens. While B cell SAg

Table 5.2. V_H family distribution in the antibody phage-display libraries

Library	V_H1	V_H2	V_H3	V_H4	V_H5	V_H6	Total
JM-0	19	0	22	39	0	7	87
JM-pFv1	13	0	19	22	2	15	71
JM-pFv2	0.5	0	47	9	0	28	84.5

V_H Family distribution in the combinatorial libraries was assayed by hybridization of bacterial colony membrane lifts with family specific probes. JM-0 represents the unselected library and JM-pFv1 and JM-pFv2 are the libraries obtained after one or two sequential rounds of selection by the pFv protein. The data represents the percentage of colonies that hybridized with each oligonucleotide probe. These data show that members of the V_H3 and V_H6 families are preferentially selected for by pFv in this in vitro human Ab phage-display system. Adapted from Silverman et al.[25]

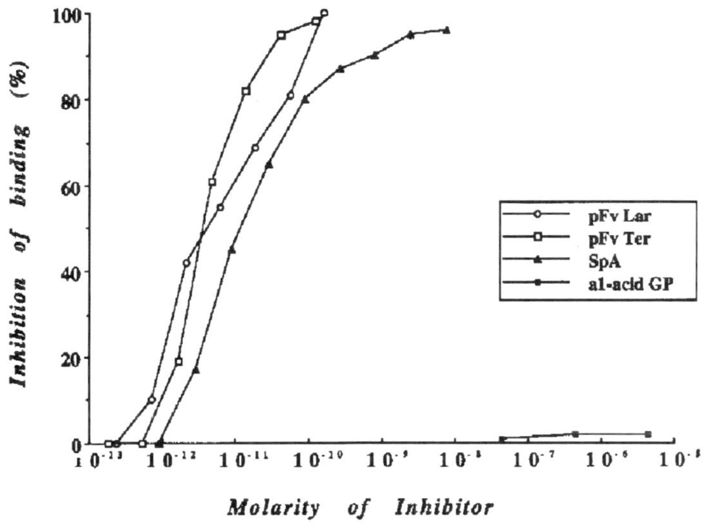

Fig. 5.6. Inhibition of IgM binding to pFv-coated plates by soluble pFv or SpA. In this example, following coating of pFv Ter on wells, a fixed concentration of the monoclonal V_H3-$V_\kappa1$ IgM, 18/2 was preincubated with a range of concentrations of SpA or pFv from two donors (Lar and Ter).[26] Under these conditions, pFv and SpA both inhibited pFv binding to the IgM. A1-acid GP represents a control sialoprotein. Adapted from Silverman and Bouvet (submitted for publication).

contact sites have not been completely localized, it is now commonly accepted that the V_H surface responsible for these interactions is distinct from the conventional Ag binding pocket created by the hypervariable loops. Available data suggests that the best characterized B cell SAg, SpA, interacts with a binding site that is equivalent to the site on TcR localized for staphylococcal T cell SAg, which is heavily dependent on the HV4 loop of the FR3 subdomain.[57] Comparable to evidence that SpA affinity can be "fine-tuned" by the associated L chain in the B cell receptor,[16] optimal T cell SAg interactions can also involve specific TcR a chains,[58] although this likely reflects the influence of the α chain on T cell SAg binding of Class II molecule and not direct effects on TcR-SAg affinity.

Although from very different biologic sources, a retroviral (MMTV from SHN mice) and a bacterial (SEB) T cell SAg can have very comparable TcR V_β specificities.[59] Similarly, we have recently demonstrated that B cell SAgs of diverse origins can also have overlapping V_H family specific binding sites, as demonstrated by SpA and pFv. Other putative B cell SAgs may also share related BcR binding specificities.[60,61]

These observations raise the question of why these unconventional sites on lymphocyte Ag receptors are such common targets for high affinity binding interactions. Even though all currently known T cell SAgs are of viral or bacterial origin, it seems doubtful that SAg binding sites have been conserved during evolution solely to aid the pathogenicity of microbes. However, if protein Fv is confirmed to be produced by the healthy human liver, then the interactions of pFv with BcR will be the first instance in which a SAg system is part of the physiologic immune system (see below).

While the fundamental bases for the binding of both types of SAgs appear to be comparable, there are also several very important differences in the molecular correlates of their receptor interactions. Importantly, the properties of B cell superantigens are highly influenced by the unique personality of the B cell Ag receptor (BcR). For example, although the frequency of lymphocytes that can bind a B cell SAg in the preimmune IgM B cell repertoire is many orders of magnitude more frequent than occurs for a conventional Ag, SpA binding is much less frequent among IgG-bearing B cells.[17] Similar findings in IgG Fab and IgM Fab libraries[16,25] also strongly argue that these binding differences are not due to valency/avidity effects that might be responsible for the differential binding of native IgM, IgA and IgG.[10,15] Significantly, every Ab with a germline configuration V_H3 gene studied to date has displayed SpA binding capacity,[19] while only about 60% of hypermutated V_H3 IgG Fab bind SpA.[16] These data indicate that B cell SAg binding is often adversely influenced by somatic hypermutation, which has much greater effects on the IgG repertoire. Another important difference from the properties of T cell SAgs is that at many anatomic sites (e.g., blood) interactions of Ag with the BcR may involve a competition with a B cell's own soluble receptors, e.g., Ig. Finally, the ability to switch heavy chain constant regions is uniquely associated with the BcR. Although B cell SAg binding does not appear to be directly influenced by Ig isotype, the outcome can be differentially affected by the associated H chain constant region of the Ab that is responsible for effector functions, e.g., only certain isotypes can fix complement, IgE trigger mast cells, etc. None of these processes is relevant to TcR.

The role of pFv in the immune system has not been directly examined. However, our studies of the molecular V_H preferences of Abs with optimal pFv binding activity revealed selection for rearrangements of specific V_H genes that are known to be overexpressed during early human ontogeny.[25] Even more provocative was the remarkably consistent pattern discerned in the V_H CDR3 sequences of Fab selected by B cell SAgs from the IgG and IgM phage-display libraries. While there were no recurrently utilized sequence motifs or charge-hydrophilicity distributions, there was evidence of selection based on the size of the CDR3. This trend was even more pronounced among the V_H genes that were preferentially selected by pFv. The CDR3 size of these 15 sequences exhibit a restricted size range of 7-11 codons (mean 9.1 ± S.D. 1.8),[25] which are all smaller than the mean size of V_H CDR3 expressed in the adult repertoire.[62,63] Significantly, V_H CDR3 of such smaller sizes are also more common in the human fetal repertoire compared to the adult repertoire. While the developmental regulation of CDR3 size has been primarily attributed to molecular biases in the mechanisms responsible for Ab gene rearrangements,[64] we have speculated that if pFv is produced at sites of early B cell lymphogenesis, it is possible that the early B cell repertoire is molded by binding preferences of a SAg that translates into differential B cell receptor-mediated selection of the immune repertoire.[25]

We speculate that the compartmentalization of pFv to the gut, especially in later development, may control and focus the influence of this endogenous SAg on the immune system. The impact of the multiple Fab-binding sites of protein Fv may then be limited to immune cells in the gut-associated lymphoid tissue, and avoid immune dysregulation that might result from uncontrolled exposure to pFv. pFv may contribute to the mucosal immune response by augmenting the effector functions of secretory Abs[30] and complexes of secretory Ig (and enteric Ags) with pFv have also been postulated to aid the passage of microbes from the body. These interactions with soluble Ig may also act as a necessary mechanism to dampen the effect of pFv on B cells. However, even a limited effect on B cells is not trivial, as greater than 80% of all mature B cells have transited through the gut and most adult B cells reside in gut-associated lymphoid tissue.[65] Confirmation of this proposed mechanism of regulating pFv activity will provide a unique insight into the relationship of the gut-associated system to overall immune responsiveness.

The demonstration that SpA interacts with a site on both human B cells and Abs that is also involved in pFv binding is consistent with the hypothesis that the Fab-binding activity of the bacterial membrane protein, SpA, likely was developed to disrupt physiologic immunoregulatory pathways.[25,21] Similarly, the Fcγ binding activity of SpA also resembles a separate binding interaction that is integral to the physiologic immune response. In fact, the exact IgG Fc site that interacts with SpA is also the primary site recognized by most rheumatoid factors (RF), and SpA and RF have been shown to compete for Fcγ binding.[66] While RF is present at high levels in certain diseases, such as rheumatoid arthritis, RF can also represent a type of natural auto-Ab that is produced in health. RF are produced during secondary Ab responses and may aid the Ag-presentation function of B cells.[67] Therefore, although it is not required for bacterial metabolism, SpA appears to have several functions useful for interfering with host defenses.

In conclusion, SAg mimic and amplify the receptor-mediated interactions of conventional Ags. For T cell SAgs, their biologic activities are intimately linked to their capacity for promiscuous molecular binding interactions with MHC and TcR molecules. Although B cell SAgs are less well understood, in their native states all proteins currently evaluated as possible B cell SAgs display multivalent binding sites. This is likely required for BcR cross-linking in a manner equivalent to conventional TI-2 (T helper cell independent) Ags. In vitro SpA stimulation studies suggest that, despite the unique broad V_H family binding interactions, even B cell SAg-mediated stimulation still conforms to the two signal model of B cell activation.[68,69] These in vitro studies[70] appear to predict that B cell SAg-mediated in vivo effects will likely require a T cell (or cytokine) signal. We believe that the most important lessons to be learned from the study of B cell SAgs are what they can tell us about the cellular and molecular features of lymphocyte activation in the immune response. Future investigations of the in vivo activities of B cell SAgs should provide valuable insights into the mechanisms responsible for tolerance, effective immune responsiveness, and the regulation of clonal heterogeneity in the B cell repertoire.

Acknowledgments

Our early studies were performed in collaboration with Eric Sasso and Mark Mannik (U. of Washington). Work in my laboratory has been greatly aided by the contributions of Susan Wormsley, Minoru Sasano, Paul Roben, Klaus Warnatz and Jayakar Nayak. This work was supported in part by NIH grants AI34001 and AR07567, and by grants from the Crohn's and Colitis Foundation and UCAIDS, and Biomedical Sciences Awards from the Arthritis Foundation.

References

1. White J, Herman A, Pullen AM et al. The V beta-specific superantigen staphylococcal enterotoxin B: stimulation of mature T cells and clonal deletion in neonatal mice. Cell 1989; 56:27-35.
2. Pullen AM, Wade T, Marrack P et al. Identification of the region of T cell receptor beta chain that interacts with the self-superantigen MIs-1a. Cell 1990; 61: 1365-1374.
3. Herman A, Kappler JW, Marrack P et al. Superantigens: mechanism of T cell stimulation and role in immune responses. Annu Rev Immunol 1991; 9:745-772.
4. McCormack JE, Kappler J, Marrack P. Stimulation with specific antigen can block superantigen-mediated deletion of T cells in vivo. Proc Natl Acad Sci U S A 1994; 91:2086-2090.
5. He XW, Goronzy J, Weyand C et al. Selective induction of rheumatoid factors by

superantigens and human helper T cells Evidence for the effects of a superantigen in rheumatoid arthritis. Science 1991; 253:325-329.
6. Bohach GA, Fast DJ, Nelson RD et al. Staphylococcal and streptococcal pyrogenic toxins involved in toxic shock syndrome and related illnesses. Crit Rev Microbiol 1990; 17:251-272.
7. Abe J, Kotzin BL, Jujo K et al. Selective expansion of T cells expressing T cell receptor variable regions V beta 2 and V beta 8 in Kawasaki disease. Proc Natl Acad Sci U S A 1992; 89:4066-4070.
8. Paliard X, West SG, Lafferty JA et al. Evidence for the effects of a superantigen in rheumatoid arthritis. Science 1991; 253:325-329.
9. Sasso EH, Silverman GJ, Mannik M. Human IgM molecules that bind staphylococcal protein A contain VHIII H chains. J Immunol 1989; 142:2778-2783.
10. Silverman GJ. Human antibody responses to bacterial antigens: studies of a model conventional antigen and a proposed model B cell superantigen. Int Rev Immunol 1992; 9:57-78.
11. Silverman GJ, Sasano M, Wormsley SB. The variable-region specificity of bacterial Fab-binding proteins:The search for B cell superantigens. Immunomethods 1993; 2:17-23.
12. Langone JJ. Protein A of Staphylococcus aureus and related immunoglobulin receptors produced by streptococci and pneumonococci. Adv Immunol 1982; 32:157-252.
13. Inganas M. Comparison of mechanisms of interaction between protein A from Staphylococcus aureus and human monoclonal IgG, IgA and IgM in relation to the classical FC gamma and the alternative F(ab')2 epsilon protein A interactions. Scand J Immunol 1981; 13:343-352.
14. Young WW, Tamura Y, Wolock DM et al. Staphylococcal protein A binding to the Fab of mouse monoclonal antibodies. J Immunol 1984; 133:3163-3166.
15. Sasso EH, Silverman GJ, Mannik M. Human IgA and IgG F(ab')2 that bind to staphylococcal protein A belong to the VHIII subgroup. J Immunol 1991; 147: 1877-1883.
16. Sasano M, Burton DR, Silverman GJ. Molecular selection of human antibodies with an unconventional bacterial B cell antigen. J Immunol 1993; 151:5822-5839.
17. Silverman GJ, Sasano M, Wormsley SB. Age-associated changes in binding of human B lymphocytes to a VH3-restricted unconventional bacterial antigen. J Immunol 1993; 151:5840-5855.
18. Roben P, Salem A, Silverman GJ. VH3 antibodies bind domain D of staphylococcal protein A. J Immunol 1995; 154: 6437-6446.
19. Hillson JL, Karr NS, Oppliger IR et al. The structural basis of germline-encoded VH3 immunoglobulin binding to staphylococcal protein A. J Exp Med 1993; 178:331-336.
20. Ibrahim S, Seppala IJ, Sarvas H et al. Proportion of protein A bindable molecules in human IgM and IgA antibodies to seven antigens. Microb Pathog 1993; 15:159-168.
21. Ibrahim S, Seppala I, Makela O. V-region-mediated binding of human Ig by protein A. J Immunol 1993; 151:3597-3603.
22. Hakoda M, Hayashimoto S, Yamanaka H et al. Molecular basis for the interaction between human IgM and staphylococcal protein A. Clin Immunol Immunopathol 1994; 72:394-401.
23. Kozlowski LM, Kunning SR, Zheng Y et al. Staphylococcus aureus Cowan I-induced human immunoglobin responses: Preferential IgM rheumatoid factor production and VH3 mRNA expression by protein A-binding B cells. J Clin Immunol 1995; 15: 145-151.
24. Randen I, Potter KN, Li Y et al. Complementarity-determining region 2 is implicated in the binding ostaphylococcal protein A to human immunoglobulin VHIII variable regionsf. Eur J Immunol 1993; 23:2682-2686.
25. Silverman GJ, Roben P, Bouvet J-P et al. Superantigen properties of a human sialoprotein involved in gut-associated immunity. J Clin Invest 1995; 96:417-426.
26. Bouvet JP, Pires R, Lunel-Fabiani F et al. Protein F. A novel F(ab)-binding factor, present in normal liver, and largely released in the digestive tract during hepatitis. J Immunol 1990; 145:1176-1180.
27. Bouvet JP, Pires R, Charlemagne J et al. Non-immune binding of human protein Fv to immunoglobulins from various mamma-

lian and non-mammalian species. Scand J Immunol 1991; 34:491-496.

28. Ruffet E, Pires R, Pillot J et al. Activation of the classical pathway of complement by non-immune complexes. Scand J Immunol 1994; 40:359-362.
29. Patella V, Bouvet JP, Marone G. Protein Fv produced during viral hepatitis is a novel activator of human basophils and mast cells. J. Immunol. 1993; 151:5685-5689.
30. Bouvet JP, Pires R, Iscaki S et al. Non-immune macromolecular complexes of Ig in human gut lumen. Probable enhancement of antibody functions. J Immunol 1993; 151:2562-2571.
31. Silverman GJ, Carson DA. Structural characterization of human monoclonal cold agglutinins: evidence for a distinct primary sequence-defined VH4 idiotype. Eur J Immunol 1990; 20:351-356.
32. Silverman GJ, Goni F, Fernandez,J et al. Distinct patterns of heavy chain variable region subgroup use by human monoclonal autoantibodies of different specificity. J Exp Med 1988; 168:2361-2366.
33. Silverman GJ. Unconventional antigen-antibody binding interactions and B cell superantigens. The Immunologist 1994; 2:51-57.
34. Schroeder HWJ, Hillson JL, Perlmutter RM. Structure and evolution of mammalian VH families. Int Immunol 1990; 2:41-50.
35. Schroeder HW,Jr., Mortari F, Shiokawa S et al. Developmental regulation of the human antibody repertoire. Ann N Y Acad Sci 1995; 764:242-260.
36. Myhre EB. Interaction of bacterial immunoglobulin receptors with sites in the Fab region. In: Boyle MDP, ed. Bacterial Immunoglobulin-Binding Proteins, Volume I. San Diego, CA: Academic Press, Inc., 1990:243-256.
37. Kirkham PM, Mortari F, Newton JA et al. Immunoglobulin VH clan and family identity predicts variable domain structure and may influence antigen binding. EMBO J 1992; 11:603-609.
38. Silverman GJ. Unconventional B cell antigens and human immune repertoires. Annals New York Academy of Sciences 1995; 764:566-585.
39. Padlan EA. Anatomy of the antibody molecule. Mol Immunol 1994; 31:169-217.
40. Hakoda M, Kamatani N, Kurumanda S et al. Involvement of framework region 3 of VH3 IgM in the binding of the B cell superantigen, staphylococcal protein A. Arthritis Rheum 1995; 38:S190.
41. Silverman GJ, Lucas AH. Variable region diversity in human circulating antibodies specific for the capsular polysaccharide of Haemophilus influenzae type b. Preferential usage of two types of VH3 heavy chains. J Clin Invest 1991; 88:911-920.
42. Sjodahl J. Structural studies on the four repetitive Fc-binding regions in protein A from Staphylococcus aureu. Eur J Biochem 1977; 78:471-479.
43. Lofdahl S, Guss B, Uhlen M et al. Gene for staphylococcal protein A. Proc Natl Acad Sci U S A 1983; 80:697-701.
44. Uhlen M, Guss B, Nilsson B et al. Complete sequence of the staphylococcal gene encoding protein A. A gene evolved through multiple duplications. J Biol Chem 1984; 259:1695-1702.
45. Moks T, Abrahmsen L, Nilsson B et al. Staphylococcal protein A consists of five IgG-binding domains. Eur J Biochem 1986; 156:637-643.
46. Romagnani S, Giudizi MG, del Prete G et al. Demonstration on protein A of two distinct immunoglobulin-binding sites and their role in the mitogenic activity of Staphylococcal aureus Cowan II on human B cells. J Immunol 1982; 129:596-602.
47. Inganas M, Johansson SG, Sjoquist J. Further characterization of the alternative protein-A interaction of immunoglobulins: demonstration of an Fc-binding fragment of protein A expressing the alternative reactivity. Scand J Immunol 1981; 14:379-388.
48. Erntell M, Myhre EB, Kronvall G. Non-immune F(ab')2- and Fc-mediated interactions of mammalian immunoglobulins with S. aureus and group C and G streptococci. Acta Pathol Microbiol Immunol Scand [B] 1986; 94:377-385.
49. Deisenhofer J, Jones TA, Huber R et al. Crystallographic refinement and atomic models of a human Fc fragment and its complex with fragment B of protein A from Staphylococcus aureus at 2.9- and 2.8- resolution. Hoppe Seylers Z Physiol Chem 1978; 359:975-985.

50. Gouda H, Torigoe H, Saito A et al. Three-dimensional solution structure of the B domain of staphylococcal protein A: comparisons of the solution and crystal structures. Biochemistry 1992; 31:9665-9672.
51. Crowley JJ, Mageed RA, Silverman GJ et al. The incidence of a new human cross-reactive idiotype linked to subgroup VHIII heavy chains. Mol Immunol 1990; 27:87-94.
52. Klein U, Kuppers R, Rajewsky K. Human IgM+IgD+ B cells, the major B cell subset in the peripheral blood, express V kappa genes with no or little somatic mutation throughout life. Eur J Immunol 1993; 23:3272-3277.
53. Pascual V, Liu YJ, Magalski A et al. Analysis of somatic mutation in five B cell subsets of human tonsil. J Exp Med 1994; 180:329-339.
54. Bouvet JP, Pires R, Quan C et al. Nonimmune VH-binding specificity of human protein Fv. Scand J Immunol 1991; 33:381-386.
55. Middaught CR, Litman GW. Atypical glycosylation of an IgG monoclonal cryoimmunoglobulin. J Biol Chem 1987; 262:3671-3673.
56. Spiegelberg HL, Abel CA, Fishkin BG et al. Localization of the carbohydrate within the variable region of light and heavy chains of human gammaG myeloma proteins. Biochemistry 1970; 9:4217-4223.
57. Pullen AM, Bill J, Kubo RT et al. Analysis of the interaction site for the self superantigen Mls-1a on T cell receptor V beta. J Exp Med 1991; 173:1183-1192.
58. Alam SM, Sim BC, Gascoigne NR. Selection of TCR V alpha by MHC class II predicts superantigen reactivity. Int Immunol 1995; 7:1311-1318.
59. Luther S, Shakhov AN, Xenarios II et al. New infectious mammary tumor virus superantigen with V beta-specificity identical to staphylococcal enterotoxin B (SEB). J Immunol 1994; 24:1757-1764.
60. Berberian L, Goodglick L, Kipps TJ et al. Immunoglobulin VH3 gene products: natural ligands for HIV gp120. Science 1993; 261:1588-1591.
61. Lenert P, Kroon D, Spiegelberg H et al. Human CD4 binds immunoglobulin. Science 1990; 248:1639-1642.
62. Yamada M, Wasserman R, Reichard BA et al. Preferential utilization of specific immunoglobulin heavy chain diversity. J Exp Med 1991; 173:395-407.
63. Sanz I. Multiple mechanisms participate in the generation of diversity of human H chain CDR3 regions. J Immunol 1991; 147: 1720-1729.
64. Feeney AJ, Victor KD, Vu K et al. Influence of the V(D)J recombination mechanism on the formation of the primary T of B cell repertoires. Semin Immunol 1994; 6: 155-163.
65. Brandtzaeg P, Halstensen TS, Kett K et al. Immunobiology and immunopathology of human gut mucosa: humoral immunity. Gastroenterology 1989; 97:1562-1584.
66. Nardella FA, Teller DC, Barber CV et al. IgG rheumatoid factors and staphylococcal protein A bind to a common molecular site on IgG. J Exp Med 1985; 162:1811-1824.
67. Roosnek E, Lanzavecchia A. Efficient and selective presentation of antigen-antibody complexes by rheumatoid factor B cells. J Exp Med 1991; 173:487-489.
68. Bretscher P, Cohn M. A theory of self-nonself discrimination: Paralysis and induction involve the recognition of one or two determinants on antigen, respectively. Science 1970; 163:1042-1049.
69. Lafferty KJ, Cunningham AJ. A new analysis of allogeneic interactions. Aust J Exp Biol Med Sci 1975; 53:27-42.
70. Kristiansen SV, Pascual V, Lipsky PE. Staphylococcal protein A induces biased production of Ig by VH3-expressing B lymphocytes. J Immunol 1994; 153:2974-2984.
71. Dersimonian H, Schwartz RS, Barrett KJ et al. Relationship of human variable region heavy chain germ-line genes to genes encoding anti-DNA antibodies. J Immunol 1987; 139:486-501.

CHAPTER 6

Staphylococcal Protein A and Staphylococcal Enterotoxins: Two Model B Cell Superantigens

Rana Domiati-Saad and Peter E. Lipsky

INTRODUCTION

Superantigens have been implicated in the pathogenesis of diverse disease processes.[1] Moreover they have been suggested to play a role in the selection of the T cell repertoire.[2] Recently, superantigens have also been proposed to play a role in shaping the B cell repertoire.[3] Here, we describe evidence in support of this hypothesis and propose a novel mechanism involving superantigen-regulated B cell apoptosis in this selection process.

B and T cells are both critical elements in regulating the normal immune response. They allow the immune system to recognize and respond to a host of foreign antigens. The comparison between antigen presentation to B cells and T cells points to the difference in their recognition of antigen. B cells utilize surface immunoglobulins (Ig) to recognize the three-dimensional configuration of intact molecules, whereas T cells employ the T cell receptor (TcR) to recognize a complex of peptides processed by other specialized antigen presenting cells and presented in association with major histocompatibility complex molecules (MHC).

In addition to their capacity to recognize antigenic peptides, T lymphocytes are also known to interact with superantigens. The term superantigen was initially employed to describe a group of molecules that have an immunostimulatory activity for T cells.[4-6] The unique features of T cell superantigens are the capacity to bind MHC class II molecules on the surface of a variety of cell types and to interact with specific

Human B Cell Superantigens, edited by Moncef Zouali. © 1996 R.G. Landes Company.

variable regions of the β chains (Vβ) of the TcR. Moreover, superantigens are not processed to yield peptides that bind into the peptide binding groove of MHC molecules, but rather the intact superantigen is thought to bind both MHC and TcR molecules outside the regions normally required for peptide recognition.[7-10] The hallmark of superantigen stimulation of T cells is that only T cells expressing a TcR that contains the β chain bound by the superantigen is activated. Although the interaction sites on the TcR and MHC class II are different from that used to recognize antigenic peptides, it is in association with MHC class II that superantigens are usually presented to T cells. Although presentation of superantigen is not restricted by MHC class II molecules as is recognition of nominal antigenic peptides, several of the superantigens show differential binding to MHC class II alleles.[11-12]

The superantigen concept for T cells might also be applicable for B cell responses. Thus, a number of materials from microbial origin have been suggested to stimulate B cells in a superantigenic manner. Staphylococcal protein A (SpA), for example, has been described to induce variable heavy chain (V_H) specific B cell responses.[13] As V_H of Ig is homologous to the β chain of the TcR, the stimulatory capacity of SpA for B cells has features of superantigenic activity. B cell activation by SpA is thought to require the binding of the superantigen to the appropriate V_H gene segment and the influence of costimulatory molecules to induce B cell responses, although no apparent interaction with other cells of the immune system is required. Therefore, one difference between T cell superantigens and B cell superantigens may be the absence of a requirement for MHC class II interaction for the latter. This parallels the absence of a requirement for an MHC class II restricted antigen presenting cell in B cell antigen recognition of conventional antigens.

Endogenous T cell superantigens are self proteins that have been suggested to play a role in shaping the T cell repertoire by interacting with the appropriate Vβ region independently of the α chain of the TcR.[2] An example of such T cell superantigens is the minor lymphocyte stimulatory antigen (Mls) encoded by mouse mammary tumor virus.[14] Mls has been postulated to shape the mature T cell repertoire by expansion of superantigen-reactive T cells followed by T deletion or anergy.[15,16] In parallel, an in vivo action of a yet unidentified B cell superantigen has been suggested to play a role in shaping the expression of V_H gene families within the B cell repertoire by interacting with V_H gene segments independent of the light chain. Analysis of the immature and mature murine B cell repertoires indicates that in the immature repertoire there is a more diverse representation of V_H genes within a family, whereas small overlapping sets of germline genes are dominantly expressed in the mature repertoire.[17] This bias in the mature repertoire appears to operate at the level of V_H and is independent of complementarity determining regions 3 (CDR3) or light chains. These findings, therefore, have suggested that selection of B cells into the peripheral B cell pool is mediated through selection by unknown internal and/or external ligands with superantigenic properties. The study of the human B cell repertoire has yielded further evidence for the potential selective influences of putative B cell superantigens. Comparison of the productive and nonproductive V_HDJ_H rearrangements in peripheral blood shows that certain members of the V_H4 family are found more frequently in the nonexpressed repertoire than in the expressed. This observation suggests the presence of negative selection, a process that may function by a V_H specific superantigen-like mechanism.[18]

A number of other observations have suggested the possibility that a variety of microbial products might directly bind to specific regions of the V_H segment of Ig and thereby function as B cell superantigens. SpA, which is not a typical T cell superantigen, has been recently described to be a putative B cell superantigen.[13,19-21] Besides its ability to bind the Fc fragment of IgG, SpA also binds to the heavy chain of the immunoglobulin molecule[22] containing V_H3 gene segments independently of the light chain, D or J utilization.[23,24] Another microbial product that has been seen suggested to be a B cell superantigen is HIV gp120. HIV gp120 has been shown to bind to B cells through surface Ig containing V_H3 gene segments, regardless of light chain utilization[25] and subsequently activate these B cells. This has been suggested to play a role in the deletion of V_H3-expressing B cells in HIV-infected individuals.[26,27] Thus, proteins with the ability to bind to the V_H domain appear to have the capacity to activate B cells or induce their deletion, as has been shown for T cell superantigens.

The crystal structure of the extracellular portion of β chain of the TcR shows structural similarity to the heavy chain of Ig.[28] The binding site for T cell superantigens has been suggested to lie in the so-called fourth hypervariable region (HV4).[29-32] This region is located in the center face of the β chain of TcR and forms a loop that is directed toward the solvent. The Ig molecule also possesses a region homologous to HV4 in the solvent exposed surface that does not interact directly with antigen, but could potentially bind superantigen. The structural similarity of Ig V_H and TcR Vβ gene segments[28,33] lead to the hypothesis that staphylococcal enterotoxins (SE), which are T cell superantigens, might also function as B cell superantigens.

STAPHYLOCOCCAL PROTEIN A

The interaction of SpA and Ig has been extensively studied and has been suggested to be a model of a B cell superantigen. SpA has been shown to bind to various isotypes of the heavy chain of Ig molecules containing V_H3 gene segments.[22,34] Studies using EBV transformed B lymphoblastoid cell lines from V_H3-enriched B cells showed that *S. aureus* Cowan I strain (SAC) preferentially bound to V_H3-expressing cells.[24] In vitro studies have demonstrated that SAC is a mitogenic stimulator of human B cells and that B cell stimulation of SpA is characterized by B cell proliferation and differentiation into Ig secreting cells and rheumatoid factor (RF) producing cells.[35,36] In these studies SpA was shown to be one of the major mitogenic components of SAC, although the V_H specificity of the Ig produced had not be delineated.

Studies from our laboratory have shown that SpA preferentially activated V_H3-expressing human B cells and induced the production of V_H3 specific IgM molecules.[13] Only IgM producing cells were analyzed to avoid bias that might be introduced by stimulation of IgG by direct binding of SpA to the Fc portion of this molecule. Human B cells from normal donors, rheumatoid arthritis or systemic lupus erythematosus patients and umbilical cord blood were stimulated in the presence of T cells and recombinant SpA (rSpA), formalized Cowan I strain of *S. aureus* (Pansorbin), Sansorbin (Wood 46 strain of *S. aureus* that lacks SpA) or SpA-linked to sepharose beads. The analysis of V_H families contained in IgM mRNA showed that the initial B cell activation in the culture was polyclonal as a result of features of *S. aureus* other than SpA. This feature of SpA is shared with Sansorbin that lacks SpA. After initial activation, however, subsequent maintenance of the response by SAC was related to an ongoing engagement and stimulation of V_H3 expressing B cells by SpA (Fig. 6.1). Thus, the Wood 46 strain of *S. aureus* as well as SAC induced initial polyclonal activation of B cells, whereas only SAC or SpA-linked to sepharose beads caused subsequent V_H3 specific stimulation.

To determine whether SpA stimulation of B cells had features of superantigenic stimulation, the sequences of V_H3 gene segments expressed by SpA-stimulated IgM-secreting B cells were examined. The analysis revealed the use of different members of the V_H3 gene family, each of which utilized different CDR3 regions. These results are consistent with the conclusion that under certain circumstances, specific engagement of V_H segments by an appropriate ligand can lead to functional stimulation of B cells expressing that Ig determinants, regardless of D_H and J_H utilization. In this regard SpA stimulation of B cells had features of superantigenic activity. The data, therefore, are consistent with the conclusion that SpA might function as a B cell superantigen by interacting with surface IgM molecules containing V_H3 segments and, thereby induce secretion of V_H3 containing IgM specifically.

Several studies have investigated the specific portions of V_H3 accounting for SpA binding. The study by Hillson et al[37] used 27 human IgM monoclonal proteins derived from fetal B cells. Analysis of the IgM V_H sequences suggested that conserved

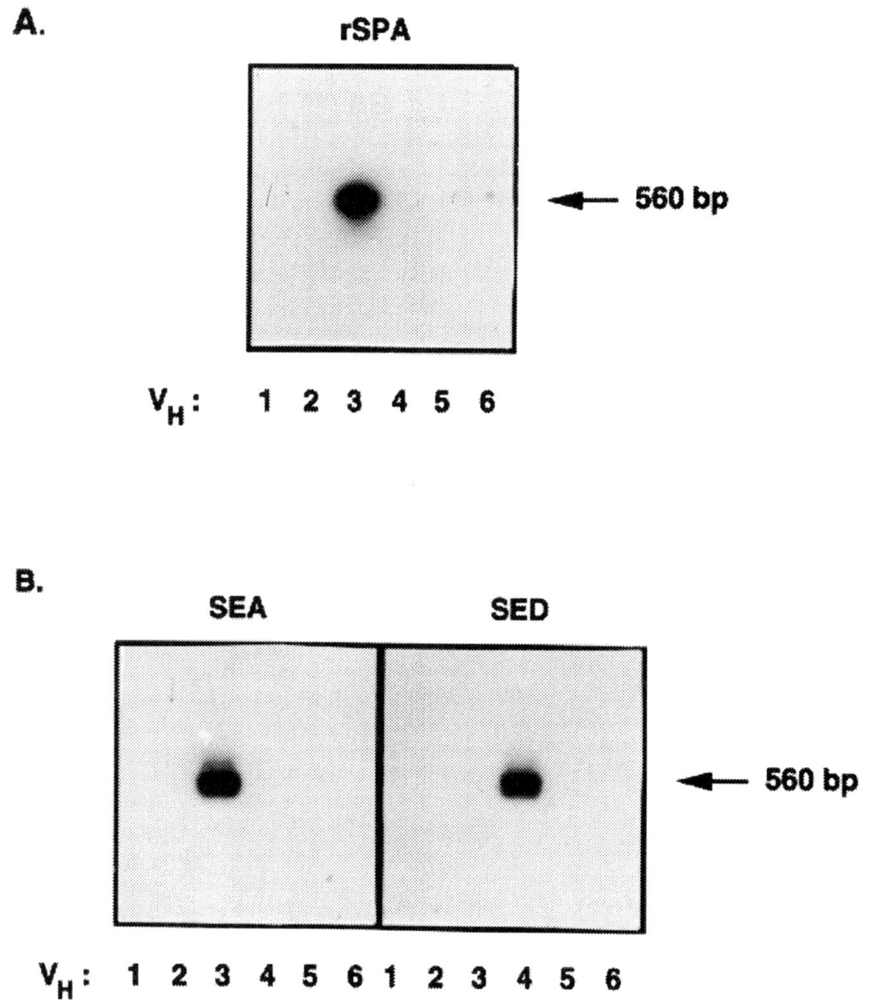

Fig. 6.1. V_H specific responses to staphylococcal proteins. (A) B cells were stimulated in the presence of mitomycin C treated T cells with recombinant SpA and IL2. After 12 days the cells were harvested and analyzed for the V_H families contained in IgM mRNA by RT-PCR. Fresh B cells expressed IgM mRNA from all V_H families before stimulation. (B) B cells alone were stimulated either with SEA or SED and IL2. After 9 days the cells were harvested and analyzed for the V_H families contained in IgM mRNA by RT-PCR.

residues in framework region (FR1), 3'CDR2 and FR3 were likely to play a role in SpA binding. Another study by Randen et al[38] showed that position 57 in CDR2 is critical for SpA binding. A single amino acid substitution from glutamic acid to lysine at this position changed a V_H3 family member from a nonbinder to a binder. Another study that used a phage-display library showed that the region critical for SpA binding is likely to be in FR3.[21] In our study, the region involved in SpA stimulation was deduced by analyzing the sequences of V_H3 genes expressed by SpA-stimulated B cells. The regions identified were similar to these identified by Hillson et al[37] and were centered in FR1, the 3' end of CDR2 and FR3. Together the above studies suggest that the binding of SpA and its capacity to activate B cells reside in residues in the solvent exposed loop of Ig in FR1, the 3' end of CDR2 or FR3 outside the conventional paratope of the hypervariable loops. This observation implies that SpA may activate V_H3-expressing B cells through binding to an unconventional site analogous to that used by T cell superantigens.

STAPHYLOCOCCAL ENTEROTOXINS

Other proteins that are produced by *S. aureus* include the staphylococcal enterotoxins (SE). These toxins are small basic proteins responsible for food poisoning and toxic shock syndrome in humans.[1] These enterotoxins are well characterized as being T cell superantigens in that they have potent T cell stimulatory activity. They have been shown to stimulate T cells expressing particular Vβ segments preferentially. We were interested in determining whether these same enterotoxins could induce B cell responses by a V_H specific mechanism. Our recent studies shows that SEA and SED might function as unique B cell superantigens by inducing survival of B cells expressing particular V_H gene segments. The results indicated, as was previously shown,[39] that in the presence of T cells SE induced B cell proliferation and differentiation. The T cell influence appeared to be partially accounted for by the activity of the CD40 ligand expressed by activated T cells as recombinant CD40 ligand and IL2 supported responses of purified B cells to SED.[40] In the absence of T cells, B cells stimulated with SEA and SED did not proliferate. However, highly purified B cells stimulated with SE and IL2 were noted to have enhanced survival potential compared to B cells supported by IL2 alone. Of note, this survival was V_H specific in that B cells stimulated with SEA expressed only V_H3 gene segments, whereas B cells stimulated with SED uniquely expressed V_H4 gene segments (Fig. 6.1). This implies that SE induced a V_H specific response. Here, it must be emphasized, however, that this bias in V_H expression was seen in the absence of T cells in the cultures, even though there was no obvious B cell activation or proliferation.

In order to determine whether the SED-driven B cell responses exhibited the characteristics of an antigenic or superantigenic response, V_H4 IgM cDNAs expressed by SED-activated B cells, were cloned and sequenced.[40] The analysis of V_H4 gene segments stimulated with SED revealed the usage of six of the ten functional V_H4 genes with different CDR3 regions including different D_H and J_H gene segments, a characteristic of a superantigenic response (Table 6.1). Moreover, detailed sequence analysis revealed possible regions of the Ig molecule that were potentially important for SED stimulation. Thus, regions in FR1 and 3' end of CDR2 and FR3 were conserved in the V_H4 genes of SED-stimulated B cells.

Analysis of the mechanism by which SED induced survival of the V_H4 specific B cells indicated that SED induced apoptosis of purified B cells presumably by binding HLA-DR. We speculated, therefore, that the maintenance of V_H4-expressing B cells was related to the induction of apoptosis of B cells expressing other V_H segments, thus permitting only V_H4^+ B cells to survive in the culture. Since SED is known to bind HLA-DR, the data suggest that the non-V_H4 B cells that bind SED may receive a signal via MHC class II

Table 6.1. Characteristics of SED-stimulated V_H4 containing IgM gene products

V_H4	J_H	D_H
4-34/DP-63	4	D21/9
4-39/DP-79	5	DXP'1, DLR2
4-59/DP-71	3	DK4
4-31/DP-65	6,2	DN1
4-61/DP-66	1	DM2, DN4
4-4 /DP-70		DIR1, DIR2, DΨA1, other

Elements used are listed in descending order of frequency.

molecule alone that stimulates programmed cell death. Consistent with this observation is the finding that mAb to HLA-DR also induce apoptosis.[41-43] One explanation for the finding that V_H4^+ B cells survived SED stimulation could be related to the potential of SED to bind both IgM and HLA-DR, leading to selective rescue of the B cells from apoptosis. Further studies with mAb to HLA-DR and IgM showed that engagement of either of HLA-DR or surface IgM alone induced apoptosis, whereas simultaneous crosslinking of these molecules or HLA-DR alone failed to induce B cell apoptosis. This indicates that crosslinking of HLA-DR and Ig containing V_H4 gene segments by SED may rescue B cells from apoptosis, whereas ligation of MHC class II alone on non-V_H4-expressing B cells delivers a signal for programmed cell death (Fig. 6.2).

DISCUSSION

We have analyzed the capacity of the staphylococcal proteins, SpA and SEs, to stimulate B cells through a superantigen-like mechanism by inducing specific responses of V_H-expressing B cells. SpA stimulated V_H3-expressing B cells in the presence of T cells, presumably by the interaction of the protein with V_H3 determinants on the Ig molecule. Binding studies have demonstrated that SpA interaction with Ig is through the V_H3 gene segments of the

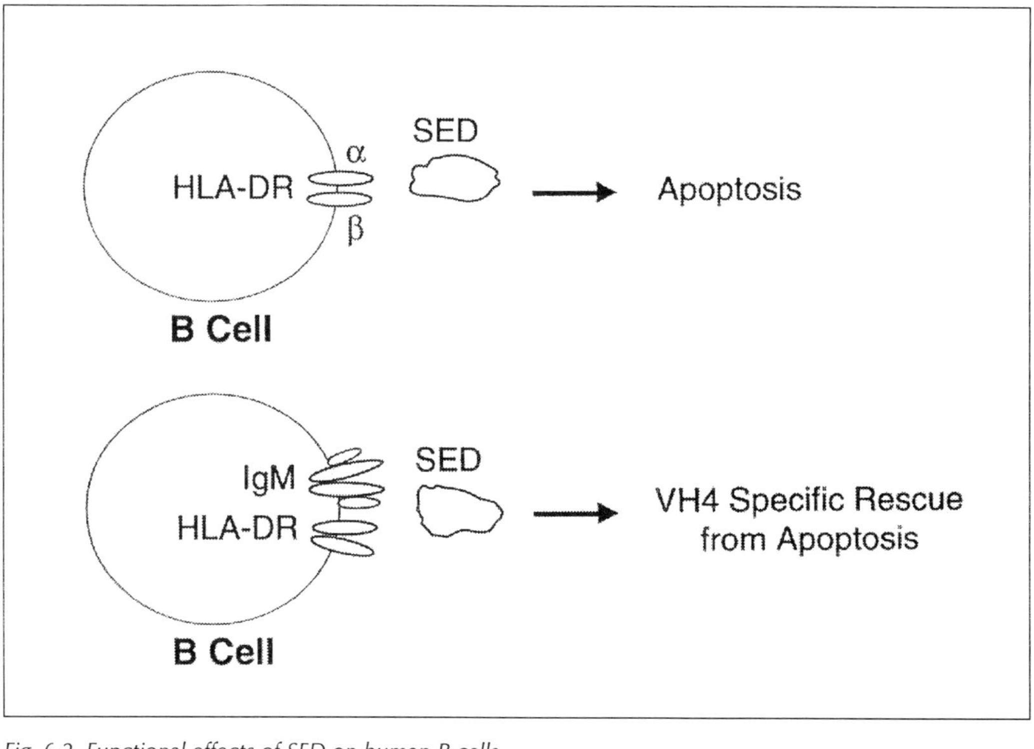

Fig. 6.2. Functional effects of SED on human B cells.

molecule. Analysis of sequences of monoclonal IgM have shown that SpA binding includes V_H3 residues in FR1, FR3 and 3' end of CDR2. In our studies the structural basis of SpA stimulation was defined following analysis of sequences generated from SpA-activated V_H3^+ B cells. Our results identified the region that is necessary for SpA activation and localized it to the same sites previously implicated as involved in SpA binding.[37] Thus, the sites critical for SpA activation, as well as binding, lie in FR1 and the 3' end of CDR2/FR3, in the solvent exposed surface of Ig. Taken together, these observations indicate that SpA binding to V_H3 determinants outside the antigen binding site is involved in stimulation of IgM expressing B cells. SpA stimulation of B cells, therefore, is analogous to the activity of superantigens on T cells, resulting from binding to a comparable region of the immune receptor distinct from the classic antigen binding region.

SAC has been found to induce T cell dependent polyclonal activation of B cells.[22] Proteins other than SpA and IL2, were found to contribute to the induction of the polyclonal response indicating that this response was not solely the result of binding of SpA. Thus, intact T cells or additional components of *S. aureus* are required for SpA to induce B cell activation.[44] These influences are nonspecific, however, and lead to polyclonal activation of B cells. It is the SpA moiety of SAC that has specificity for V_H3 segments and has the capacity to induce V_H3 specific B cell responses. Recent studies by Levinson et al[45] showed that SpA elicited IgM RF production by B cells enriched in V_H3-expressing cells. Taken together, these observations and the binding studies of others indicate that SpA is a model B cell superantigen because it interacts with V_H3 gene determinants outside the antigen binding site and induces V_H3 specific B cell responses.

The other model B cell superantigens we have described are SEs. It is known that SEs interact with specific regions of Vβ segments of TcR and induce stimulation of T cells bearing the appropriate Vβ chain. Our data indicate that SEs might also interact with the V_H domain of specific Ig by a superantigen-like binding which can lead to selective protection from apoptosis. SEs have the capacity to bind HLA-DR on B cells.[7-10] We hypothesized that SEs might bind HLA-DR alone and induce apoptosis. However, if SEs bound HLA-DR and surface Ig bearing the appropriate V_H segments, B cells would be rescued from apoptosis. The conclusions were confirmed by the studies reported herein. In this manner, SEs function as V_H dependent modulators of apoptosis and not classical superantigens, since they elicit minimal B cell proliferation even though both HLA-DR and surface Ig are putatively engaged.

Superantigen killing of B cells by apoptosis has been previously demonstrated in the presence of T cells. SED-responsive TH0 but not TH2 clones were found to trigger B cell apoptosis.[46] Furthermore, Stohl et al[47] reported that in the presence of T cells and high doses of SED, B cell differentiation did not occur. Moreover, in the presence of low doses of SED, the degree of apoptosis was reduced, and B cell differentiation was enhanced. In these studies, however, the direct role of the SED in inducing apoptosis was not examined and many of the effects could be explained by the action of other cellular interactions, including those mediated by Fas and Fas ligand.[48] The current observations provide additional insight into the complex role of T cells in regulating SED responses. Beyond the induction of apoptosis, for example, T cells can also overcome direct SED-induced apoptosis caused by HLA-DR ligation by engaging CD40.

Analysis of the sequences expressed by SED-stimulated B cells indicated that they utilized a variety of different CDR3 regions, including various D_H and J_H gene segments. This observation points to the possibility that there is a direct interaction between SED and V_H4 segments independent of D_H and J_H that induces the survival of B cells expressing that Ig product. This finding leads to the conclusion that SED has the capacity to recognize

B cells expressing the particular V_H gene segments independently of the rest of the elements of Ig and therefore, has the features of a B cell superantigen. However, the superantigenic influence of SED is unique in that it does not result in B cell activation, but rather V_H specific rescue from apoptosis.

T cell superantigens have been used as a tool to investigate the development of the T cell repertoire. Recently, Zouali[2] has suggested that B cell superantigen might play a role in shaping the overall expression of human V_H-gene families within the repertoire. Moreover, we have proposed a novel mechanism of B cell repertoire selection by a superantigen-induced regulation of B cell apoptosis. This mechanism may play a role in shaping the V_H genes found in the expressed B cell repertoire. Such findings may contribute to our current understanding of the selection of the normal B cell repertoire. Further insight into superantigen-mediated selection of V_H-expressing B cells may lead to recognition of diseases involving biased V_H expression.

References

1. Kotzin BL, Leung DM, Kappler J et al. Superantigens and their potential role in human diseases. Adv Immunol 1993; 54:99-166.
2. Janeway CA Self-superantigens? Cell 1990; 63:659-661.
3. Zouali M. B cell superantigens: implications for selection of the human antibody repertoire. Immol Today 1995; 16:399-405.
4. Marrack P, Kappler J. The staphylococcal enterotoxins and their relatives. Science 1990; 248:705-711.
5. Herman A, Kappler JW, Marrack P et al. Superantigens: mechanisms of T cell stimulation and role in immune responses. Ann Rev Immunol 199; 9:745-772.
6. Irwin MJ, Hudson KR, Ames KT et al. T cell receptor β-chain binding to enterotoxin superantigens. Immunol Rev 1993; 131:61-78.
7. Dellabona P, Peccoud J, Kappler et al. Superantigens interact with MHC class II molecules outside the antigen groove. Cell 1990; 62:1115-1121.
8. Jorgensen JL, Reay PA, Ehrich EW et al. Molecular components of T cell recognition. Ann Rev Immunol 1992; 10:835-873.
9. Karp DR, Long EO. Identification of HLA-DR1α chain residues critical for binding staphylococcal enterotoxins SEA and SEE. J Exp Med 1992; 175:415-424.
10. Jardetzky TS, Brown JH, Gorga JC et al. Three dimensional structure of a human class II histocompatability molecule complexed with superantigen. Nature 1994; 368:711-718.
11. Herman A, Croteau G, Sekaly RP et al. HLA-DR alleles differ in their ability to present staphylococcal enterotoxins to T cells. J Exp Med 1990; 172:709-717.
12. Herrmann T, Accolla RS, MacDonald HR. Different staphylococcal enterotoxins bind preferentially to distinct major histocompatibility complex class II isotypes. Eur J Immunol 1989; 19:2171-2174.
13. Vasquez Kristiansen S, Pascual V, Lispky PE. Staphylococcal protein A induces biased production of Ig by V_H3-expressing B lymphocytes. J Immunol 1994; 153: 2974-2982.
14. Marrack P, Winslow GM, Choi Y et al. The bacterial and mouse mammary tumor virus superantigens; two different families of proteins with the same functions. Immunol Rev 1993; 131:79-82.
15. Kappler JW, Staerz U, White J et al. Self-tolerance eliminates T cells specific for Mls-modified products of the major histocompatibility complex. Nature 1988; 332: 35-40.
16. Huang L, Crispe IN. Superantigen-driven peripheral deletion of T cells. Apoptosis occurs in cells that lost the α/β T cell receptor. J Immunol 1993; 151:1844-1851.
17. Gu H, Tarlington D, Müller W et al. Most peripheral B cells in mice are ligand selected. J Exp Med 1991; 173:1357-1371.
18. Brezinschek HP, Brezinschek RI, Lipsky PE. Analysis of the heavy chain repertoire of human peripheral B cells using single cell polymerase chain reaction. J Immunol 1995; 155:190-202.
19. Sasso EH, Silverman GJ, Mannik M. Human IgA and IgG $F(ab')_2$ that bind to staphylococcal protein A belong to the V_HIII

subgroup. J Immunol 1991; 147: 1877-1883.
20. Silverman GJ. Human antibody responses to bacterial antigens: studies of a model conventional antigen and a proposed model B cell superantigen. Int Rev Immunol 1992; 9:55-78.
21. Sasano M, Burton DR, Silverman GJ. Molecular selection of human antibodies with an unconventional bacterial B cell antigen. J Immunol 1993; 151:5822-5839.
22. Romagnani S, Giudizi MG., Del Prete G et al. Demonstration on protein A of two distinct immunoglobulin-binding sites and thier role in the mitogenic activity of *Staphylococcal aureus* Cowan II on human B cells. J Immunol 1992; 129:596-602.
23. Sasso EH, Silverman GJ, Mannik M. Human IgM molecules that bind staphylococcal protein A contain V_HIII H chains. J Immunol 1989; 142:2778-2783.
24. Shokri F, Maged RA, Maziak BR et al. Expression of V_HIII-associated cross-reactive idiotype on human B lymphocytes. Association with staphylococcal protein A binding and Staphylococcal aureus Cowan I stimulation. J Immunol 1991; 146:936-940.
25. Berberian L, Goodligck L, Kipps TJ et al. Immunoglobulin V_H3 gene products: natural ligands for HIV gp120. Science 1993; 261:1588-1591.
26 Berberian L, Shukla J, Jefferis R et al. Effects of HIV infection on V_H3 (D12 idiotope) B cells in vivo. J AIDS 1994; 7:641-646.
27. David D, Demaison C, Bani L et al. Selective variations in vivo of V_H3 and V_H1 gene family expression in peripheral B cell IgM, IgD and IgG during HIV infection. Eur J Immunol 1995; 25:1524-1528.
28. Bently GA, Boulot G, Karjalainen K et al. Crystal structure of the β chain of a T cell antigen receptor. Science 1995; 267: 1984-1987.
29. Pullen AM, Wade T, Marrack P et al. Identification of the region of the T cell receptor β chain that interacts with the self superantigen Mls-1[a]. Cell 1990; 61:1365-1374.
30. Pontzer C, Irwin MJ, Gascoigne RJ et al. T cell antigen receptor binding sites for microbial superantigen staphylococcal enterotoxin. A Proc Natl Acad. USA 1992; 89:7727-7731.
31. Choi Y, Herman A, DiGusto D et al. Residues of the T cell-receptor β chain that interact with *S. aureus* toxin superantigens. Nature 1990; 346:471-473.
32. Malchiodi EL, Eisenstein E, Fields B et al. Superantigen binding to a T cell receptor β chain of known three-dimensional structure. J Exp Med 1995; 182:1833-1845.
33. Chothia C, Boswell DR, Lesk AM. The outline structure of the T cell αβ receptor. EMBO J 1988;7:3745-3755.
34. Inganas M. Comparison of mechanisms of interaction between protein A from *Staphylococcal aureus* and human monoclonal IgG, IgA and IgM in relation to the classical Fc gamma and the alternative F(ab')2 protein A interactions. Scand J Immunol 1981; 13:343-352.
35. Levinson AI, Tar L, Carafa C et al. *Staphylococcal aureus* Cowan I. Potent stimulus of immunoglobulin M rheumatoid factor production. J Clin Invest 1986; 78:612-617.
36. Hirohata S, Inoue T, Miyamoto T. Frequency analysis of human peripheral blood B cells producing IgM-rheumatoid factor: Differential effects of stimulation with monoclonal antibodies to CD3 and *Staphylococcal aureus*. J Immunol 1990; 145: 1681-1686.
37. Hillson JL, Karr NS, Oppliger NR et al. The structural basis of germline-encoded V_H3 immunoglobulin binding to staphylococcal protein A. J Exp Med 1993; 178:331-336.
38. Randen I, Potter K, Li Y et al. Complementarity determining region 2 is implicated in the binding of staphylococcal protein A to human immunoglobulin VHIII variable regions. Eur J Immunol 1993; 23:2682-2686
39. Stohl W, Elliot EJ, Linsley PS. Human T cell-dependent B cell differentiation induced by staphylococcal superantigens. J Immunol. 1994:153:117-127.
40. Domiati-Saad R, Attrep JA, Brezinschek HP et al. Staphylococcal enterotoxin D functions as a human B cell superantigen by rescuing

V_H4-expressing B cells from apoptosis. J Immunol 1996; 156:3608-3620.
41. Truman JP, Ericson ML, Choqueux-Séébold CJM et al. Lymphocyte programmed cell death is mediated via HLA class II DR. Intern Immunol 1994; 6:887-896.
42. Higaki Y, Hata D, Kanazashi S et al. Mechanism involved in the inhibition of growth of a human B lymphoma cell line, B104, by anti-MHC class II antibodies. Immunol Cell Biol 1994; 72:205-214.
43. Newell KM, VanderWaal J, Beard KS et al. Ligation of major histocompatibility complex class II molecules mediates apoptotic cell death in resting B lymphocytes. Proc Natl Acad Sci USA 1993; 90:10459-10463.
44. Lipsky PE. Staphylococcal protein A, a T cell regulated polyclonal activator of human B cells. J Immunol 1980; 125: 155-162.
45. Kozlowski LM, Roman Kunning S, Zheng Y et al. *Staphyloccoccus aureus* Cowan I-induced human immunoglobulin responses: preferential IgM rheumatoid factor production and VH3 mRNA expression by protein A-binding B cells. J Clin Immunol 1995; 15:145-151.
46. He X, Zhong W, Goronzy JJ et al. Induction of B cell apoptosis by TH0, but not TH2, $CD4^+$ T cells. J Clin Invest 1995; 95:564-570.
47. Stohl W, Elliot JE. Differential human T cell-dependent B cell differentiation induced by staphylococcal superantigens (SAg). Regulatory role for SAg-dependent B cell cytolysis. J Immunol 1995; 155: 1838-1850.
48. Shigekazu N, Golstein P. The Fas death factor. Science 1995; 267:1449-1456.

CHAPTER 7

Staphylococcal Protein A: Functional Properties of a Model B Cell Superantigen

Arnold I. Levinson and Lisa M. Kozlowski

INTRODUCTION

Staphylococcal Protein A (SpA), a cell wall component of *Staphylococcus aureus*, binds to the Fc fragment of IgG. The site that binds the IgG Fc region is termed the classical binding site on SpA.[1,2] In addition, an alternative site on SpA has been defined that binds to the Fab fragments of immunoglobulins (Igs) independent of heavy chain isotype.[1-6] Studies have mapped the Fab determinants to framework regions (FR) 1 and 3 in the variable heavy chain (V_H) region[7-9] with a possible contribution of residues in the second complementarity-determining region (CDR2).[8] Binding of this alternative site on SpA is restricted to human Igs utilizing V_H3 heavy chains[9,10] and mouse Igs utilizing J606 and S107 heavy chains.[11] The alternative binding site endows SpA with the ability to crosslink membrane IgM on B cells and thereby induce their activation in what was previously considered to be a non-V_H-selective manner.[5,6] More recent work suggests that SpA, in the presence of a source of T cell help, causes a restricted pattern of Ig production, namely immunoglobulins enriched for usage of V_H3 heavy chains.[12,13] These properties are reminiscent of those of a T cell superantigen and have led SpA to be characterized as a B cell superantigen.[10,14-19] Recently, several other proteins have also been defined as B cell superantigens, including HIV gp120, protein Fv (a human liver sialoprotein), and protein L (a coat protein of *Peptostreptococcus magnus*).[20-22]

In this communication, we review our studies on SpA that illustrate two potential functional properties of a B cell superantigen, namely the elicitation of autoantibody production and activation of the complement cascade. Both of these properties highlight mechanisms by which this novel class of antigens may contribute to inflammation and disease.

Human B Cell Superantigens, edited by Moncef Zouali. © 1996 R.G. Landes Company.

BINDING OF SPA TO B CELLS EXPRESSING V_H3+ IGS

Our interest in SpA grew out of the observation that SpA-rich *Staphylococcus aureus* Cowan I (SAC) was demonstrated to be a potent T cell dependent polyclonal B cell activator of human lymphocytes.[23] This property is conferred by SpA which delivers an activation signal to B cells by cross-linking the Fabs of their membrane Igs.[5,6] The activated B cells respond by differentiating into immunoglobulin secreting cells in what was considered to be an unrestricted manner. However, the unrestricted nature of this response had to be reevaluated when it became obvious that the alternative site of SpA binds to V_H3 Igs.

To this end, we sought to determine if SpA-binding (PA^+) B cells would be enriched for the expression of V_H3 heavy chains. Because the total population of V_H3-expressing B cells from any source cannot be identified phenotypically with antibody probes, we utilized an RT-PCR technique which allowed us to determine if the B cells from the PA^+ and SpA-nonbinding (PA^-) B cell populations were enriched for or depleted of V_H3 heavy chain mRNA expression.[24] The RT-PCR was performed on total RNA from unfractionated cells, PA^+ B cells, and PA^- B cells. The amplified IgM cDNA products were probed on Southern blots (representative blots are shown) with a V_H3 specific oligonucleotide (Fig. 7.1A) or a V_H4 specific oligonucleotide (Fig. 7.1B). The PA^+ fraction showed marked enrichment of V_H3 mRNA expression whereas the PA^- fraction showed a marked reduction of V_H3 mRNA (Fig. 7.1A). By contrast, V_H4

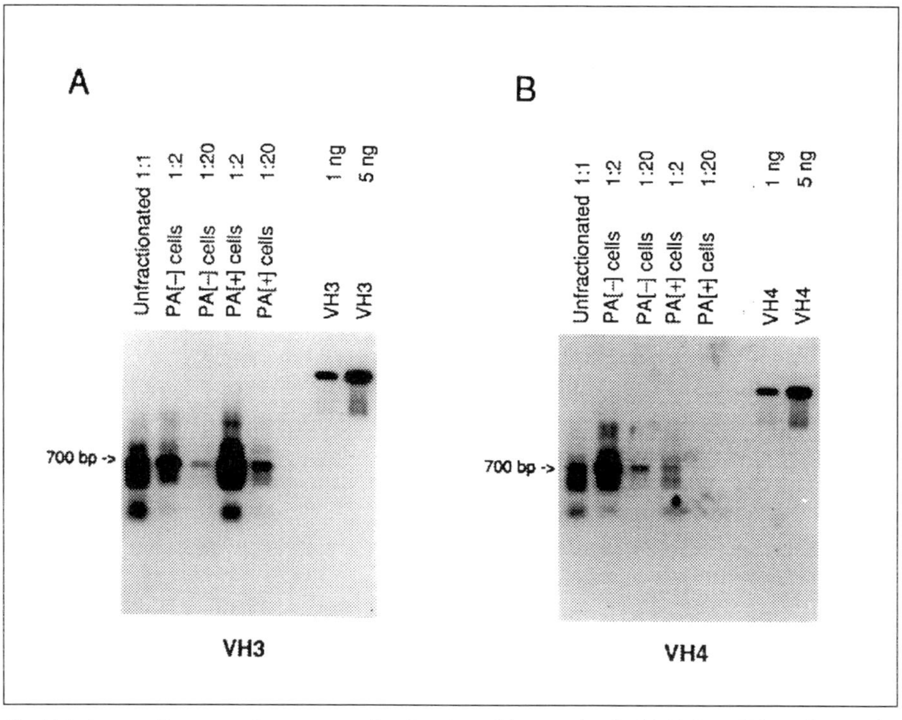

Fig. 7.1. Autoradiograms of representative Southern blots probed with V_H3 and V_H4 oligonucleotides. Two dilutions of cDNA aliquots for each cell population were run on duplicate agarose gels and transferred to nylon membranes. A known amount of V_H3 cDNA was run as a standard on one of the duplicates and this blot was probed with our V_H3-specific oligonucleotide (Fig. 7.1A). A known amount of V_H4 cDNA was run as a standard on the other duplicate and this blot was probed with our V_H4-specific oligonucleotide (Fig. 7.1B). The intensity of the hybridization signal emitted by the appropriately sized band (700 bp) was then quantified by densitometry. (Reprinted with permission from Kozlowski LM et al. J Clin Immunol 1995; 15:145-151.)

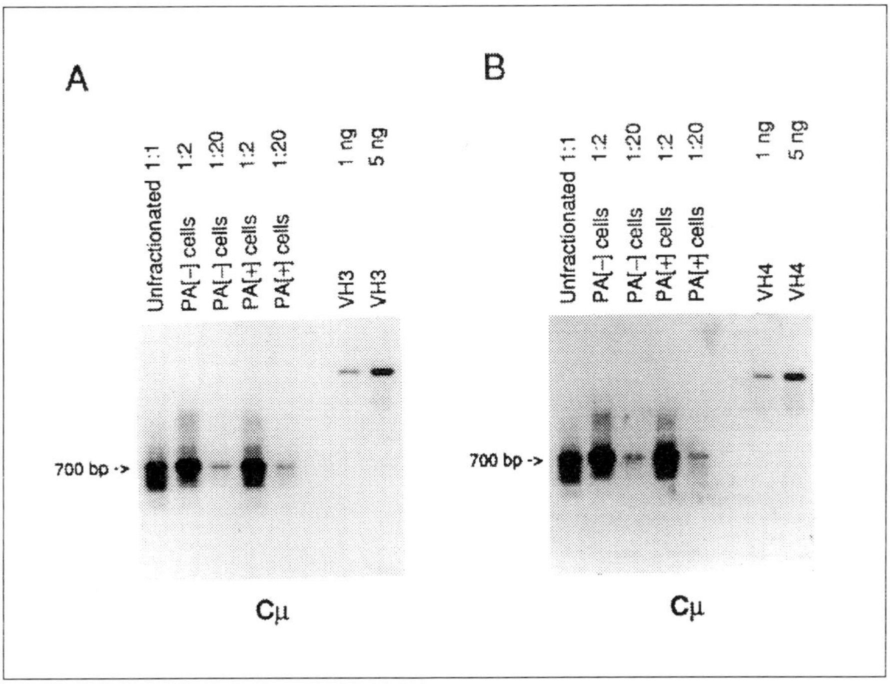

Fig. 7.2. Autoradiograms of Southern blots from Fig. 7.1 reprobed with an IgM constant region oligonucleotide (Cμ). The Southern blots in Fig. 7.1 were stripped of the V_H-specific oligonucleotide probes and reprobed with an IgM constant region-specific oligonucleotide (Figs. 7.2A and 7.2B) and the signals quantified by densitometry. (Reprinted with permission from Kozlowski LM et al. J Clin Immunol 1995; 15:145-151.)

mRNA expression was enriched in the PA^- fraction (Fig. 7.1B) and reduced in the PA^+ B cell fraction. The enrichment or reduction in each fraction was also notable when compared to the unfractionated cell population.

By stripping the blots and re-probing with an IgM constant region oligonucleotide, we demonstrated that equal amounts of cDNA had been loaded into the wells of the duplicate gels for each cell population (Figs. 7.2A & 7.2B). This IgM constant region probe, in conjunction with the V_H3 and V_H4 cDNA standards, was also used to normalize the intensity of the signal generated from the V_H3 and V_H4 oligonucleotide probes when quantified by scanning phosphorimaging. In Table 7.1, the phosphorimager values are represented as relative contributions of the particular V_H sample compared to the total IgM for the respective sample. The values were normalized to the V_H/IgM constant region ratios of the appropriate V_H cDNA standards. In each of the two representative experiments, the V_H3 mRNA expression of the PA^+ B cells was greater than threefold the expression of the PA^- B cells. By contrast, V_H4 mRNA expression of the PA^- B cells was greater than four-fold the expression of the PA^+ B cells. Thus, PA^+ B cells are enriched for expression of V_H3 mRNA and are depleted of V_H4 mRNA, whereas, the PA^- B cell population is enriched for V_H4 mRNA and is depleted of V_H3 mRNA.

INDUCTION OF AUTOANTIBODY PRODUCTION BY SPA

The interaction of a B cell superantigen like SpA with self-reactive V_H3^+ B cells could lead to the production of autoantibodies. This possibility is highlighted by our previous finding that SAC is a powerful in vitro trigger of IgM rheumatoid factor (IgMRF) production by the peripheral blood mononuclear cells (PBMC) of normal hosts. We found that

Table 7.1. Relative contribution of V_H3 and V_H4 cDNAs to amplified IgM cDNAs

	Unfractionated	PA^+ cells	PA^- cells
EXP 1			
V_H3comp	0.98	1.29	0.39
V_H4comp	0.26	0.19	2.27
EXP 2			
V_H3comp	0.42	0.63	0.17
V_H4comp	0.28	0.17	2.40

To assess the relative contributions of a particular V_H to the total IgMcDNAs amplified from each cell population, a V_H/IgM C-region ratio was determined. These values were then normalized to the V_H/IgM C-region ratios of the respective VH cDNA standard and expressed as the relative V_H composition ($V_H$comp) where $V_H$comp equals: (counts from V_H sample/counts from total IgM of V_H sample)/(counts from V_H standard/counts from total IgM of V_H standard); PA^+: SpA-binding cells; PA^-: SpA-non-binding cells. (Reprinted with permission from Kozlowski LM et al. J Clin Immunol 1995; 15:145-151.)

SpA-enriched-SAC induced IgMRF production by the PBMC of healthy donors via a T cell dependent mechanism (Fig. 7.3).[25] Our experimental results indicated that this autoantibody response was elicited by the SpA component of SAC. First, we observed that the Wood strain of *S. aureus,* whose cell wall lacks SpA, elicited polyclonal B cell differentiation but little to no IgMRF production (Fig. 7.3). Secondly, we found that IgMRF production could be elicited by SpA insolubilized on sepharose beads (Fig. 7.4). We also observed that SAC stimulated even greater amounts of IgMRF by the mononuclear cells obtained from the blood of umbilical cord veins of full term infants (Fig. 7.5).[26] Indeed, on the average, 16% of the total polyclonal IgM response to SAC of cord blood mononuclear cells could be attributed to this autospecificity.

The experiments described above implied that precursors of SAC-induced

Fig. 7.3. IgMRF production induced by SAC, S. aureus *Wood strain (SAW), and PWM. Peripheral blood mononuclear cells from 15 healthy donors were incubated for 7 to 8 days with varying concentrations of the designated culture additives and supernatants analyzed for IgMRF by ELISA. Values represent peak responses to each additive. IgMRF was not detected when cells were incubated with media alone. The dashed line signifies the lower threshold of IgMRF detection. (Reprinted with permission from The Journal of Clinical Investigation, 1986; 78:6122-617, ©1986, the American Society for Clinical Investigation.)*

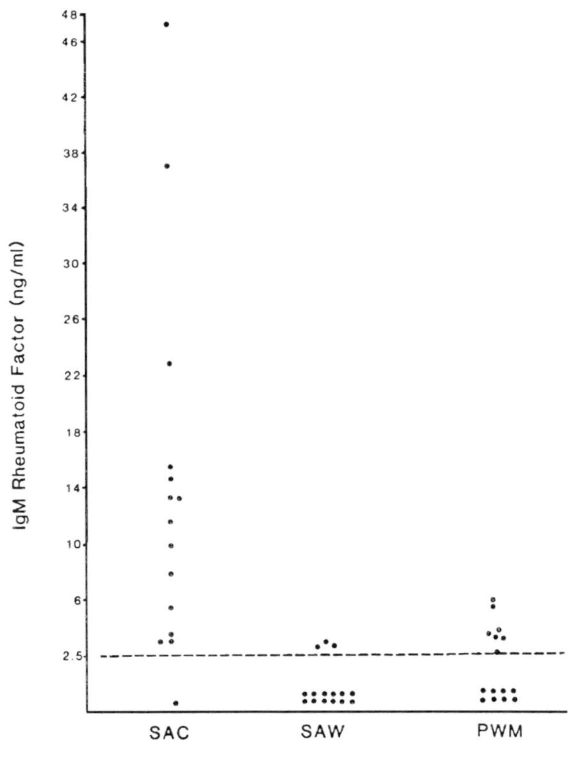

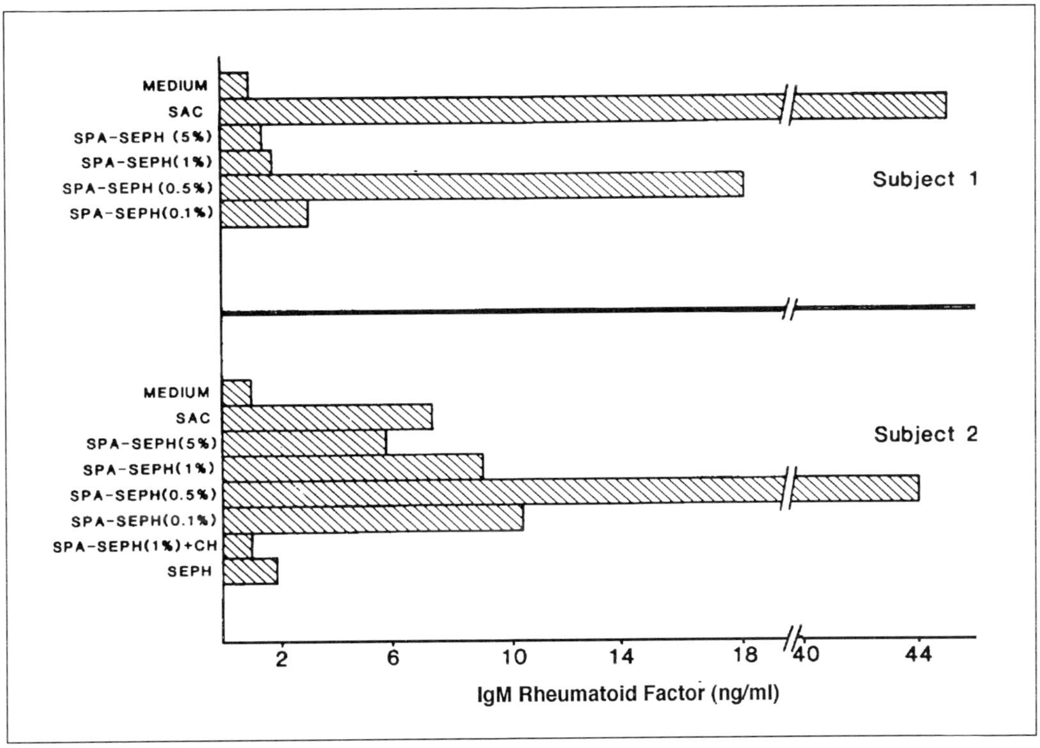

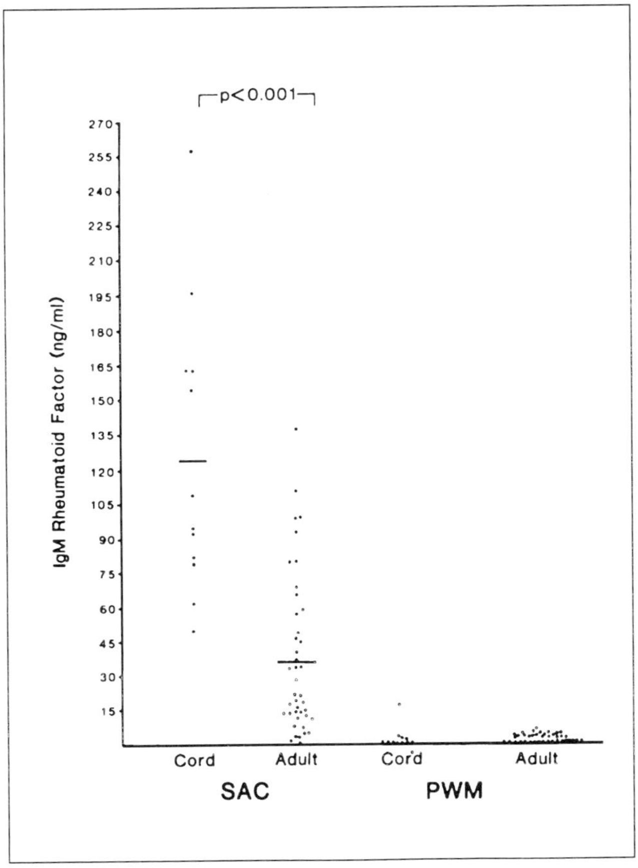

Fig. 7.4. (Top) Soluble SpA coupled to sepharose beads induces IgMRF production. Peripheral blood mononuclear cells were incubated with the designated culture additives and supernatants analyzed for IgMRF by ELISA. SpA-Seph, sepharose beads conjugated with soluble SpA; CH, cycloheximide; Seph, unconjugated sepharose beads. (Reprinted with permission from The Journal of Clinical Investigation, 1986; 78:6122-617, ©1986, the American Society for Clinical Investigation.)

Fig. 7.5. (Left) IgMRF production of cord blood cells stimulated with SAC and PWM. Cord blood cells from 12 full-term infants were incubated with SAC or PWM and IgMRF was measured in the supernatants after 7 to 8 days of culture. Values represent peak responses to each additive, and the mean responses are signified by horizontal bars. Results of similarly stimulated adult peripheral blood mononuclear cells are shown for comparison. IgMRF was not detected when cord blood cells were incubated in media alone. (Reprinted with permission from Levinson AI et al. The Journal of Immunolology 1987; 139:2237-2241. ©1987, the American Association of Immunologists.)

Table 7.2. SAC-induced IgMRF production by SpA-binding and SpA-non-binding B cells

	ng/ml Ig in Supernatant			
	IgG	IgM	IgMRF	%IgMRF/total IgM
Exp 1				
PBMC	1236	1204	43	3.6
B cells	18	34	0	0.0
B + T cells	985	2659	96	3.6
PA⁺ B + T cells	102	450	45	10.0
PA⁻ B + T cells	6945	6850	3	0.04
Exp 2				
PBMC	597	1043	92	8.8
B cells	8	40	0	0.0
B + T cells	1110	2314	78	3.4
PA⁺ B + T cells	300	1610	110	6.8
PA⁻ B + T cells	1943	9996	0	0.0

PBMC, 2×10^5 ; B cells, 5×10^4; T cells, 1×10^5; SpA-binding: PA^+; SpA-non-binding: PA^-. (Reprinted with permission from Kozlowski LM et al. J Clin Immunol 1995; 15:145-151.)

IgMRF secreting cells are confined to the subset of B cells that binds SpA. To test this hypothesis, T and B cell fractions were prepared from the PBMC of healthy donors.[24] The B cell enriched fraction was further segregated into PA^+ and PA^- B cells. We observed (Table 7.2) that SAC-induced IgMRF production was largely confined to cultures containing PA^+ B cells. Cultures of PA^- B cells produced little, if any, IgMRF (0-3 ng/ml). The greater production of IgMRF by PA^+ B cells did not reflect a greater capacity to produce total IgM in response to SAC. Indeed, the total IgM and IgG responses were consistently higher in cultures containing PA^- B cells than in cultures containing PA^+ B cells. Therefore, the ratio of IgMRF/total IgM was much higher for the PA^+ B cell population than for the PA^- population. These results indicate that SAC-induced IgMRF production is limited to a subset of B cells that bind SpA, likely via their membrane IgM. Since this B cell subset is enriched for usage of V_H3 heavy chains, our results strongly suggest that IgMRF produced in response to SAC are similarly enriched for usage of V_H3 elements.

ACTIVATION OF COMPLEMENT BY SPA

Unlike T cell superantigens, a B cell superantigen has the ability to react with potentially large amounts of its receptor (Ig) in the serum as well as on B cells. For example, the B cells reactive with HIV gp120[20] and the Fab binding site on SpA are restricted to those that express V_H3 gene family products. Since this family is the largest of seven human V_H gene families and is expressed by 30-60% of peripheral B cells,[27-29] it is possible that a large proportion of human serum Igs utilize V_H3 heavy chains. The encounter of a B cell superantigen with such a large reservoir of reactive serum Igs could have deleterious effects on the host, particularly if this interaction led to the formation of immune complexes with subsequent activation of the complement cascade. Such complement activation could result in prominent tissue inflammation and damage.

Using SpA as a model B cell superantigen, we have initiated studies to determine if the interaction of a B cell superantigen and its reactive V_H-restricted immunoglobulins leads to complement activation.[30-32] Prior studies demonstrated that addition of SpA to serum leads to activation of the complement cascade.[33] This outcome was attributed to the interaction of the classical site on SpA with the Fc fragment of serum IgG. However, recent reports on the B cell superantigen properties of SpA led us to postulate that the interaction of its alternative binding site with the Fabs of reactive (V_H3^+) Igs leads to activation of the complement cascade. We compared the ability of SpA hyperiodinated to abrogate its Fc binding ability (mod-SpA) with that of unmodified SpA to cause complement consumption when added to normal human serum. Using a hemolytic complement assay, we observed greater than 60% inhibition of CH_{50} activity in SpA and mod-SpA treated serum (62 ± 12%, mean ± SD vs 62 ± 13%, $p > 0.1$, paired t-test).[30-32] More recently, we have demonstrated that this mod-SpA induced complement consumption is associated with the appearance of sizable amounts of C3a in treated sera.[32] Thus, we established that although SpA activates complement, mod-SpA (SpA abrogated of its IgG Fc binding activity) retains its ability to activate the complement cascade. These results strongly suggested that the Fab binding site on SpA is important for complement consumption.

To directly determine if complement activation was (1) dependent on an interaction between the Fab binding site on SpA and V_H3^+ Igs and (2) proceeded via the classical complement pathway, we assessed the ability of human polyclonal IgM and a panel of monoclonal IgM proteins to bind C1q following their interaction with SpA in an ELISA. We observed that polyclonal IgM and only V_H3^+, SpA-reactive IgM proteins bound C1q following their interaction with SpA (Fig. 7.6).[30-32] Therefore, we concluded that binding of the first component of the classical complement pathway and, presumably, the activation of the complement cascade, are byproducts of the superantigenic properties of SpA.

To formally determine if the binding of SpA to V_H3^+ IgM proteins can lead to comple-

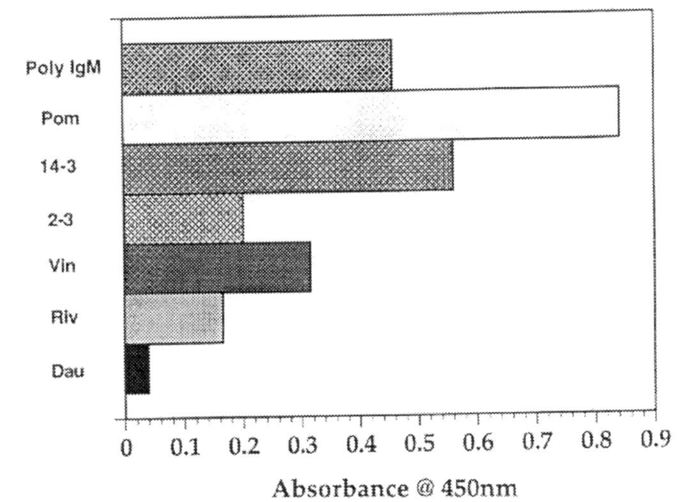

Fig. 7.6. Binding of SpA-reactive IgM/SpA to C1q as detected by peroxidase conjugated anti-IgMFc. The binding of IgM/SpA reaction mixtures to C1q was analyzed in an ELISA. Polyclonal IgM, or monoclonal V_H3+ IgM proteins Pom, 14-3, Vin, 2-3, Riv, and Dau, pre-incubated with SpA (1 μg/ml), were added to C1q-fixed ELISA plates. Background absorbance was subtracted from the raw data. The background absorbance was determined in C1q-coated wells in which IgM proteins and SpA were sequentially incubated and the ELISA then developed by standard protocol. All of the V_H3^+ monoclonal proteins bound SpA in a separate ELISA except for Dau. The ODs represent means of duplicate determinations from a representative experiment; similar results were obtained in three separate experiments.

ment activation, we utilized serum (reconstituted with selected monoclonal IgM proteins) from a severely hypogammaglobulinemic patient.[32] Addition of mod-SpA to hypogammaglobulinemic serum reconstituted with an SpA-nonreactive, V_H3^+ IgM did not alter the CH_{50} activity of the serum. By contrast, addition of mod-SpA to hypogammaglobulinemic serum reconstituted with an SpA-reactive, C1q-binding, V_H3^+ IgM did support complement consumption and C3a gneration. In addition, incubation of mod-SpA alone with the hypogammaglobulinemic serum did not cause any complement consumption. The latter observation eliminated the possibility that direct activation of the alternative complement pathway contributed to the findings observed with the mod-SpA-treated, normal serum. Taken together with the C1q binding data, the above results provided formal proof that the interaction of V_H3^+ Igs with the Fab binding site on SpA leads to binding of C1q and activation of the classical complement cascade.

DISCUSSION

Superantigens have been extremely helpful tools in exploring fundamental questions in immunobiology including mechanisms of cell activation, tolerance and autoimmunity. Until recently, attention has been focused exclusively on T cell superantigens. However, new data suggest that there are agents that may qualify as B cell superantigens.[7-10,14-22]

Amongst the B cell superantigens reported to date, SpA is the best characterized with regard to structure and function. The studies reviewed herein add to the body of information that the alternative binding site of SpA selectively interacts with Igs containing V_H3 elements. Sasso et al were the first to make this association in man when they studied the binding of human monoclonal proteins to SpA.[10] All binders shared usage of V_H3 heavy chains and almost all V_H3^+ monoclonal proteins tested were positive in their binding assay. Binding appeared to be independent of the source of light chain. They subsequently reported that SpA bound to roughly 22% of human polyclonal IgA and 15% of polyclonal human IgG $F(ab')_2$ fragments.[9] Similar observations were made by Ibrahim et al who found that 32% of polyclonal human IgM, 13% of IgA1 and 22% IgA2 had SpA binding activity.[34] In addition these investigators reported that 14% of polyclonal human IgG_3 bound SpA (the Fc of IgG_3 will not bind to the conventional SpA binding site unless the IgG_3 bears the Gm3(s,+) allotype).[34] Using a phage combinatorial IgG Fab display library, Sasano reported that 17% of Ig-producing clones bound SpA.[16] The apparent K_D of Fab binders ranged from 2.5×10^{-7} to 10^{-5} M. Binding was restricted to V_H3-producing clones. Moreover, 60% of V_H3^+ clones in the unselected library had SpA binding activity. Binding was not skewed towards usage of particular V light chains although binding activity showed a four-fold variation with substitution of particular light chains.

Using a molecular approach, we provided direct evidence that SpA-binding B cells are enriched for expression of V_H3 heavy chains.[24] We observed that the SpA-binding (PA^+) B cells preferentially expressed V_H3 mRNA. SpA binding of human B cells has also been directly examined by multiparameter flow cytometry. Silverman et al reported that 14-54% of human B cells bound SpA that had been chemically modified to abrogate IgGFc binding activity.[14] Binding was a feature of V_H3^+ B cells since it was inhibited by a V_H3 but not a V_H4 monoclonal protein. Binding activity was influenced by the age of the donor and the anatomic compartment of the B cells. The percentage of positive B cells was higher in umbilical cord vein blood (mean, 46%) than in the peripheral blood of adults (mean, 30%) with a shift to adult levels occurring around 10 months of age. Interestingly, $CD5^+$ B cells showed greater binding than $CD5^-$ B cells. This population of B cells is enriched in the neonate where it accounts for upwards of 70% of the circulating B cells versus 25% in adult peripheral blood.[37] The more prominent binding of SpA by (1) newborn

B cells than adult B cells, (2) IgM than IgG, and 3) IgA2 than IgA1, have been taken as evidence that SpA binds preferentially to ontogenically less developed B cells and their immunoglobulin products. Binding of SpA to V_H3^+ Fabs has therefore been viewed as a primitive host defense characteristic of the preimmune repertoire.

From a functional standpoint, a B cell superantigen could have a major impact on immune and inflammatory responses. Our studies on the model B cell superantigen, SpA, provide evidence for two types of effects, namely elicitation of autoantibody production and activation of the complement cascade. As noted above, the SpA component of SAC is a powerful stimulant of IgMRF production of normal PBMC.[25] In the studies reviewed herein, we demonstrated that the production of IgMRF was largely limited to SpA-binding (PA^+) B cells, which produced copious amounts of IgMRF compared to the SpA-nonbinding (PA^-) B cell preparations. This production was not a reflection of an enhanced capacity of PA^+ B cells to produce IgM. In fact, the PA^- B cells consistently produced a greater total Ig response than the PA^+ B cells. The Ig produced by the PA^- B cell population is likely induced by stimulating components of the staphylococcal cell wall other than SpA, in conjunction with T cell help.[25] Our findings suggested that SAC-induced IgMRF production requires direct interaction of the alternative binding site of SpA with the Fabs of reactive B cells, presumably via surface IgM molecules. Since the binding of SpA to B cells is restricted to those B cells that express V_H3^+ surface Igs, our results establish that SAC-induced IgMRF production represents a superantigenic property of SpA.

Our results provide insight into the prominent RF stimulating properties of SpA. Prior studies have demonstrated that SAC-induced IgMRF is a product of $CD5^+$ B cells.[37] As already mentioned, cord blood cells, enriched for $CD5^+$ B cells, make a particularly striking IgMRF response to SAC.[26] Moreover, $CD5^+$ B cells are enriched for SpA-binding B cells, i.e. V_H3 heavy chain expressing B cells.[14] Taken together, these results lead us to hypothesize that the proclivity of SpA for inducing IgMRF production relates to its capacity to preferentially stimulate V_H3-bearing, $CD5^+$ B cells. Interestingly, studies of monoclonal RFs generated from the peripheral blood and synovium of rheumatoid arthritis patients and from the peripheral blood of normal donors have underscored the frequent utilization of V_H3 heavy chains.[38,39] This frequent usage could merely reflect the apparent high prevalence of this V_H family in the adult peripheral B cell repertoire.[27-29] However, an appealing alternative is that the frequent utilization of V_H3 heavy chains could reflect selection by an exogenous or endogenous agent, namely a superantigen.

A major difference between T cell and B cell superantigens is the ability of the latter to react with potentially large amounts of soluble antigen receptor molecules in the serum. The interaction of conventional antigens with the CDRs of IgG and IgM antibodies leads to activation of the complement cascade with attendant release of potent mediators of inflammation. Deposition of complement containing antigen/antibody complexes can cause inflammation at the sites of immune complex deposition. A B cell superantigen could have deleterious effects on the host by virtue of its ability to bind relatively large amounts of serum immunoglobulin if the complexes formed activated the complement cascade.

The studies described herein show unequivocally that the interaction of the alternative site of SpA and serum Ig leads to consumption of complement. Indeed mod-SpA and untreated SpA were equally efficient in causing complement consumption, implying that the Fab binding site of this B cell superantigen is a key element in mediating this activity. Complement consumption was due to complement activation as evidenced by the generation of C3a in mod-SpA treated sera. Moreover, our C1q binding results clearly indicated that mod-SpA-induced complement activation in serum required the interaction of this B cell superantigen with V_H3^+ immunoglobulins and proceeded by the classical cascade. The reliance on V_H3^+ immunoglobulins was further demonstrated with a hypogammaglobulinemic serum reconstituted with selected IgM monoclonal proteins. In addition, the fact that incubation of mod-SpA alone with the hypogammaglobulinemic serum did not cause any complement consumption eliminated the possibility that direct activation of the alternative complement pathway contributed to the findings observed with the mod-SpA-treated, normal serum.

Taken together, our results provide formal proof that the interaction of V_H3^+ Igs with the Fab binding site on SpA leads to binding of C1q and activation of the classical complement cascade. Complement activation by protein Fv has also recently been described.[40] However, our results provided direct evidence for the first time that the interaction of a model B cell superantigen, mod-SpA, with its reactive (V_H3^+) Igs leads to activation of the classical complement cascade. Complement activation by a B cell superantigen is also being examined in the HIV gp120 system. Townsley-Fuchs and co-workers have suggested that gp120 and V_H3^+ Igs may form immune complexes and activate complement, which may sequester HIV to phagocytic cells.[41] They found that serum IgM could inhibit binding of gp120 to T cells, but only in the presence of complement. They suggested that the interaction between gp120, V_H3^+ Igs, and complement may cause phagocytic cells to more readily take up HIV.

The interaction of a B cell superantigen with the Fabs of reactive Igs in vivo could lead to the formation of complement-activating immune complexes, which may have profound clinical significance. For example, patients with SpA^+, *Staphylococcus aureus*-induced endocarditis and patients treated with autologous plasma perfused through a SpA-immunoabsorbent column develop immune complex-mediated glomerulonephritis and vasculitis, respectively.[42,43] These manifestations may be a result of an interaction between SpA and V_H3^+ Igs with the formation of immune complexes and resultant complement activation. Moreover, some cases of glomerulonephritis, arthritis, and thrombocytopenia in HIV-infected patients may be caused by deposition of complexes containing HIV gp120 and Igs containing V_H3 heavy chains.[44-46] Unlike a conventional antigen, a B cell superantigen can react with a large fraction of serum Igs. This interaction can lead to activation of the classical complement cascade and thus has the potential to elicit prominent tissue inflammation in a host.

In summary, the studies reviewed herein underscore two potential consequences of the host's encounter with a B cell superantigen, i.e., elicitation of autoantibody production and activation of the complement cascade. When considered along with the reported ability of a B cell superantigen to degranulate mast cells and basophils,[47-49] it is clear that this novel class of unconventional antigens may evoke inflammatory responses and contribute to the pathogenesis of autoimmune and allergic diseases.

Acknowledgments

This work was supported in part by N.I.H. Training grant 2T32CA09140, a Merit Review grant from the Veterans Administration, and a grant from the University of Pennsylvania Research Foundation.

References

1. Inganas M, Johansson SGO, Benninch HH. Interaction of human polyclonal IgE and IgG from different species with protein A from *Staphylococcus aureus*: demonstration of protein A-reactive sites located on the $F(ab')_2$ fragments of human IgG. Scand J Immunol 1980; 12:23-31.
2. Inganas M. Comparison of mechanisms of interaction between protein A from *Staphylococcus aureus* and human monoclonal IgG, IgA, and IgM in relation to the classical Fcγ and the alternative $F(ab')_2$ protein A interactions. Scand J Immunol 1981; 13:343-352.
3. Young WW Jr, Tamura Y, Wolock DM, et al.

Staphylococcal protein A binding to the Fab fragments of mouse monoclonal antibodies. J Immunol 1984; 133: 3163-3166.
4. Vidal MA, Conde FP. Alternative mechanism of protein A-immunoglobulin interaction: The V_H-associated reactivity of a monoclonal human IgM. J Immnuol 1985; 135:1232-1238.
5. Romagnani S, Guidizi MG, Biagiotti R, et al. Surface immunoglobulins are involved in the interaction of protein A with human B cells and in the triggering of B cell proliferation induced by protein A-containing *Staphylococcus aureus*. J Immunol 1981; 127:1307-1313.
6. Romagnani S, Guidizi MG, Del Prete G, et al. Demonstration on protein A of two distinct immunoglobulin-binding sites and their role in the mitogenic activity of *Staphylococcus aureus*. J Immunol 1982; 129:596-602.
7. Hillson J, Karr NS, Oplinger I, et al. The structural basis of germline encoded V_H3 immunoglobulin binding to staphylococcal protein A. J Exp Med 1993; 178:331-336.
8. Randen I, Potter K, Li Y, et al. Complementarity-determining region 2 is implicated in the binding of staphylococcal protein A to human immunoglobulin V_HIII variable regions. Eur J Immunol 1993; 23:2682-2686.
9. Sasso EH, Silverman G, Mannik M. Human IgA and IgG F(ab')$_2$ that bind to staphylococcal protein A belong to the V_HIII subgroup. J Immunol 1991; 147:1877-1883.
10. Sasso EH, Silverman GJ, Mannik M. IgM molecules that bind staphylococcal protein A contain V_HIII H chains. J Immunol 1989; 142:2778-2783.
11. Seppala I, Kaartinen M, Ibrahim S, et al. Mouse Ig coded by V_H families S107 and J606 bind to protein A. J Immunol 1990; 145:2989-2993.
12. Shokri F, Mageed RA, Maziak BR, et al. Expression of V_HIII-associated cross-reactive idiotype on human B lymphocytes. Association with staphylococcal protein A binding and *Staphylococcus aureus* Cowan I stimulation. J Immunol 1991; 146:936-940.
13. Vasquez Kristianson S, Pascual V, Lipsky PE. Staphylococcal protein A induces biased production of immunoglobulin by V_H3 expressing human B lymphocytes. J Immunol 1994; 150:2974-2982.
14. Silverman GJ, Sasano M, Wormsley SB. Age-associated changes in binding of human lymphocytes to a V_H3-restricted unconventional bacterial antigen. J Immunol 1993; 151:5840-5855.
15. Silverman GJ. Human antibody response to bacterial antigens: studies of a model conventional antigen and a proposed model B cell superantigen. Inter Rev Immunol 1992; 9:57-78.
16. Sasano M, Burton D, Silverman G. Molecular selection of human antibodies with an unconventional bacterial B cell antigen. J Immunol 1993; 151:5822-5839.
17. Silverman GJ. B cell superantigens and the spectrum of unconventional antigens. The Immunologist 1994; 2:51-.58
18. Levinson AI, Kozlowski L, Zheng Y, et al. B cell superantigens: Definition and potential impact on the immune response. J Clin Immunol 1995; 15:26S-36S.
19. Zouali M. B cell superantigens:implications for selection of the human antibody repertoire. Immunol Today 1995; 16:399-405.
20. Berberian L, Goodglick L, Kipps T, et al. Immunoglobulin V_H3 gene products: Natural ligands for HIV gp 120. Science 1993; 261:1588-1591.
21. Silverman GJ, Roben P, Bouvet J-P, et al. Superantigen properties of a human sialoprotein involved in gut-associated immunity J Clin Invest 1995; 96:417-426.
22. Bjorck L. Protein L, a novel cell wall protein with affinity for Ig L chains. J Immunol 1988; 140:1194-1197.
23. Muraguchi A, Kehrl J, Butler JL et al. Regulation of human B cell activation, proliferation and differentiation by soluble factors. J Clin Immunol 1984; 4:337-347.
24. Kozlowski LM, Kunning SR, Zheng Y, et al. *Staphylococcus aureus* Cowan I-induced human immunoglobulin responses: Preferential IgM rheumatoid factor production and V_H3 mRNA expression by protein A binding cells. J Clin Immunol 1995; 15:145-151.

25. Levinson AI, Tar L, Carafa C, et al. *Staphylococcus aureus* Cowan I: A potent stimulus of IgM rheumatoid factor production. J Clin Invest 1986; 78:612-617.
26. Levinson AI, Dalal NF, Haidar M, et al. Prominent IgM rheumatoid factor production by human cord blood lymphocytes stimulated in vitro with *Staphylococcus aureus* Cowan I. J Immunol 1987; 139:2237-2241.
27. Zouali M, Theze J. Probing V_H gene-family utilization in human peripheral B cells by in situ hybridization. J Immunol 1990; 146:2855-2864.
28. Huang C, Stewart AK, Schwartz RS, et al. Immunoglobulin heavy chain gene expression in peripheral blood B lymphocytes. J Clin Invest 1992; 89:1331-1343.
29. Guigou V, Cuisinier AM, Tonnelle C, et al. Human immunoglobulin V_H and V_K repertoire revealed by in situ hybridization. Mol Immunol 1990; 27:935-940.
30. Kozlowski LM, Lambris JD, Levinson AI. Effect of a putative B cell superantigen on complement. Ann NY Acad Sci 1995; 764:356-358.
31. Kozlowski LM, Lambris JD, Levinson AI. B cell superantigen-mediated complement activation in mouse and man. FASEB J 1995; 9:A518.
32. Kozlowski LM, Soulika AM, Silverman GJ, et al. Complement activation by a B cell superantigen. J Immunol 1996; 157:1200-1206.
33. Kronvall G, Gewurz H. Activation and inhibition of IgG-mediated complement fixation by staphylococcal protein A. Clin Exp Immunol 1970; 7:211-220.
34. Ibrahim S, Seppala I, Makela O. V-region-mediated binding of human Ig by protein A. J Immunol 1993; 151:3597-3603.
35. Ibrahim S, Kaartinen M, Seppala I, et al. The alternative binding site for Protein A in the Fab fragment of immunoglobulins. Scand J Immunol 1993; 37:257-264.
36. Antin, JH, Emerson SG, Marin P, et al. Leu 1^+ ($CD5^+$) B cells. A major lymphoid subpopulation in human fetal spleen: phenotypic and functional studies. J Immunol 1986; 136:505-510.
37. Hardy RR, Hayakawa K, Shimizu M, et al. Rheumatoid factor secretion from human LEU 1^+ B cell. Science 1987; 236:81-83.
38. Randen I, Thompson KM, Pascual V, et al. Rheumatoid factor V genes from patients with rheumatoid arthritis are diverse and show evidence of an antigen-driven response. Immunol Rev 1992; 128:49-71.
39. Thompson KM, Randen I, Natvig JB, et al. Human monoclonal rheumatoid factors derived from the polyclonal repertoire of rheumatoid synovial tissue: incidence of cross-reactive idotypes and expression of V_H and V_k subgroups. Eur J Immunol 1990; 20:863-868.
40. Ruffet E, Pires R, Pillot J, et al. Activation of the classical pathway of complement by non-immune complexes of immunoglobulins with human protein Fv (Fv fragment-binding protein). Scand J Immunol 1994; 40:359-362.
41. Townsley-Fuchs J, Goodglick L, Braun J. V_H3 immunoglobulins of the natural antibody repertoire bind gp120, activate complement and sequester gp120 away from T cells. J Cell Biochem 1995; S21B:227.
42. Glassock RJ, Cohen AH, Adler SG, et al. Secondary glomerular diseases. In: Brenner BM and Rector FC, eds. The Kidney. Vol 1. WB Saunders Co., 1986: 1052-1053.
43. Sculley RE, EJ Mark, McNeely WF, et al. Case Records of the Massachusetts General Hospital, Case #35-1994. N Engl J Med 1994; 331:792.
44. Glassock RJ. Renal pathology of human immunodeficiency virus (HIV) infection and the kidney. Ann Int Med 1990; 112:35-49.
45. Kaye BR. Rheumatologic manifestations of infection with human immunodeficiency virus (HIV). Ann Int Med 1989; 111: 158-167.
46. Karpatkin S, Nardi M. Autoimmune anti-HIV-1gp120 antibody with anti-idiotype-like activity in sera and immune complexes of HIV-1 related immunologic thrombocytopenia. J Clin Invest 1992; 89:356-364.
47. Marone G, Tamburini M, Giudizi G, et al. Mechanism of activation of human basophils by *Staphylococcus aureus* Cowan I. Infect

Immun 1987; 55:803-809.

48. Patella V, Casolaro V, Bjorck L, et al. A bacterial Ig-binding protein that activates human basophils and mast cells. J Immunol 1990; 145:3054-3061.

49. Patella V, Bouvet J-P, Marone G. Protein Fv produced during viral hepatitis is a novel activator of human basophils and mast cells. J Immunol 1993; 151:5685-5698.

CHAPTER 8

Low-Affinity Binding of Human Immunoglobulin Variable Domains: A New Superantigen in *Escherichia coli*?

Mats Ohlin, Christina Furebring and Carl A. K. Borrebaeck

INTRODUCTION

Antigen-specifically induced molecules are able to act alone or in concert with other components of the immune system to protect the human body against potentially harmful molecules, bacteria and viruses. Over the last couple of years it has become increasingly apparent that many invading organisms also produce molecules specifically interacting with various parts of the immune system and which use this function to evade its destructive powers. Consequently, many bacteria are able to bind to the constant regions of immunoglobulins (Ig) thus camouflaging their surface to appear less foreign to the host organism. Furthermore, the bound Ig are unable to evoke biological effector functions in the format they are presented to the immune system thus evading protective immune responses.[1] Similarly, recent reports show that certain viruses are able to pick up cellular molecules which block the complement fixation cascade, consequently reducing the ability of antibodies to enforce their protective effector mechanisms.[2,3] Some intracellular parasites are also able to downregulate the expression of major histocompatibility complex (MHC) class II reducing cytotoxic cellular responses.[4] Similarly, bacteria and viruses are known to produce components which interact with T cell receptors (TcR) in a polyclonal manner thus evoking a general immune stimulation and possibly diverting the power of the immune system from the specific response towards the invading organism as such.[5]

Furthermore, these reactivities may result in clonal exhaustion of the responding T cell repertoire. To what extent these organisms are able to exploit these superantigens in their survival strategy is a matter which deserves further studies.

Lately, several lines of investigation have proved the existence of not only T cell-specific but also B cell-specific superantigens (SAg), which interact with the variable regions of B cell antigen-specific receptors in an antigen-nonspecific manner.[6-11] These reactivities have also been suggested to affect the available antibody repertoire by expanding or deleting particular subsets of B cells. This activity has been particularly well documented for the B cell SAg activity of the human immunodeficiency virus type 1 (HIV-1)-encoded surface molecule gp120.[6,7] In addition to known SAg activities, some antibody responses have been suggested to be restricted in the usage of variable regions of the developing repertoires.[12-16] Some of these restricted responses might be expected to result from the simple structure exposed by certain antigens, in analogy with certain hapten-responses seen in mice. Other responses of this type against complex protein epitopes might be associated with B cell SAg activities affecting the developing repertoire. Such effects have also been attributed to an endogenous SAg found in certain tissues.[17] Below we describe the presence and features of an apparent, new antibody variable domain-binding component found in *Escherichia coli*,[18] and some of the possible implications of this activity. In particular, the low affinity but potentially high avidity associated with the antibody-SAg interaction points towards a possibly new concept of SAg action.

IDENTIFICATION OF AN *E. COLI* IG-BINDING SAG COMPONENT.

We used a new immunoassay format based on electrochemiluminescence (ORIGEN analyzer; IGEN Inc., Rockville, MD, USA).[19] This technique involves detection of a fluorescent-labeled component captured on a magnetic bead as an immune complex. In these studies the labeled compound was an anti-human-Ig antibody which binds to and crosslinks the primary antibody being studied. When investigating the binding of antibodies to magnetic bead-immobilized *E. coli*-derived recombinant proteins by use of this immunoassay format, unexpected levels of binding of otherwise highly monospecific antibodies of the IgG isotype were observed.[18] In particular, it was noted that the SAg-IgG interaction was undetectable unless the crosslinking agent was present during the incubation of the SAg with the antibody. In contrast, high-affinity antigen-specific interactions were, as expected, not dependent on any cross linking agent as schematically outlined in Figure 8.1.

Antibodies were also shown to bind the SAg-like component without additional crosslinking agents if they had been previously aggregated by light heat treatment (56°C for 30 min). Thus, the interaction between the putative *E. coli*-derived SAg and antibodies displayed low affinity, but crosslinking promoted a detectable high avidity interaction. Further investigations of these reactivities firmly confirmed that we were dealing with a new Ig variable domain-specific binding activity with several interesting properties (Table 8.1).[18]

Briefly, knowing that the SAg activity was recognizing antibody structures we were interested in delineating the exact specificity of this reactivity. Using a set of diverse,

***Table 8.1. Summary of the characteristics of the Ig-specific binding activity found in* E. coli*, as determined by Ohlin and Borrebaeck*[18]**

Low-affinity interaction
Specificity for Ig variable domains
Recognition of several V_H families ($V_H1,4>V_H3,5$).*
Inhibition of interaction by antigen
Protease sensitivity of the activity

* V_H2 and V_H6 genes have not been investigated

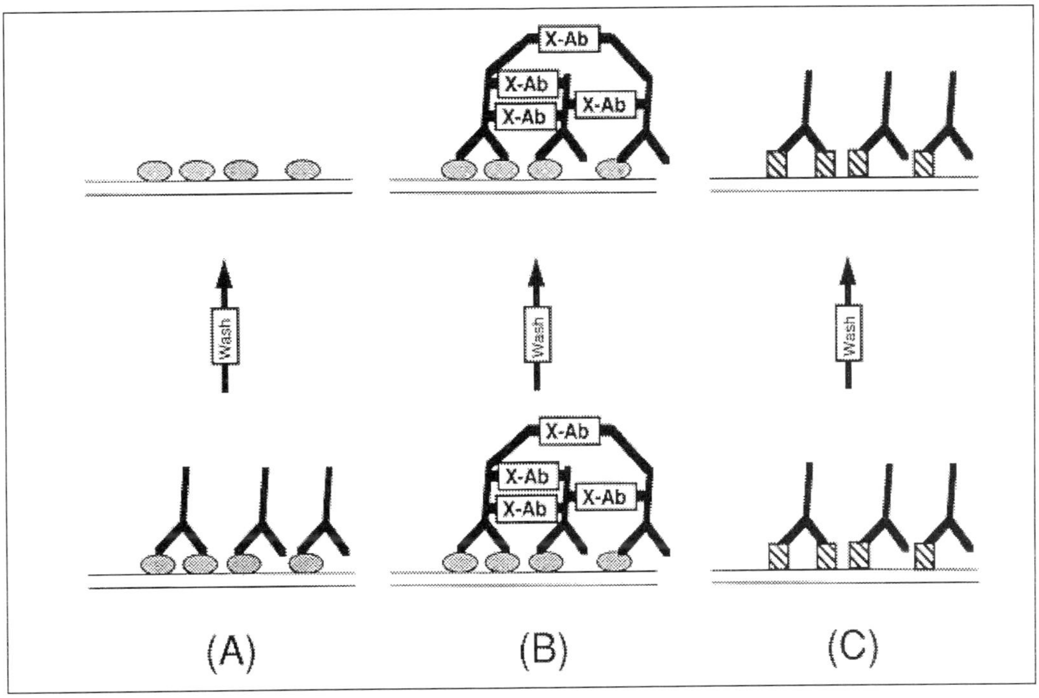

Fig. 8.1. Schematic description of the outcome of the low affinity interaction between Ig and SAg (grey ovals) and/or the interaction of Ig and its conventional antigen (hatched boxes) under the various assay conditions employed by the ORIGEN analyzer. (A) SAg-specific binding of Ig is not detectable if the primary reaction is performed in the abscence of a crosslinking antibody (X-Ab). (B) In contrast the superantigen/antibody complexes remain intact if the crosslinker is present when the primary superantigen/antibody interaction occurs. (C) High affinity antigen-antibody interactions are not dependent on the presence of the crosslinking reagent under these conditions.

high affinity monospecific monoclonal antibodies with known variable region gene sequences it was observed that the SAg recognized antibodies using different variable region germline genes. However, the binding of the SAg to antibodies encoded by genes of the V_H1 and V_H4 families was somewhat ($p = 0.12$) stronger than the interaction with antibodies encoded by V_H3 and V_H5 family genes (Fig. 8.2). Together with the fact that antigen bound to the variable domain strongly inhibited the SAg-binding capacity of antibodies, this finding strongly supports the fact that the *E. coli*-derived SAg is specific for antibody variable domains.[18]

DISCUSSION

These data describe to our knowledge for the first time an Ig-binding component in *E. coli*. Its discovery was made possible through the use of an analytical technique which allows low affinity interactions to be detected through a crosslinking procedure which adds an avidity component to the interaction. Although it is not yet possible to exactly determine the site which the Ig-binding component binds in the variable domain, mutation studies utilizing the known differences between the described antibodies (Fig. 8.3) will shed light on the exact specificity of this Ig variable domain binding activity. Another, as yet unexplored, possibility which might explain the ability of this Ig variable domain-binding capacity to interact with antibodies originating from highly diverse germline sequences is that the binding moiety may actually consist of several different molecular species each binding different antibody families. Further studies will be required to resolve these issues.

In general, low affinity interactions strengthened by multiple contact points promoting a high total avidity is a common

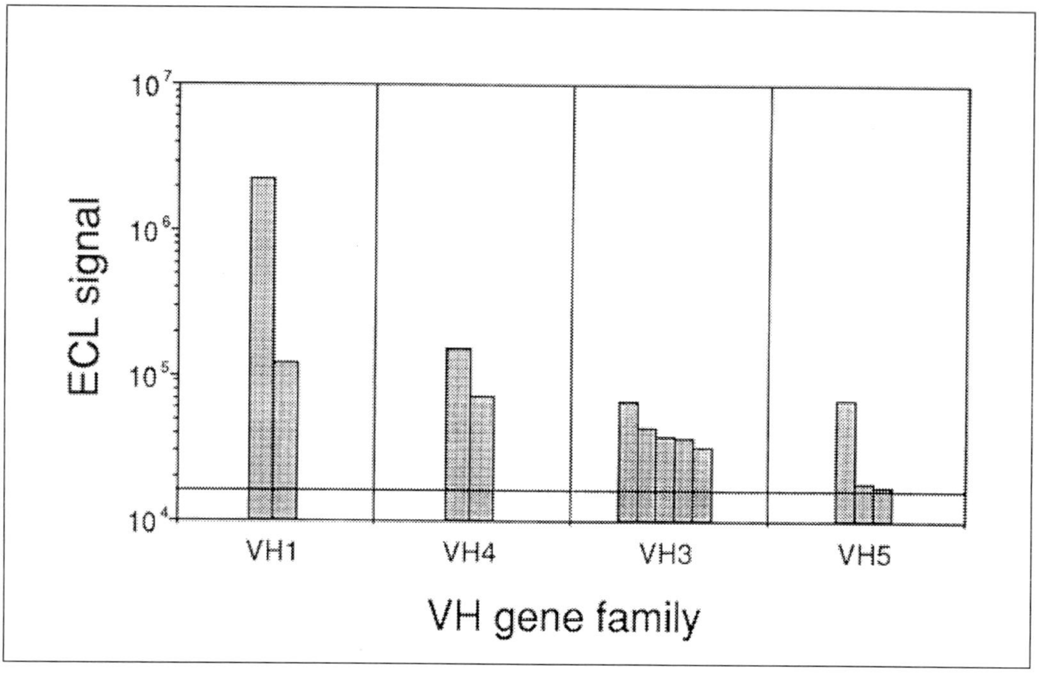

Fig. 8.2. Binding of twelve human monoclonal IgG encoded by known variable region genes to the E. coli-*derived, immobilized SAg contained in recombinant UL57/2-GST (fragment of CMV UL57 fused to glutathione-S-transferase)*[20] *in the presence of crosslinking, constant domain-specific antibodies. Background ECL signal in the absence of human antibody is indicated by a horizontal line. Some antibodies which are marginally positive at this concentration show positive signal at higher Ig concentrations. The analysis was performed by electrochemiluminescence (ECL) using the ORIGEN analyzer technology.*[18-19] *All antibodies were added at a final concentration of 33 ng IgG/ml. (Reprinted in a modified form from Ohlin M, Borrebaeck CAK. FEMS Immunol Med Microbiol 1996; 13:161-168. ©1996, Elsevier Science)*

feature of many biological systems. For instance, certain adhesion molecules[22,23] display such characteristics. Similarly, the T cell SAg staphylococcal enterotoxin A and related molecules exhibit a low affinity for the TcR.[24] However, after being captured by MHC class II molecules displayed on cell surfaces efficient binding of the SAg to TcR is made possible through the multiplicity of the interaction.

We have not yet evaluated the possible in vivo effects of the *E. coli*-derived SAg activity described here. It is, however, tempting to speculate on the possibility of this, or other molecules displaying similar binding features, to interact with antibody-expressing cells and modify their level of activation either directly or together with other stimulating agents. Such interactions would add binding strength to the interaction of low affinity antibodies found in previously nonimmunized individuals and multivalent or aggregated antigens. If such low affinity SAg-activities are not directed specifically towards the antigen-binding site of the antibody (as is the case with the SAg activity described here) but rather to the V region framework they may also strengthen low affinity binding of antibodies to epitopes found within the very same molecule. Consequently, the repertoire responding towards such antigens may be skewed towards an overrepresentation of particular variable segment genes depending on the specificity of the SAg activity. It is also conceivable that the availability of efficient T cell help at any given time might affect the outcome of such interactions resulting in either stimulation, deletion or anergy of the SAg-reactive clones. Such effects have, as indicated above, previously been observed in the case of the well documented variable domain binding activity of HIV-1 gp120 which expands or

```
                                                                                                                 1                      1    VH
                    1          2           3           4           5           6           7          8           9           0                      1    fa-
                    0          0    ABC    0           0           0 A         0           0          0  ABC      0           0 ABCDEFGHIJKLM        0    mily
(A)
cons.          *VQL**SG** **K******* *C**S---G**** *******W*R** *G*G**W*G* *********Y* *****R**** *D*S****** *L******DTAVY *C******** **************WGQGTLV* VSS
cons. (75%)    QVQL**SG** **KP****** *C**S---G*S** *******W*RQ* PG*GLEW*G* I****CS**Y* *****RVTM* *DTS****** *LS*****DTAVY YC*R****** *****---------**WGQGTLVT VSS
LuNm03         RVQLMQSGAE VRKHGASVKV SCKAS---GYSFG NYFMH--WLRQA PGQGPEWMGM INPRDNKANYA QKFRGRVTMT KDTSTSIFYM ELSRLRSDDTAVY FCARDMGSHD FWAVGINLPGSLFDNWGQGTLVT VSS  1
MO81           QVQLQVSGPG LVKPSQTLSL TCTVS---GGSIS TSGHCWSWLRRP AGKGLEWIGR IC-SRGSTNYI PSLKSRVVMS VDSSKNQFSL RLSSVTAADTAVY YCARAPPGDY FF-----------DFWGQGTLVA VSS  4
MO58           QVQLVQSGAE VKKPGASVKV SCKAS---GYTFS SHYMH--WVRQA PGQGLEWMGI MIPSRGSATYA ERFQGRVTMT SDTSTDTVYI ELRSLRSEDTAVY YCVREDEYYD ISGYF---------NYWGQGTLVT VSS  1
ITC48          QVQLQESGPG LVKPSQTLSL TCTVS---GGSIN TGGYYWSWIRQH PGKGLKWIGY II-YSGSTSYN PSLQSRITIS ADTSKSQFSL RLSAVTAADTAVY YCVGKGINTA RGNF---------EYWGQGTLVT VSS  4
                                                   #                                    ##         # #    #          ##

(B)
cons.          ****V*SG** ***PG**L** SC**S***G**F* *****--WVRQ* PG*G**W*** *********** *S*******S *D*******I ***SL***D*A*Y YC******** ***********--D*WGQG**** VSS
cons. (75%)    *VQLV*SG** V**PG*SLR* SC**S---G*TF* *Y*I*--WVRQ* PGKGLEW*** I****S***Y* *S**G**TIS *D*S*NT**L Q**SL***DTA*Y YCAR****** *******------D*WGQGT*V* VSS
ITC52          EVQLVQSGAE VKKPGDSLRI SCKGS---GYTFG GYWIA--WVRQM PGRGLEWMGI IYPGDSDTTYS PSFQGQVSIS ADKSINTAYL QWSSLRASDTAMY YCARKGLRDV EWYDPREDVL---DVWGQGTMVI VSS  5
MO53           QV-LVQSGGG VVQPGRSLRL SCVTS---GFTFS NFGID--WVRQA PGKGPEWVAY ISNDGTNINYA DSVKGRFTVS RDTSKNTLSL AMNSLRLEDTAVY YCARQPRYFD SGGYYI-------DYWGQGTLVI VSS  3
ITC88          QLQLVESGGG VVQPGRSLRL SCAAS---GFIFS EYDMH--WVRQA PGKGLQWVAV ISVDGSDKHYA DSVKGRFTIS RDNSQNMLFL QMDSLRGDDTAVY YCARDGKSLN GYSGII-------DYWGQGSLVT VSS  3
ITC39          QVQLVESGGG VVQPGRSLRL SCAAS---GFTFN SYAIH--WVRQV PGKGLEWVAV VSYDGSNKYFA DSVKDRFTIS RDNSKNTLFL QLNSLTTEDTAVY YCVRGPDPIV VTGPFYF------DSWGQGTLVT VSS  3
B715A2         QVQLVESGGG VVQPGRSLRL SCAAS---GFTFN NYAIH--WVRQA PGKGLEWVAF ISYDGSKNYYA DSVKGRFTIS RDNSKNTLFL QMNSLRPEDTAIY YCARVLFQQL VLYAPF-------DIWGQGTMVT VSS  3
MO61           EVQLVESGGG LVKPGGSLRL SCAAS---GFTFS SYSMN--WVRQA PGKGLEWVSL IRSSSSHIYYA DSVKGRFTIS RDNAKNSLYL QMNSLRAEDTAVY YCAVSAIEAQ L------------DYWGQGTLVT VSS  3
ITC63B         EVQLVQSGAE VKKPGEALKV SCKGS---GYTFS TYWIA--WVRQL PGKGLEWMGI IYPGDSDTNYS PSFQGQVTIS VDKSISTAYL EWSSLKASDTAIY YCARWSVVIP AAIEVEGNYGM--DVWGQGTTVT VSS  5
ITC33          EVKVVQSGAE VKKPGESLHI SCQISADGGDDFT TLWIG--WVRQM PGKGLEWMGI IWPGDSDTTYS PSFQGHVSIS ADKSTSTAYL QWSSLKASDSAMY YCATNSGYYP GDGF---------DYWGQGTLII VSS  5
                                                ..CDR1.              ........CDR2.......                                          .........CDR3.........
```

Fig. 8.3. Amino acid sequences of heavy chain variable domains used by the antibodies used in this study.[18] The numbering is according to Kabat et al.[21] Sequences are grouped with the more reactive V_H1 and V_H4 (A) and the somewhat less reactive V_H3 and V_H5 Ig (B). In each group they are shown according to their binding activity in descending order (Fig. 8.2). Above each group a consensus sequence and a sequence with residues shared by at least 75% of all sequences in the group are shown. Asterisks (*) indicate variability between the sequences in each group and dashes (-) indicate absence of that particular residue in a sequence. Some residues which apparently differ between the two groups are highlighted (#). The locations of complementarity determining regions (CDR) are indicated below the sequences.

deletes SAg reactive clones dependent on the availability of T cell help at different stages of the disease.[7]

Another aspect of the Ig-binding activity of this *E. coli*-derived component is its potential to interfere in immunological analysis. In fact, this reactivity was detected using an analytical approach where antibodies were crosslinked when incubated with immobilized antigen. This binding activity is not a general feature of the crosslinking system as such, since a number of other assay systems not employing immobilized *E. coli*-derived antigens do not display any nonantigen specific binding of antibodies. Rather, our results might explain instances of false positive results encountered when assessing various reactivities in samples containing rheumatoid factors (RF). Such RF might, much like our crosslinking antibody, provide a sufficient degree of multivalency to assure a high avidity interaction with the *E. coli* SAg. Analysis of specific IgM might be particularly prone to this reactivity since this molecule is, by itself, already multivalent.

In conclusion, we have demonstrated the presence of a low affinity Ig-binding activity in extracts of *E. coli*. Further evaluation of this phenomenon as well as of similar potential reactivities produced by other pathogens will shed light on their biological significance during developing antibody responses occurring as a consequence of infection.

Acknowledgments

We gratefully acknowledge the support of IGEN Inc. for allowing access to the ORIGEN analyzer.

References

1. Boyle MDP. Bacterial immunoglobulin binding proteins. San Diego: Academic Press Inc. 1990.
2. Schmitz J, Zimmer JP, Kluxen B et al. Antibody-mediated complement-mediated cytotoxicity in sera from patients with HIV-1 infection is controlled by CD55 and CD59. J Clin Invest 1995; 96:1520-1526.
3. Spear GT, Lurain NS, Parker CJ et al. Host cell derived comlement control proteins CD55 and CD59 are incorporated into the virions of two unrelated enveloped viruses. Human T cell leukemia/lymphoma virus type 1 (HTLV-1) and human cytomegalovirus (HCMV). J Immunol 1995; 155: 4376-4381.
4. Warren AP, Ducroq DH, Lehner PJ et al. Human cytomegalovirus-infected cells have unstable assembly of major histocompatibility complex class II complexes and are resistant to lysis by cytotoxic T lymphocytes. J Virol 1994; 68:2822-2829.
5. Marrack P, Kappler J. The staphylococcal enterotoxins and their relatives. Science 1990; 248:705-711.
6. Goodglick L, Zevit N, Neshat MS et al. Mapping the Ig superantigen-binding site of HIV-1 gp120. J Immunol 1995; 155: 5151-5159
7. Berberian L, Shukla J, Jefferis R et al. Effects of HIV infection on VH3 (D12 idiotope) B cells in vivo. J Acquir Immune Defic Syndr 1994; 7:641-646.
8. Berberian L, Goodglick L, Kipps TJ et al. Immunoglobulin VH3 gene products: natural ligands for HIV gp120. Science 1993; 261:1588-1591.
9. Sasso EH, Silverman GJ, Mannik M. Human IgA and IgG $F(ab')_2$ that bind to Staphylococcal proteinA belong to the VHIII subgroup. J Immunol 1991; 147: 1877-1883.
10. Kristiansen SV, Pascual V, Lipsky PE. Staphylococcal protein A biased production of Ig by VH3-expressing B lymphocytes. J Immunol 1994; 153:2974-2982.
11. Zouali M. B cell superantigens: implications for selection of the human antibody repertoire. Immunol Today 1995; 16:399-405.
12. Ohlin M, Owman H, Rioux JD et al. Restricted variable region gene usage and possible rheumatoid factor relationship among human monoclonal antibodies specific for the AD-1 epitope on cytomegalovirus glycoprotein B. Mol Immunol 1994; 31: 983-991.
13. Ikematsu H, Harindranath N, Ueki Y et al. Clonal analysis of a human antibody response. II. Sequences of the VH genes of human IgM, IgG, and IgA to rabies virus

reveal preferential utilization of VHIII segments and somatic hypermutation. J Immunol 1993; 150:1325-1337.

14. Lucas AH, Azmi FH, Mink CM et al. Age-dependent V region expression in the human atibody response to the Haemophilus influenzae type b polysaccharide. J Immunol 1993; 150:2056-2061.
15. Silverman GJ, Lucas AH. Variable region diversity in human circulating antibodies specific for the capsular polysaccharide of Haemophilus influenzae type b. Preferential usage of two types of VH3 heavy chains. J Clin Invest 1991; 88:911-920.
16. Ohlin M, Borrebaeck CAK. Characteristics of human antibody repertoires following active immune responses in vivo. Mol Immunol 1996; 13:583-592.
17. Silverman GJ, Roben P, Bouvet JP et al. Superantigen properties of a human sialoprotein involved in gut-associated immunity. J Clin Invest 1995; 96:417-426.
18. Ohlin M, Borrebaeck CAK Low affinity, antibody binding of an *Escherichia coli*-derived component. FEMS Immunol Med Microbiol 1996; 13:161-168.
19. Yang H, Leland JK, Yost D et al. Electrochemiluminescence: a new diagnostic and research tool. Bio/Technology 1994; 12:193-194.
20. Vornhagen R, Hinderer W, Sonneborn H-H et al. The DNA-binding protein pUL57 of human cytomegalovirus is a major target antigen for the immunoglobulin M antibody response during acute infection. J Clin Microbiol 1995; 33:1927-1930.
21. Kabat EA, Wu TT, Perry HM et al. Sequences of proteins of immunological interest. 5th ed. Bethesda: National Instititutes of Health, 1991.
22. van der Merwe PA, Barclay AN, Mason DW et al. Human cell-adhesion molecule CD2 binds CD58 (LFA-3) with a very low affinity and an extremely fast dissociation rate but does not bind CD48 or CD59. Biochemistry 1994; 33:10149-10160.
23. Lasky LA. Selectin-carbohydrate interactions and the initiation of the inflammatory response. Annual Rev Biochem 1995; 64: 113-139.
24. Malchiodi EL, Eisenstein E, Fields BA et al. Superantigen binding to a T cell receptor β chain of known three-dimensional structure. J Exp Med 1995; 182:1833-1845.

CHAPTER 9

Genetic Basis and Somatic Evolution of a Human Polysaccharide-Specific Antibody Repertoire

Alexander H. Lucas

INTRODUCTION

Polysaccharide (PS) capsules are common among many gram-positive and gram-negative bacterial pathogens, such as pneumococci, streptococci, staphylococci, meningococci, *Haemophilus*, *Escherichia coli*, *Pseudomonas*, and *Klebsiella*. The capsule inhibits complement binding and phagocytosis, and thereby functions as a major virulence determinant by conferring the property of invasiveness.[1-3] The surface expression of PS capsules makes them accessible to humoral attack, and indeed, antibodies (Abs) specific for capsular PS antigens play a central role in protection against invasive bacterial diseases.[1]

Because of their importance in protective immunity anti-PS Abs are of adaptive significance, and presumably, they have been subjected to strong evolutionary selection pressures. Therefore, PS-specific Ab repertoires represent a good model for studying the genetic basis of protective immune responses. In addition, Ab responses to PS Ags possess several distinctive features, such as delayed ontogenic expression, isotype restriction, and T cell-independence, that make them an attractive model for studying immune system development and regulation.

The Ab response to the caspular PS of *Haemophilus influenzae* type b (Hib) has been the subject of intense scrutiny for the past two decades. The impetus for these investigations stemmed from the desire to develop an effective pediatric vaccine against Hib, which causes meningitis, epiglottitis, and

Human B Cell Superantigens, edited by Moncef Zouali. © 1996 R.G. Landes Company.

other serious invasive diseases. Efforts focused upon the Hib capsular PS as a potential vaccine since the protective function of these Abs had been firmly established.[2-5] The PS could be isolated in relatively pure form and was chemically well-defined, consisting of repeating units of 3-β-D-ribose-(1-1)-ribitol-5-phosphate. The purified PS was found to be a poor immunogen in infants, a finding which necessitated the development of alternate vaccine strategies.[6,7] Based upon the early work of Goebel, Avery and their colleagues,[8,9] protein conjugated forms of the Hib PS were developed, and these so-called conjugate vaccines were shown to be capable of inducing protective anti-Hib PS Ab responses in infants.[10-13] A dramatic decline in invasive Hib disease has occurred since the use of Hib PS-protein conjugates for the routine vaccination of infants.[14] Thus, the development of Hib conjugates represent a major advance in pediatric vaccination, and the strategy of coupling carrier proteins to increase PS immunogenicity is being applied to other encapsulated bacterial pathogens.[15,16]

During these vaccine investigations it became apparent that the Hib model provided an opportunity to dissect at the molecular level a human anti-PS Ab response. Initial studies demonstrated the oligoclonal nature of the serum anti-Hib PS Ab population[17,18] and the expression of cross-reactive idiotypes (Ids),[19] findings indicating that the repertoire may be of limited heterogeneity and tractable to molecular definition. This has proven to be true. At present, the Hib PS model represents one of the best characterized human Ab repertoires to a foreign Ag.

Table 9.1. V region gene segments used by anti-Hib PS antibodies§

H Chain:	V_HIIIa	VH26; DP77
	V_HIIIb	LSG6.1; LSG12.1 (9.1)
L Chain:	VκI	08/018; L11; O12
	VκII	A2; A1/A17; A3
	VκIII	A27; L16
	VκIV	B3
	VλII	2.1
	VλIII	3.1
	VλVII	4A

§Compiled from refs. 20-29. Includes V regions identified by partial amino acid sequence analysis of clonally purified serum Abs and by nucleotide sequence analysis of hybridoma cDNA.

GENETIC BASIS OF THE ANTI-HIB PS REPERTOIRE

Definition of the variable (V) gene elements used in the human Hib PS repertoire has been accomplished by determining partial amino acid sequences of clonally purified serum Abs[20-22] and by determining nucleotide sequences of hybridoma cDNA.[23-29] Table 9.1 lists the V_H and V_L segments used by anti-Hib PS Abs. V_H regions are derived from a small set of closely related genes from the V_HIIIa and V_HIIIb families. V_L usage is more complex with as many as 12 distinct V_κ and V_λ gene segments contributing to the repertoire. V_L regions derived from the same V gene segment pair with different VH regions. For example, the A2 and the λ2.1 V_L regions can pair with either the VH26 or the LSG6.1 V_H region (Table 9.2). Forty-eight V_H-V_L combinations can be assembled from the random assortment of these V_H and V_L gene segments. Thus, potential diversity is considerable, but as discussed below the expressed repertoire appears to be dominated by only a few H-L combinations.

Sequence analyses of Hib PS-specific hybridoma cDNA has provided information concerning D/J usage, H-L chain pairing and the extent of somatic mutation. Table 9.2 summarizes the V regions of 21 Hib PS-specific hybridomas. Eight hybridomas use the V_H26 gene segment, one uses the DP77 V_H gene and the remainder use either the LSG6.1 or LSG12.1 genes which are close relatives of the 9.1 V_H gene.[26] In the absence of germline sequence information from each donor, the definitive assignment of germline counterparts and the estimate of somatic mutation can be problematic since the observed deviation from the candidate germline gene could be due to germline-encoded polymorphisms or to the existence of other V gene segments. Nonetheless, it is likely that the actual germline gene has been identified in many cases as shown by the high degree of similarity between the sequences of the hybridoma V_H gene segment and the candidate germline gene (Table 9.2), and therefore, reasonable estimates of somatic mutation can be made.

Some anti-Hib PS monoclonal Abs use V_H genes in near germline configuration. For example, the hybribomas ED8.4 and CB6 use a V_H26 gene segment that has 98% overall identity with the germline sequence, and hybridomas SB5/D6 and RAY4 use V_H genes that are 99% and 98% identical, respectively, to the LSG6.1 germline gene segment (Table 9.2). Other V_H segments appear to be mutated versions of the assigned germline gene, and replacement to silent ratios exceeding 9:1 in complementarity-determining regions (CDRs) have been observed. Diversity is present in V_H CDR-3 as shown by the variation in the length of the D region and in the usage of five J_H genes. The recurrence of the same D-J junctional residues in independently-derived hybridomas suggests that particular CDR-3 configurations may be favored.

V_L usage is more complex than V_H usage. Twelve V_L gene segments can encode anti-Hib PS Abs, and they derive from both κ and λ loci (Table 9.1). Several of the V_L genes identified by partial amino acid sequencing of purified serum Abs, e.g., κI-08, κII-A1/A17, and κIV-B3, have

Table 9.2. Anti-Hib PS hybridomas and their V regions†

Hybridoma	[H isotype]	V_H V	V_H [%]§	V_H D (bp)	V_H J	V_L V	V_L [%]¶	V_L J
ED8.4	[M]	IIIa-VH26	98	1	6	κII-A2	100	
D3F3	[M]	IIIa-VH26	91	3	6	κII-A2	96	
Gar6E8	[G4]	IIIa-VH26	93	3	6	κII-A2	96	
Ann2	[A1]	IIIa-VH26	96	1	4	κII-A2	98	κ1
16M3C8	[G2]	IIIa-VH26	85	34	4b	λII-2.1	89	
CB6	[A]	IIIa-VH26	98	1	6	NK*		
SD15	[A2]	IIIa-VH26	90	1	6	NK		
Ann6	[A]	IIIa-VH26	94	1	4	NK		
CA4	[G2]	IIIa-DP77	96	39	4b	κIII-A27	94	κ1
LSF2	[A1]	IIIb-LSG6.1	94	3	4	λVII-4A	89	λ2/3
SB5/D6	[A1]	IIIb-LSG6.1	99	10	4	λVII-4A	90	λ2/3
RAY4	[A2]	IIIb-LSG6.1	98	10	4	λVII-4A	90	λ2/3
JB32	[A1]	IIIb-LSG6.1	94	14	5a	λVII-4A	88	λ2/3
CB20	[A2]	IIIb-LSG6.1	95	28	1	λIII-3.1		
JB21	[G2]	IIIb-LSG6.1	94	14	5a	λII-2.1	91	
RC3	[A]	IIIb-LSG6.1	94	3	4	κII-A2	100	κ3
ED6.1	[G2]	IIIb-LSG12.1	93	18	4	κI-012	95	κ4
SB1/D8	[G1]	IIIb-LSG12.1	94	34	3	NK		
BA3	[G2]	IIIb-9.1	78	24	4	κI-L11	95	
SC6	[A2]	IIIb-9.1	85	33	4	κII-A3	97	
LD21	[A2]	NK				κIII-L16		

†Compiled from refs. 23-29.
§% overall identity to candidate germline VH gene segment
¶% overall identity to candidate germline VL gene segment
*Not known

not yet been found in hybridomas (Tables 9.1 and 9.2). Of the 17 hybridomas where V_L usage has been defined, 10 use V_κ genes and 7 use V_λ genes. This κ/λ ratio differs with what is seen from analysis of serum Abs where κ Abs predominate. These findings raise the possibility that the B cells contributing to the serum may comprise a population that is distinct from those clones which enter the peripheral circulation following vaccination and which are immortalized as hybridomas.

V_κ genes are expressed in association with 4 J_κ regions and V_λ genes recombine with either $J_\lambda2$ or $J_\lambda3$ (Tables 9.2 and 9.3). Interestingly, an arginine occurs at the V-J junction (residue 95a) in 18 of 20 monoclonal anti-Hib PS Abs (Table 9.3).[21,24] The recurrence of this junctional arginine in Abs using different V_L gene segments suggests that it serves an important role in Hib PS binding. A similarly placed arginine occurs in murine anti-phenylarsonate Abs and is essential for hapten binding activity.[30] Preliminary evidence from chain recombination experiments suggests that the presence of an arginine and its precise location at position 95a are critical determinants of Hib PS binding since a V_L region lacking an insertional residue at 95a but having an arginine at position 96 does not form a Hib PS-specific combining site (D. Reason and A. Lucas, unpublished observation). The positively charged arginine may bond to the negatively charged phosphate residues of Hib PS and serve to anchor the epitope at the base of the combining site. The majority of junctional arginine residues which occur in anti-Hib PS Abs at position 95a cannot be accounted for by alternative recombination between bases at the 3' end of V of the 5' end of J but rather must result from addition of nontemplated nucleotides or from mutation.

Initial results from partial amino acid sequence analyses of serum anti-Hib PS Abs indicated that the extent of V_L somatic hypermutation may vary depending upon the particular V_L gene.[22] The κII-A2 V region, which comprises the most common V_L region in the serum repertoire (see below) was expressed in germline form, whereas non-A2 V_L regions Abs appeared to have acquired mutations. This pattern may not be uniform however, since as more sequences have become available it appears that the A2 V region may undergo mutation and that non-A2 V genes such as O12 and A3 may be expressed in near germline configuration (Table 9.2).

Based upon patterns of D region usage, Adderson and colleagues[25] and more recently Pinchuk and colleagues[29] have suggested that Hib PS Abs may derive from two distinct B cell lineages: the $CD5^+$ (B-1B) subset characteristic of fetal or neonatal repertoires that have short D segments with a paucity of N-region additions, and adult-like $CD5^-$ B cells that typically have longer D regions. Furthermore, from their examination of hybridoma V gene usage, Pinchuk et al observed two predominant configurations: fetal-like Abs with short D regions that use the V_HIIIa-26 gene segment, J_H6 and the A2 Vκ gene segment, and adult-like Abs with longer D regions that use V_HIIIb genes, J_H4 and non-A2 VL gene segments (Table 9.3). Although not absolute, these configurations are nonetheless striking, and they may determine paratope geometry and epitope specificity (see below).

As shown in Table 9.4, the V_H genes and many of the V_L genes used by anti-Hib PS Abs are also used by Abs reactive with both foreign PS and protein Ags as well as self carbohydrate, nucleic acid and protein Ags. As with Hib PS Abs, self-reactive Abs may use both mutated and nonmutated copies of germline genes. The recurrent utilization of closely related V gene segments amongst Abs of disparate specificities points to the importance of combinatorial diversity and chain pairing in generating Ab diversity.[62]

SPECIFICITY

Two fine-specificity patterns have been observed with Hib PS Abs: reactivity with the structurally related capsular PS of *E. coli* K100 (3-β-D-ribose-(1-2)-ribitol-5-phosphate),[63] and reactivity with DNA.[25] Usage of the λVII-4A V region and possibly some κIII V regions appears to correlate

Table 9.3. V_L junctions of anti-Hib PS antibodies§

Ab	Source ¶		89	90	91	92	93	94	95	95A	J
		κA2	M	Q	S	I	Q	L	P		
DG1	S		-	-	-	-	-	-	-	R	κ1
WG1-II	S		-	-	-	-	-	-	-	R	κ3
DG2b	S		-	-	-	-	-	-	-	R	κ1
C-G1	S		-	-	-	-	-	-	-	R	κ1
B-G1	S		-	-	-	-	-	-	-	R	κ1
B-G2a	S		-	-	-	-	-	-	-	R	κ2
E-G1	S		-	-	-	-	-	-	-	R	κ1
A-E1	S		-	-	-	-	-	-	-	R	κ1
RC3	H		-	-	-	-	-	-	-	R	κ3
ED8	H		-	-	-	-	-	-	-	R	κ4
		λ2.1	S	Y	A	G	S	S	T		
JB21	H		-	-	T	T	-	T	V	R	λ2/3
16M3C8	H		-	-	R	S	D	T	-	R	λ2/3
		λ4A	L	L	Y	Y	G	G	A		
RAY4	H		-	-	S	-	S	-	-	R	λ2/3
SB5/D6	H		-	-	S	-	S	-	-	R	λ2/3
LSF2	H		-	-	S	-	T	-	-	R	λ2/3
JB32	H		-	-	S	-	S	A		R	λ2/3
		κA27	Q	Q	Y	G	S	S	P		
CA4	H		-	-	-	-	-	-	-	P	κ1
		κO12	Q	Q	S	Y	S	T	P		
ED6.1	H		-	-	-	-	T	L	-		κ4

§Compiled from refs. 20-28.
¶Ab derived from serum (S) or hybridoma(H).

Table 9.4. The V gene segments used by anti-Hib PS Abs are used by other Abs reactive with foreign and self antigens*

Gene segment	Foreign	Self
V_HIII-9.1	Hib PS;[23,25] MenB PS[31]	DNA;[32] Sm ribonucleoprotein[33]
V_HIII-26	Hib PS;[23] α-galactosyl;[34] *Cryptococcus neoformans* PS;[38] HSV;[41] streptococcal M protein[39]	DNA;[35] myelin;[36] thyroglobulin;[37] cardiac myosin;[39] IgG; [40] thyrotropin receptor[42]
VκI-O12	Hib PS;[24,31] MenB PS[31]	rbc i oligosaccharide;[43] thyroid peroxidase[44]
VkII-A3	Hib PS[29]	thyroid peroxidase;[44] cardiolipin;[45] ssDNA[45]
VκIII-A27 (kv325)	Hib PS;[20,28] CMV;[46] HIV gp120;[47] lipid A;[54] Rh(D)[55]	DNA;[48] LDL;[49] IgG;[50,51] polyreactive;[52] insulin[53]
VκIII-L16 (kv328)	Hib PS[20]	rbc I oligosaccharide;[43] IgG;[56] insulin[57]
VλII-2.1	Hib PS[24]	rbc i oligosaccharide;[58] DNA;[59] hepatitis A;[60] GM1 ganglioside[61]

*Abbreviations: MenB, *Neisseria meningitidis* Group B ; HSV, herpes simplex virus; CMV, cytomegalovirus; LDL, low-density lipoprotein; HIV, human immunodeficiency virus; rbc, red blood cell;

with K100 reactivity. This observation when taken with the finding that a limited number of V_H regions may pair with several different V_L regions to generate Hib PS-specific paratopes, has led to the suggestion that the V_H region may play a dominant role in determining Hib PS binding whereas the V_L region may determine fine-specificity. Similar associations between V_L usage and fine specificity have been observed with Abs to other carbohydrate determinants such as bacterial levan[64] and red blood cell N-acetyl-lactosamine I/i Ags.[43]

The Hib PS-specific hybridomas, Ann2 and CB20 (Table 9.2), react with single-stranded DNA, double-stranded DNA and polynucleotides, but this binding appears to be of low affinity.[25] The similarity in charge distribution between the phosphodiester groups in Hib PS and DNA may contribute to this cross-reactivity as has been suggested for other Abs cross-reactive with anionic structures such as bacterial polysaccharides, DNA and phospholipids.[65] The molecular basis of this cross-reactivity is not readily apparent as Ann2 and CB20 use different V_H gene segments, D regions and V_L genes (Table 9.2).

Kabat and colleagues have distinguished two types of anti-carbohydrate combining site geometries based upon immunochemical analyses: cavity-type which accommodate terminal, nonreducing epitopes, and groove-type which lie across the length of the polymer and recognize internal epitopes.[66,67] Modeling studies of several anti-carbohydrate Ab specificities suggest that cavity-type sites have long H chain CDR3 and that groove-type sites have short H chain CDR3.[68,69] If Hib PS Abs follow this general rule then the two gene configurations discussed above should correlate with paratope type: V_HIIIa-A2 Abs with short D regions will have groove sites which recognize an internal Hib PS epitope, and V_HIIIb-non-A2 Abs with long D regions will have cavity sites which recognize a terminal Hib PS epitope. Experiments performed by Nahm and colleagues examining the reactivities of clonal Abs with Hib PS ligands varying in size agree with this model.[70]

AGE-RELATED V EXPRESSION

Sequence analysis of V region usage in the infant has not been possible since the techniques applicable to the adult repertoire, namely purification of serum Abs and construction of hybridomas, are not easily performed with infants. However, the use of anti-Id reagents of defined specificity provides a means to study V_L expression in early ontogeny. Furthermore, unlike hybridoma technology and serum purification schemes which are necessarily limited in scope, Id analyses permit the evaluation of V region expression in large populations, defined by age or vaccine type. Two anti-Hib PS associated Ids have been defined: HibId-1 which is a marker for the κII-A2 V region[71,72] and HibId-2, which is a marker for a subset of Abs using the λVII-4A V region.[73] HibId-1 and HibId-2 expression were examined in three age groups, 2-month-old infants, 18-month-olds and adults, following vaccination with the conjugate vaccine consisting of Hib PS coupled to the outer membrane complex of *Neisseria meningitidis* (Hib PS-OMPC).[74] Hib PS-OMPC vaccine was used in this study because unlike the other Hib conjugates, it is uniquely capable of stimulating serum Ab responses after a single injection at 2 months of age, thus permitting examination of the primary repertoire.[75,76] Also in this study, κIII anti-Hib PS Abs were monitored using a monoclonal Ab specific for this κ subgroup.[77]

Figure 9.1 shows the distribution of HibId-1, HibId-2 and κIII Hib PS-specific Abs in these three age groups. HibId-1 Abs are prevalent in all age groups and comprise a substantial proportion of the total serum Ab. HibId-2 Abs are expressed in 2 month-olds at a frequency similar to HibId-1, minimally represented in 18 months-olds, and undetectable in adults. The κIII component of the serum anti-Hib PS response shows a pattern inverse to that seen with HibId-2 Abs; They are undetectable in 2 month-olds, slightly represented in 18

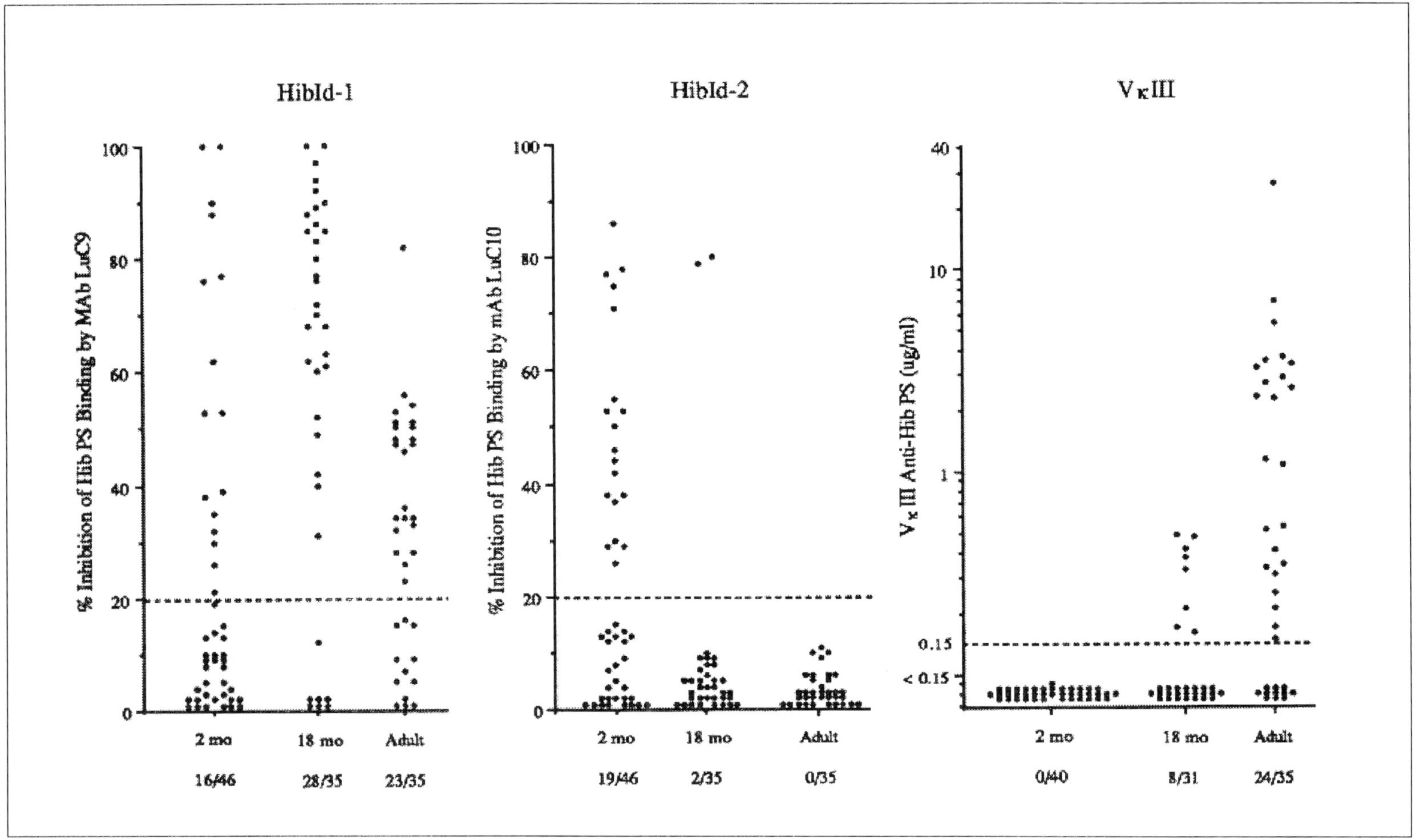

Fig. 9.1. Age-related V region expression in the serum Ab response elicited by Hib PS-OMPC vaccine. Each circle represents the result for a single responder subject selected based on the presence of ≥ 0.9 μg/ml anti-Hib PS Ab. (Reprinted with permission from Lucas AH et al. J Immunol 1993; 150: 2056-2061. ©1993 by The American Association of Immunologists.)

month-olds, but readily detectable in adults. These results show that the relative contributions of κIII and λVII-4A V regions to the serum Hib PS repertoire vary as a consequence of age, whereas Abs using the κII-A2 gene are prevalent in both the adult repertoire and in the infant primary repertoire.

V_H expression by Hib PS-specific Abs has not been examined in infants, but other studies have shown that the V_H26, 9.1 and DP77 gene segments are rearranged and expressed in fetal and perinatal life.[78-80] Therefore, V_H gene expression in the infant probably does not differ substantially from the adult. Infant Abs could have short H CDR3 regions since fetal and neonatal repertoires have shorter D regions and limited N-region nucleotide additions as compared to adult repertoires.[81,82] This potential difference could be magnified if $CD5^+$ B cells, which purportedly have fewer N sequences than conventional B cells, are more preponderant in infants than in adults. However, N-region additions can be present as early as 130 days of gestation in the human,[79] and adult Hib PS-specific hybridomas have both short and long D regions, suggesting that presence of infant-(or $CD5^+$) and adult-like configurations.

OLIGOCLONALITY AND PREDOMINANCE OF κII-A2 ABS

Despite the potential to assemble a large repertoire by pairing numerous V_L regions with a smaller set of V_H regions, the Hib PS-specific serum Ab population appears to be highly restricted. Isoelectric focusing analyses have shown that the response is oligoclonal; only a few distinct spectrotypes are present and unrelated individuals frequently share similar spectrotypes.[17,18] Remarkably, in many individuals the Hib PS-specific Ab population appears to be monoclonal. Id analyses are consistent with these findings. Table 9.5 shows the representation of serum anti-Hib PS Abs using the A2 V region (HibId-1 positive) in children and adults following vaccination with either Hib PS or Hib PS-diphtheria toxoid conjugate.[72] A2 Abs are prevalent in these populations, and they comprise 55% to nearly 70% of the total serum anti-Hib PS Ab. Thus, Abs using a single V_κ gene segment dominate the serum Ab repertoire. Interestingly, the representation of A2 Abs did not differ significantly between vaccine groups, in that both plain PS as well as diphtheria toxoid-conjugated PS elicited similar distributions of HibId-1 Abs. This finding contrasts with what is seen in infants where different molecular forms of

Table 9.5. Expression of HibId-1 (κII-A2) serum anti-Hib PS Abs following vaccination[§]

Vaccine	Age Group years	No. of Subjects	HibId-1 (κII-A2) Abs[¶] Mean % of total anti-Hib PS (range)	% of subjects positive for
Hib PS-DT*	1.4- 2.1	47	58 (1- 97)	75
Hib PS-DT	21- 45	25	69 (12-95)	96
Hib PS	1.7- 6.3	22	56 (1- 90)	82
Hib PS	13- 57	66	54 (1- 92)	86

[§]Data adapted from ref. 72.

[¶]A2 anti-Hib PS Abs were measured in post-vaccination sera using the A2-specific anti-Id LuC9. Percentage of total Ab expressing A2 was determined by measuring the extent to which LuC9 inhibited ^{125}I-Hib PS binding. A subject was scored aspositive for A2 Abs if ≥20% of serum Hib PS binding could be inhibited by LuC9.

*Hib PS DT: Hib PS coupled to diphtheria toxoid.

Hib PS induce markedly distinct patterns of Hibld-1 expression (see below).

Hibld-1 Abs also are prevalent among so-called natural Abs which are presumably induced by Hib or Hib PS-cross reactive Ags. Hibld-1 is expressed on average by approximately 50% of natural Abs as determined by analysis of normal sera[71,72] and of intravenous gamma globulin preparations (A. Lucas, unpublished observation).

IMMUNOGEN STRUCTURE AFFECTS V REGION EXPRESSION AND AB FUNCTION

Several different Hib conjugate vaccines have been developed. They differ in the size of the Hib PS moiety, the type of carrier protein and in the nature of the chemical linkage between the PS and protein components.[15,83] These structural differences confer different immunological properties to these vaccines (see ref. 16 for review). For example, the Hib PS-OMPC vaccine stimulates Hib PS-specific Ab production after a single injection at 2 months of age, whereas a conjugate consisting of Hib PS oligomers coupled to a nontoxic mutant diphtheria toxin (Oligo-CRM) requires 2 or 3 injections at intervals of 2 months to generate detectable serum Ab responses.[76]

The molecular form of the Hib PS immunogen affects not only immunogenicity but also the functional quality of the Ab response. Schlesinger et al demonstrated that in infants Oligo-CRM vaccination induces higher avidity serum Abs than does vaccination with Hib PS-OMPC.[84] VL expression also is influenced by vaccine type (Table 9.6).[73] Following three injections of Hib PS-OMPC, Hibld-1 and Hibld-2 Abs were expressed in similar frequency, and both Ids comprised a substantial portion of the serum Ab. In contrast, vaccination with Oligo-CRM induced a serum Ab response dominated by Hibld-1 and with a lower representation of Hibld-2. To examine the relationship between V_L usage and Ab function, IgG1 Id-defined fractions were prepared from post-vaccination serum pools made from sera of infants vaccinated with either Oligo-CRM or Hib PS-OMPC.[85] Table 9.7 summarizes the avidities and bactericidal activities of these Ab fractions. Analysis of the starting serum pools showed that HbOC vaccination induced 3-fold higher net serum avidity Abs than did OMPC, a result confirming previous observations of individual serum samples. Of the Abs induced by HbOC vaccination, the Hibld-1 population had the highest avidity for Hib PS and higher bactericidal activity against Hib organisms. Hib PS-OMPC vaccination elicited Hibld-1 Abs that were functionally equivalent to Hibld-0 Abs (those Abs expressing neither Hibld-1 nor Hibld-2), but were more avid and bactericidal than the Hibld-2 population. Interestingly, the Hibld-1 Abs induced by HbOC were significantly more functionally active than the Hibld-1 population induced by Hib PS-OMPC.

These findings show that the Oligo-CRM vaccine elicits a serum response predominated by high avidity Hibld-1 Abs, whereas Hib PS-OMPC vaccine elicits more heterogeneous V_L expression and lower avidity Abs. Furthermore, usage of the A2 V region (Hibld-1) *per se* does not confer uniformly high affinity or optimum functional activity. Apparently, Hib conjugate vaccines differ in their capacity to either select or promote the development of high affinity Hib PS-specific B cells expressing the A2 V region.

POSSIBLE MECHANISMS OF V_H RESTRICTION

A notable characteristic of the Hib PS repertoire is the restricted usage of a small number of closely related genes from the V_H3 family. This feature is not unique to Hib PS-specific Abs. The V_H3 family appears to be prominent in human Abs reactive with foreign Ags and self Ags, as well as in some B cell malignancies (see ref. 86 for review). One V_H3 gene, variably known as V_H26, DP-47, V3-21, 30p1 and 18/2, is not only highly represented among Hib PS-specific Abs but is the most commonly expressed V_H gene in the human peripheral repertoire.[87,88] Remarkably, the V_H26 gene comprises one fourth of the 500 V_H3 genes in the data base of rearranged genes, although this exceptionally high frequency could be due in part to methodological

Table 9.6. Effect of vaccine formulation on Id expression after vaccination of infants at 2, 4, and 6 months of age[§]

			Serum cross-reactive Id expression[¶]			
			HibId-1		HibId-2	
Vaccine	**No. of subjects**	**Geo. mean serum anti-Hib PS (μg/ml)**	**% of subjects positive for**	**Mean % of total anti-Hib PS ± SD**	**% of subjects positive for**	**Mean % of total anti-Hib PS ± SD**
Hib PS-OMPC	43	10.3	33	63 ± 22	47	47 ± 17
Oligo-CRM	68	10.8	68	55 ± 22	18	44 ± 22

[§]Data adapted from ref. 73.

[¶]Serum was obtained one month after the third vaccination. HibId-1 and HibId-2 were measured using LuC9 and LuC10 anti-Id Abs, respectively. Percentage of total serum Ab expressing HibId-1 and HibId-2 were determined by measuring the extent to which the respective anti-Id inhibited ^{125}I-Hib PS binding. A subject was scored Id positive if > 20% of serum Hib PS binding could be inhibited by anti-Id.

Table 9.7. Relationship between idiotype expression, anti-Hib PS avidity and bactericidal activity[§]

	Mean Avidity ± SE (nM^{-1})			Mean Bactericidal Activity[¶] ± SE, μg/ml		
Sample	**Oligo-CRM**	**Hib PS-OMPC**	**P***	**Oligo-CRM**	**Hib PS-OMPC**	**P**
Serum Pool	3.24 ± .16	1.10 ± .15	< 0.01	not done	not done	
HibId-1	4.36 ± .21	2.07 ± .17	< 0.01	0.02 ± .02	0.27 ± .03	< 0.002
HibId-2	1.49 ± .03	1.26 ± .11	> 0.10	0.38 ± .03	0.62 ± .12	> 0.10
HibId-0	2.58 ± .22	2.17 ± .34	> 0.10	0.12 ± .00	0.28 ± .05	≤ 0.06

[§]Data adapted from ref. 85. Idiotypically-defined IgG1 fractions were isolated from two post-vaccination pools prepared from serum samples of infants vaccinated with Oligo-CRM at 2, 4 and 6 months of age, or Hib PS-OMPC at 2 and 4, or 2, 4, and 6 months of age.

[¶]Anti-Hib PS concentration killing 50% of Hib organisms in the presence of 20% agammaglobulinemic serum as a complement source.

*Significance testing by t test.

biases.[89] The recurrent usage of particular V_H3 genes in the Hib PS repertoire therefore may represent a specific case of a general phenomenon.

The mechanisms that may account for the biased expression of V_H3 genes in the Hib PS repertoire might operate during Ig gene rearrangement and assembly of the primary repertoire. Over-expression of V_H3 genes and of V_H26 in particular could be related to abundance in the genome. V_H3 is the largest V_H family and multiple copies of V_H26 can be present in the germline.[89-91] Biased V_H expression may also be mediated by other attributes that could vary between genes such as chromosomal position and the presence of regulatory elements like promoters, enhancers or recombination sites.[86] The selective expression of V_H3 family members in the fetal repertoire suggests that skewed V_H expression is established early in development. These types of mechanisms could restrict gene usage prior to antigenic exposure and limit the available number of V_H regions with which to assemble the Hib PS repertoire.

Selective processes involving either conventional Ag or super-Ag (SAg) recognition could also be involved in V_H3 restriction. B cell SAgs such as Staphylococcal protein A interact selectively with V_H3 domains outside the conventional Ag binding site.[92] Thus, it is conceivable that restriction of Hib PS Abs to the V_H3 family could result from Hib PS functioning as a SAg.[93] However, a number of observations indicate that Ab recognition of Hib PS occurs by means of conventional Ag binding.[94] Hib PS-specific Abs use only a few particular V_H3 genes, whereas SAg would be expected to induce Abs using a variety of genes from the V_H3 family. SAgs such as protein A bind with high frequency to IgM macroglobulins having V_H3 regions whereas Hib PS does not (A. Lucas and F. Azmi, unpublished observations). The pattern of V_L gene usage, the recurrence of junctional arginine at V_L-J_L joints and the presence of configurations that resemble groove- and cavity-type binding sites are all features which point to conventional Ag recognition. Thus, while Hib PS itself probably does not function as a B cell SAg, it is possible that B cell SAgs from exogenous sources such as bacteria colonizing the gut or other mucosal surfaces or possibly endogenous SAgs could shape the early repertoire by activating V_H3 B cells in a nonclonally restricted manner and thereby bias the primary repertoire to V_H3 expression.

Another possible explanation for V_H restriction is due to structural constraints of Hib PS-specific paratopes. In this case, the primary repertoire could be diverse and include representatives from each of the V_H families, but only a few of these V_H regions have the potential when paired with an appropriate V_L region, to form Hib PS-specific binding sites of sufficient affinity to be selectable by Ag. The notion that certain V_H regions may be predisposed to forming particular binding sites is consistent with the observations of Chothia and colleagues showing that the number of main chain conformations generated from the hypervariable loops of the V_H region may be limited in number and comprise a small number of canonical structures.[95] Furthermore, Kirkham et al have proposed that V_H3 members have evolutionary conserved subdomain structures that could constrain the repertoire of Ags they recognize.[96] The validity of this proposition could be questioned by the finding that the V_H genes used in Hib PS Abs are also used by a plethora of Ab specificities, and it is unlikely that a common structural theme is shared by all the antigenic structures recognized by V_H3 domains. The fact that particular V_H3 gene segments in unmutated form are highly represented amongst Abs of different specificities underscores the importance of combinatorial diversity and chain pairing in generating Ab diversity.

V_L RESTRICTION AND CLONAL DOMINANCE

The pattern of V_L gene usage in the Hib PS repertoire contrasts to what is seen with V_H gene usage in that as many as 12 distinct V_L gene segments are utilized to assemble the repertoire. Thus, at the population level genetic restriction is not apparent. However, at the individual level the serum repertoire is pauciclonal and skewed towards the expression of only a few V_H-V_L combinations, exemplified by the predominance of Abs using a single V_κ gene segment, κII-A2. Two observations point to the likelihood that V_L restriction and oligoclonality are acquired during the development of the repertoire and result from selective events. First, although the A2 V_L region predominates the Ab repertoire from about 18 months of age through adulthood, its frequency of expression at 2 months of age following vaccination with the OMPC conjugate is similar to HibId-2 (λVII) and HibId-0 Abs. Therefore, the primary V_L repertoire appears heterogeneous and not intrinsically biased towards HibId-1 precursors. Second, different molecular forms of Hib PS stimulate markedly different frequencies of HibId-1 and HibId-2 Abs in infants, a result demonstrating that V_L expression can be influenced directly by the quality of the antigenic stimulus. This latter observation is reminiscent of studies which show that in mice one of 3 V_L regions may associate with a single V_H region to form anti-phosphorylcholine (PC) Abs.[97] Determination of which V_L region is used depends upon whether the PC epitope is presented in the context of the bacterial surface or as a hapten conjugated to a foreign carrier protein.[98]

Despite the potential to produce anti-Hib PS Abs with different V_L regions in infancy, the representation of A2 in both vaccine-induced and naturally-acquired Ab populations, increases as a consequence of aging. Clonal competition involving affinity selection might be involved in this process. If A2 B cells had higher affinity for Hib PS than non-A2 Abs, they could more effectively compete for Ag and thereby be selectively stimulated and expanded. This mechanism has been proposed to account for the dominance of T15 Id positive Abs in the murine anti-phosphorylcholine (PC) repertoire.[99-101] However, the A2 Abs induced in infants by Hib PS-OMPC vaccination do not have higher avidity than HibId-0 Abs. Furthermore, the ability of HbOC vaccination to induce A2 Abs with higher avidity and biological activity than HibId-1 Abs induced by OMPC suggests that immunogen structure rather than the A2 V region per se determines Ab quality. These findings raise doubts that affinity-based clonal competition can account for the predominance of A2 Abs, although it is possible that the determination of avidity is imprecise and does not provide an accurate measure of intrinsic affinity or of binding kinetics which may be more relevant in clonal competition and response maturation.[102]

Epitope-specific selection is another process that could drive the natural progression towards A2 dominance. Hib PS is likely to have both internal and terminal epitopes. If we assume that A2 Abs have groove-type sites which react with an internal epitope and non-A2 Abs react with terminal epitopes, then A2 Abs could be selectively stimulated if the Ags driving repertoire maturation contain a preponderance of linear epitopes. An implication of this proposition is that bacteria such as *E. coli* K100 which have a capsular PS antigenically cross-reactive with Hib PS would not play a major role in A2 dominance of the serum repertoire since K100-reactive Abs do not utilize the A2 VL region. The environmental Ags that stimulate natural Ab production would be expected to resemble, at least antigenically, the HbOC conjugate vaccine which selectively stimulates A2 Abs in infants. An association could exist between V region usage, antigenic fine-specificity and B cell subset. A2 Abs might arise from the $CD5^+$ subset, and this subset may be selectively activated by environmental Ags (or by HbOC vaccine). Dominance of A2 Abs would result from the selective clonal expansion of $CD5^+$ B cells driven by chronic exposure to environmental Ags. The self-renewing capacity of the $CD5^+$ population may further contribute to the over-representation of A2 Abs. Precedent for this type of phenomenon has been shown by Rittenberg and colleagues in their studies of the ontogeny of PC-specific B cells.[98] The Ab response to environmental forms of PC stimulates a B cell population (Group I) distinct from that stimulated by PC-protein conjugates (Group II). Group I B cells dominate the adult repertoire whereas Group I and Group II B cells are equally represented in neonatal mice. They suggest that fine specificity rather than avidity or V gene usage regulate the ontogeny of the PC repertoire. Analogously in the Hib PS model, A2 Abs would derive from Group I B cells (groove-type sites) and be stimulated by environmental Ags and by HbOC vaccine. Group II B cells would secrete non-A2 Abs (cavity type sites) and would be stimulated by Ags resembling the OMPC conjugate vaccine.

It is important to note that while Abs using the A2 V_L region comprise 50% to 60% of the serum population, the remaining 40 to 50% of the repertoire at the population level is encoded by as many as 11 V_L gene segments. At the individual level however, the non-A2 population is not heterogeneous but pauciclonal, indicating that non-A2 Abs also can be clonally dominant. One explanation for this phenomenon is that the precursor frequencies of Hib PS-specific B cells expressing non-A2 V_L genes are low, resulting in limited clonal expression of any one particular V_L gene in individual repertoires. Once a particular V_H-V_L pair is expressed in the primary repertoire, becomes selected by Ag and perhaps refined by hypermutation, this clone effectively out competes any other non-A2 Abs that may arise. Clonal depletion by means of somatic hypermutation may also influence clonal representation of non-A2 Abs.[103] The primary repertoire could be clonally heterogeneous, with a variety of V_L genes contributing to the Hib PS-specific precursor pool. Following Ag stimulation and V gene mutation, the majority lose reactivity to Hib PS, and only those mutated clones that retain Hib PS reactivity are able to contribute to the memory response. This proposal would explain why most non-A2 Abs appear to be mutated variants of germline genes.

Id recognition is a type of intrinsic selection that could bias the repertoire toward expression of particular V regions. B cell based Id interactions have been shown to influence the hierarchical expression of particular Ab specificities in the murine neonatal repertoire, and anti-Id B cells and T cells have been implicated in establishing the clonal dominance of the PC repertoire by Abs with the T15 Id (see ref. 104 for review). One could envision that Id interactions play a similar role in regulating A2 dominance. Since the primary repertoire appears not to be biased towards A2 expression, Id selection probably does not operate at the precursor cell level but more likely exerts its effect at a later stage of development (and response maturation) when A2 dominance becomes apparent. One 'Id' recognition mechanism that seems plausible in promoting A2 dominance involves the participation of T cells specific for peptides derived from the A2 V region.[105,106] In this scheme, B cells activated by Hib PS or cross-reactive Ags would endocytose the Ag-Ab complex and subsequently present A2-derived peptides on the cell surface in the context of major histocompatibility complex (MHC) class II molecules. T cells specific for these V region-derived peptides (VRDP) could then be clonally expanded and mediate direct helper effects on A2 B cells. This process also could occur at the level of professional Ag-presenting cells. Hib PS-Ab complexes generated following the primary response could be endocytosed by Ag-presenting cells and the resulting class II-A2 peptide complexes on the cell surface could then sensitize the T cell population. Whatever the pathway of induction, the resulting A2 peptide-specific T cells would selectively promote the clonal expansion of the A2 B cell population and contribute to their clonal dominance. Thus, A2-VRDPs would be treated by T cells as non-self Ags, a proposal which seems reasonable since their concentration (in association with MHC II) in the naive repertoire would be too low to result in their functioning as tolerizing self Ags. This type of 'Id' regulation does not involve the paradox of Ab-based Id network theories, namely that the destructive effector function of Abs (anti-Ids) cannot be disjoined from their nondestructive regulator function. The effector function of the VRDP-specific T cell would be to provide helper signals. Cytotoxic T cells, i.e. destructive effectors, would not be induced because VRDPs, owing to their generation through processing via the endocytotic pathway, would fail to associate with MHC class I molecules.

SOMATIC MUTATION

Studies of murine anti-hapten responses have demonstrated two general patterns of repertoire modification during progression from primary to secondary Ab responses: hypermutation and shifts in V region usage.[107] Sequence analyses of serum Abs and hybridomas have clearly established that somatic hypermutation can occur in anti-Hib PS Abs, although the extent of mutation may differ depending upon V_L usage. What is less clear is the timing of the mutation and the processes controlling mutation. Because of technical limitations, it has not been possible as has been done in the mouse, to isolate hybridomas over time that represent clonal maturation and progression from primary to secondary responses. Most of the anti-Hib PS hybridomas isolated to date probably derive from memory compartment. Only two of 20 Hib PS-specific hybridomas secrete IgM Abs that might represent products of primary B cells, and one uses mutated V regions and the other does not.

Sequences of V regions used in the primary infant repertoire are not yet available, but the findings showing that V_L Id expression changes as a consequence of aging are consistent with the processes of mutation and/or V region shifts. The diminution in HibId-2 expression as a consequence of increased age cannot be accounted for by lack of expression of the λVII V gene as HibId-2 positive hybridomas using the λVII V region have been isolated from adults. The diminished expression of HibId-2 with age more likely represents mutational modification of the amino acid residues critical for expression of the HibId-2 determinant.[73,108,109] That mutation might extinguish HibId-2 is suggested by examination of the CDR regions of 4 λVII anti-Hib PS mAbs. One of these 4 mAbs does not express HibId-2, and this mAb shows more extensive CDR sequence differences from the candidate germline VλVII segment that the three HibId-2 positive λVII mAbs. Similarly, the appearance of $V_\kappa 3$ anti-Hib PS Abs with increasing age also may be explicable in terms of mutational modification. $V_\kappa 3$ Abs might arise in the primary B cell pool in germline configuration with low affinity for Hib PS, but over time, exposure to either Hib or to Hib PS cross-reactive antigens generates a hypermutated memory B cell population that has acquired sufficient high affinity for Hib PS such that it can effectively compete for a clonal niche.

Analysis of A2 Abs elicited in infants by conjugate vaccination suggests that Ag-driven V region hypermutation may occur relatively early in development of the repertoire. HbOC induces high affinity HibId-1 Abs whereas Hib PS-OMPC induces lower affinity HibId-1 Abs. Since HibId-1 Abs use the A2 V gene segment which is thought to mutate minimally, then the differences between these two Ab populations probably occur in the V_H region. Extent of V_H mutation or possibly polymorphism in CDR-3 may underlie the marked functional differences between these Abs. The Hib conjugates vaccines apparently differ in their capacity to either support hypermutation or to select high affinity variants using the A2 V region. The possibility that different conjugate vaccines might vary in their capacity to sensitize helper T cells and thereby promote hypermutation is supported by the observations of Källberg et al showing that both the frequency and pattern of somatic mutation in a murine anti-hapten response differed depending upon the particular carrier protein.[110]

EVOLUTIONARY CONSIDERATIONS

The theory developed by Cohn and Langman provides a good conceptual basis for considering the evolution of the Hib PS V region repertoire.[111-113] With the risk of over-simplification, a few general principles of the Cohn-Langman formulation can be stated. Two repertoire stages exist. The stage I repertoire is encoded by V genes selected and maintained in the germline for their immediate survival value. These so-called 'germline-encoded' specificities do not require mutation and are expressed at birth. Stage I specificities are fixed in the germline and are biased toward PS Ags as opposed to protein Ags because PS Ags evolve much more slowly than protein Ags. In contrast, the stage II repertoire is composed of somatically mutated variants assembled from the stage I repertoire. The germline V genes thus provide the substrate for the stage II repertoire which generates protective Ab responses to highly mutable pathogenic determinants.

At first glance, the Hib model appears to agree with the Cohn-Langman formulation. The oligoclonality of the response, the limited V_H usage and the predominance of the A2 V region are features which conform to the notion that evolution has selected a small number of optimally fit V genes. The A2 V_L region and the one or two V_H regions with which it pairs have a paucity of mutations, and therefore, they appear to be products of the stage I repertoire. However, several features of the Hib PS repertoire are not so easily accommodated within this theoretical framework. The Hib PS repertoire is not expressed until approximately two years of age unless stimulated by vaccination with protein-conjugated Hib PS. This ontogenic delay is a property common to many human PS Ab repertoires. Therefore, the stage I repertoire does not conform to the requirement of early expression conferring immediate survival value. While the mechanism underlying the ontogenic delay in the expression of anti-PS Ab specificities is not well understood, it probably does not involve repertoire deficiency or V gene mechanics but rather appears to be a problem of B cell activation. This general characteristic needs to be incorporated into any evolutionary theory of PS immunity for presumably there is some selective advantage for delaying the expression of these specificities. Another prediction stemming from the Cohn-Langman theory is that the stage I Hib PS repertoire would be optimally fit for protection against Hib, hence their fixation in the germline. This does not appear to be the case as A2 Abs do not have intrinsically higher avidity or bactericidal activity than non-A2 Abs. Furthermore, the proposition that a particular gene such as A2 has been adaptively selected because of its potential fitness has as its corollary the prediction that loss of this gene would be expected to have a negative consequence. Again, the Hib PS repertoire does not fit this prediction. An individual homozygous for a deletion spanning the entire distal region of the kappa locus and including the A2 V gene was able to respond to Hib PS vaccination with high serum Ab levels, which were as expected devoid of HibId-1 Abs.[20] This finding demonstrates that loss of the A2 gene does not result in unresponsiveness to Hib PS, and that other V_L regions (stage II repertoire) are able to compensate for A2 deficiency. This kappa deletion, known as haplotype 11, may be relatively common[114,115] and evidence suggests that children who develop Hib disease despite vaccination express HibId-1 Abs in normal frequency.[116] Therefore, absence of the A2 gene does not explain their disease susceptibility.

Cohn and Langman suggest that the germline V genes encoding the stage I repertoire evolve slowly in a manner coordinate with the slow evolution of PS Ags. However it is apparent that Hib PS Abs also derive from the stage II repertoire. If we ascribe A2-V_H26 Abs as stage I then the other 11 V_L regions and their respective V_H partners, both of which are frequently mutated, comprise stage II. Not only are stage II Abs functionally active against Hib, but they also compensate quite well when A2 is absent. Apparently, evolution has selected a Hib PS repertoire which is degenerate and which encompasses both stages I and II. Thus, the proposition that PS Abs evolve more slowly and are necessarily 'hard-wired' stage I type specificities does not accurately describe the human Hib PS repertoire.

Underlying the idea of slow paced evolution is the notion of gradualism, namely that evolution proceeds over long time periods in small refining steps culling out the bad genes and retaining the good genes. Indeed, implicit in the Cohn-Langman theory is the notion that while evolution selects for protective V genes, it also selects against harmful V genes such as those encoding self-reactivity. Putting aside the larger issue of this teleology and the notion of evolution as a perfecting mechanism, V genes, at least the mouse-human sort, would more likely evolve in a punctualistic fashion, characterized by expansions and contractions expected of gene families consisting of tandemly arranged homologous genes. The not infrequent occurrence of haplotype 11 is informative in this respect, as are the findings that V_H gene copy number can vary between ethnic groups.[90] An evolutionary strategy relying upon stage I repertoire to protect against encapsulated pathogens would seem a risky business given this potential genomic instability. Thus, the stage II repertoire generated from hypermutation would seem essential in guarding against loss of particular stage I specificities. Furthermore, the idea that self-reactive genes are selected against also does not fit the observations demonstrating that many of the genes used in the Hib PS (and other anti-PS) repertoire are also used by Abs reactive with self Ags. The assignment of potential specificity (and fitness) to a stage I element is therefore problematic since combinatorial joining and chain pairing are critical determinants of specificity. Since the same V gene can encode anti-self and anti-non-self, it is difficult to envisage how selection operates under the self non-self dictum. Potential self reactivity appears to be a necessary consequence of a system relying upon multiple genes, combinatorial mechanisms and hypermutation to generate diversity. Maintenance of potential self reactivity in the germline does not appear to be a problem since somatic tolerance to self is learned and not germline encoded. Suppression, anergy, deletion etc. are mechanisms which have evolved to purge high affinity self-reactive cells arising from either the stage I or II repertoires.

Cohn and Langman maintain that combinatorial joining arose in evolution as a mechanism to ensure haplotype exclusion, i.e. avoidance of dually-specific B cells and the maintenance of the self-nonself discrimination and not as a diversity generating mechanism. Even if combinatorial joining originally arose for this purpose, it nonetheless may have been subsequently selected as a diversifier. The CDR3 region of both A2 and non-A2 Hib PS Abs is critical to forming both the putative stage I and the stage II specificities since these Abs rely upon a non-germline encoded arginine residue at 95a in order to construct a functional Ab.

SUMMARY

One might have predicted that the outbred nature of human populations combined with the high potential for generating Ab diversity would lead to repertoires of enormous complexity, uniquely patterned to each individual. For Hib PS this does not appear to be the case. A relatively small number of conserved V genes encode an oligoclonal repertoire. Studies of the Hib PS system have been largely descriptive in nature, and as is apparent from the speculative nature of the Discussion, the evolutionary and somatic forces involved in shaping the repertoire are poorly understood. Many fundamental issues remain to be explored. Little is known about PS processing, associability with MHC and the capacity to be recognized by T cells. The physiological basis underlying the ontogenic delay in the expression of PS-specific Abs remains an enigma. The mechanisms responsible for age-related V region expression and the ability of different PS immunogens to induce functionally disparate Abs are unknown. It will be of both practical and theoretical importance to examine these issues and to determine whether the immune response to Hib represents an accurate model of other human PS-specific Ab responses. In addition to their value as vaccines, PS Ags function as probes of immune system physiology, and as such, they serve as unique tools to increase our understanding.

Acknowledgments

The work in the Author's laboratory is supported by grant AI25008 from the National Institutes of Health.

References

1. Kasper DL. Bacterial capsule-old dogmas and new tricks. J Infect Dis 1986; 153; 407-415.
2. Robbins JB, Schneerson R, Pittman M. *Haemophilus influenzae* type b infections. In: Germanier R, ed. Bacterial Vaccines. Orlando: Academic Press Inc., 1984:289-316.
3. Anderson P, Peter G, Johnston RB Jr et al. Immunization of humans with polyribophosphate, the capsular antigen of *Haemophilus influenzae*, type b. J Clin Invest 1972; 51:39-33.
4. Schneerson RL, Rodrigues LP, Parke JC et al. Immunity to disease caused by *Haemophilus influenzae* type b. II. Specificity and some biologic characteristics of "natural" infection acquired, and immunization induced antibodies to the capsular polysaccharide. J Immunol 1971; 107:1081-1089.
5. Robbins JB, Parke Jr. JC, Schneerson R, Whisnant JK. Quantitative measurements of "natural" and immunization induced *Haemophilus influenzae* type b capsular antibodies. Pediatr Res 1973; 7:103-110.
6. Smith DH, Peter G, Ingram DL et al. Responses of children immunized with the capsular polysaccharide of *Haemophilus influenzae*, type b. Pediatrics 1973; 52: 637-644.
7. Peltola H, Kayhty H, Sivonen A et al. *Haemophilus influenzae* type b capsular polysacchaide vaccine in children: A double-blind field study of 100,000 vaccinees 3 months to 5 years of age in Finland. Pediatrics 1977; 60:730-737.
8. Avery OT, Goebel WF. Chemo-immunological studies on conjugated carbohydrate-proteins. II. Immunological specificity of synthetic sugar-protein antigens. J Exp Med 1929; 50:533-550.
9. Goebel WF. The immunologic properties of an artificial antigen containing cellobiuronic acid. J Exp Med 1939; 68: 469-444.
10. Schneerson R, Barrera O, Sutton A et al. Preparation, characterization and immunogenicity of *H. influenzae* b polysaccharide-protein conjugates. J Exp Med 1980; 152:361-367.
11. Anderson P. Antibody responses to *H. influenzae* type b and diphtheria toxin induced by conjugates of oligosaccharides of type b capsule with non-toxic protein CRM_{197}. Infect Immun 1983; 39:233-238.
12. Einhorn MS, Weinberg GA, Anderson EL et al. Immunogenicity in infants of *Haemophilus influenzae* type b polysaccharide in a conjugate vaccine with *Neisseria meningitidis* outer membrane protein. Lancet 1986; 2:299-302.
13. Anderson P, Pichichero ME, Insel RA. Immunization of 2-month-old infants with protein-coupled oligosaccharides derived from the capsule of *H. influenzae* type b. J Pediatr 1985; 107:346-351.
14. Murphy TV, White KE, Pastor P, Gabriel L, Medley F, Granoff DM, Osterholm MT. Declining incidence of *Haemophilus influenzae* type b disease since introduction of vaccination. J Am Med Assoc 1993; 269: 246-248.

15. Dick WE, Beurret M. Glycoconjugates of bacterial carbohydrate antigens: A survey and consideration of design and preparation factors. In: Cruse JM, Lewis RE, eds. Conjugate vaccines. Basel: Karger, 1989; 48-114.
16. Lucas AH. New approaches to polysaccharide vaccines. In: Ellis RW, Granoff DM, eds. Development and Clinical Uses of *Haemophilus* b Conjugate Vaccines, New York: Marcel Dekker, Inc., 1994; 455-487.
17. Insel RA, Kittelberger A, Anderson P. Isoelectric focusing of human antibody to the *Haemophilus influenzae* b capsular polysaccharide: restricted and identical spectrotypes in adults. J Immunol 1985; 135:2810-2816.
18. Insel RA, Anderson PW. Oligosaccharide-protein conjugate vaccines induce and prime for oligoclonal IgG antibody responses to the *H. influenzae* b capsular polysaccharide in human infants. J Exp Med 1986; 163:262-269.
19. Lucas AH. Expression of crossreactive idiotypes by human antibodies specific for the capsular polysaccharide of *Haemophilus influenzae* b. J Clin Invest 1988; 81:480-486.
20. Scott MG, Tarrand JJ, Crimmins DL et al. Clonal characterization of the human antibody repertoire to *Haemophilus influenzae* b polysaccharide. II. IgG antibodies contain VH genes from a single VH family and VL genes from at least four VL families. J Immunol. 1989; 143:293-298.
21. Scott MG, Crimmins DL, McCourt DW et al. Clonal characterization of the human IgG antibody repertoire to *Haemophilus influenzae* type b polysaccharide. III: a single VκII gene and one of several J genes are joined by an invariant arginine to form the most common L chain V region. J Immunol 1989; 143:4110-4116.
22. Scott MG, Crimmins DL, McCourt DW, et al. Clonal characterization of the human IgG antibody repertoire to *Haemophilus influenzae* type b polysaccharide. IV. The less frequently expressed VL are heterogeneous. J Immunol 1991; 147:4007-4013.
23. Adderson E E, Shackleford PG, Quinn A et al. Restricted Ig heavy chain usage in the human antibody response to *Haemophilus influenzae* type b polysaccharide. J Immunol 1991; 147:1667-1674.
24. Adderson EE, Shackelford PG, Insel RA et al. Immunoglobulin light chain variable region gene sequences for human antibodies to *Haemophilus influenzae* type b polysaccharide are dominated by a limited number of Vκ and Vλ segments and VJ recombinations. J Clin Invest 1992; 89:729-738.
25. Adderson EE, Shackelford PG, Quinn A et al. Restricted immunoglobulin VH usage and VDJ combinations in the human response to *Haemophilus influenzae* type b polysaccharide: nucleotide sequences of monospecific anti-*Haemophilus* antibodies and polyspecific antibodies cross-reacting with self antigens. J Clin Invest 1993; 91:2734-2743.
26. Adderson EA, Azmi FH, Wilson PM et al. The human VH3b gene subfamily is highly polymorphic. J Immunol 1993; 151: 800-809.
27. Carroll WL, Adderson EE, Lucas AH, et al. Molecular basis of antibody diversity. In:Ellis RW, Granoff DM, eds. Development and Clinical Uses of *Haemophilus* b Conjugate Vaccines, New York: Marcel Dekker, Inc., 1994; 207-229.
28. Lucas AH, Larrick JW, Reason DC. Variable region sequences of a protective human monoclonal antibody specific for the *Haemophilus influenzae* type b polysaccharide. Infect Immun 1994; 62:3873-3880.
29. Pinchuk GV, Nottenburg C, Milner ECB. Predominant V-region gene configurations in the human antibody response to *Haemophilus influenzae* capsule polysaccharide. Scand J Immunol 1995; 41:324-330.
30. Jeske DJ, Jarvis J, Milstein C et al. Junctional diversity is essential to antibody activity. J Immunol 1984; 133:1090-1092.
31. Azmi FH, Lucas AH, Raff HV, Granoff DM. Variable region sequences and idiotypic expression of a protective human immunoglobulin M antibody to capsular polysaccharides of *Neisseria meningitidis* group B of *Escherichia coli* K1. Infect Immun 1994; 62:1776-1786.
32. Dersimonian H, Schwart RS, Barrett KJ et al. Relationship of human variable region heavy chain germline genes encoding anti-DNA antibodies. J Immunol 1987; 139: 2496-2501.
33. Sanz I, Dang H, Takei M et al. VH se-

quence of a human anti-Sm autoantibody: evidence that autoantibodies can be unmutated copies of germline genes. J Immunol 1989; 142:883-887.

34. Wang L, Radic MZ, Galili U. Human antigal heavy chain genes: preferential use of VH3 and the presence of somatic mutations. J Immunol 1995; 155:127-1285.
35. Chen PP, Liu M, Sinha S et al. A 16/6 idiotype positive anti-DNA antibody is encoded by a conserved VH with no somatic mutation. Arthritis Rheum 1988; 31:1429-1431.
36. Spatz LA, Wong KK, Williams M et al. Cloning and sequence analysis of the VH and VL regions of an anti-myelin/DNA antibody from a patient with peripheral neuropathy and chronic lymphocytic leukemia. J Immunol 1990; 144:2821-2828.
37. Sanz I, Casali, Thomas JW et al. Nucleotide sequences of eight human natural autoantibody VH regions reveal apparent restricted use of VH families. J Immunol 1989; 142:4054-4061.
38. Pirofski L, Lui R, DeShaw M et al. Analysis of human monoclonal antibodies elicited by vaccination with a *Cryptococcus neoformans* glucuronoxylomannan capsular polysaccharide vaccine. Infect Immun 1995; 63: 3005-3014.
39. Quinn A, Adderson EE, Shackelford PG et al. Autoantibody germline gene segment encodes VH and VL regions of a human anti-streptococcal monoclonal antibody recognizing streptococcal M protein and human cardiac myosin epitopes. J Immunol 1995; 154:4203-4212.
40. Pascual V, Randen I, Thompson K et al. The complete nucleotide sequences of the heavy chain variable regions of six monospecific rheumatoid factors derived from EBV transformed B cells isolated from the synovial tissue of patients with rheumatoid arthritis: further evidence that some autoantibodies are unmutated copies of germline genes. J Clin Invest 1990; 86: 1320-1328.
41. Huang D-F, Olee T, Masuho Y et al. Sequence analyses of three immunoglobulin G anti-virus antibodies reveal their utilization of autoantibody-related immunoglobulin VH genes but not Vλ genes. J Clin Invest 1992; 90:2197-2208.
42. Shin EK, Akamizu T, Matsuda F et al. Variable regions of Ig heavy chain genes encoding antithyrotropin receptor antibodies of patients with Graves' disease. J Immunol 1994; 152:1485-1492.
43. Silberstein LE, Jefferies LC, Goldman J et al. Variable region gene analysis of pathologic human autoantibodies to the related i and II red blood cell antigens. Blood 1991; 78:2372-2386.
44. Portolano S, McLachlan SM, Rapoport B. High affinity, thyroid-specific human autoantibodies displayed on the surface of filamentous phage use V genes similar to other autoantibodies. J Immunol 1993; 151: 2839-2851.
45. Van Es KH, Aanstoot H, Gmelig-Meyling FHJ et al. A human systemic lupus erythematosus-related anti-cardiolipin/single-stranded DNA autoantibody is encoded by a somatically mutated variant of the developmentally restricted 51P1 VH gene. J Immunol 1992; 149:2234-2240.
46. Newkirk MM, Gram H, Heinrich GF et al. Complete protein sequences of the variable regions of the cloned heavy and light chains of a human anti-cytomegalovirus antibody reveal a striking similarity to human monoclonal rheumatoid factors of the Wa idiotypic family. J Clin Invest 1988; 81:1511-1518.
47. Marasco WA, Bagley J, Zani C et al. Characterization of the cDNA of a broadly reactive neutralizing human anti-gp120 monoclonal antibody. J Clin Invest 1992; 90:1467-1478.
48. Dersimonian H, McAdam KPWJ, Mackworth-Young C et al. The recurrent expression of variable region segments in human IgM anti-DNA antibodies. J Immunol 1989; 142:4027-4033.
49. Pons-Estel B, Goñi F, Solomon A et al. Sequence similarities among κIIIb chainss of monoclonal human IgMκ autoantibodies. J Exp Med 1984; 160:893-904.
50. Chen PP, Albrandt K, Orida NK et al. Genetic basis for the cross-reactive idiotypes on the light chains of human IgM anti-IgG autoantibodies. Proc Natl Acad Sci USA 1986; 83:8318-8322.

51. Goñi F, Chen PP, Pons-Stel B et al. Sequence similarities and cross-idiotypic specificity of L chains among human monoclonal IgMκ with anti-γ-globulin activity. J Immunol 1985; 135:4073-4079.
52. Kasaian MT, Ikematsu H, Balow JE et al. Structure of the VH and VL segments of monoreactive and polyreactive IgA autoantibodies to DNA in patients with systemic lupus erythematosus. J Immunol 1994; 152:3137-3151.
53. Ichiyoshi Y, Zhou M, Casali P. A human anti-insulin IgG autoantibody arises through the clonal selection from an insulin-specific "germline" natural antibody template. J Immunol 1995; 154:226-238.
54. Bhat NM, Bieber MM, Chapman CJ et al. Human antilipid A monoclonal antibodies bind to human B cells and the i antigen on cord blood red blood cells. J Immunol 1993; 151:5011-5021.
55. Bye JM, Carter C, Cui Y et al. Germline variable region gene segment derivation of human monoclonal anti-Rh(D) antibodies. J Clin Invest 1992; 90:2481-2490.
56. Chen PP, Robbins DL, Jirik FR et al. Isolation and characterization of a light chain variable region gene for human rheumatoid factors. J Exp Med 1987; 166:1900-1905.
57. Ikematsu H, Ichiyoshi Y, Schettino EW et al. VH and Vκ segment structure of anti-insulin IgG autoantibodies in patients with insulin-dependent diabetes mellitus. J Immunol 1994; 152:1430-1441.
58. Chapman CJ, Spellerberg MB, Smith GA et al. Auto anti-red cell antibodies synthesized by patient with infectious mononucleosis utilize the VH4-21 gene segment. J Immunol 1993; 151:1051-1061.
59. Paul E, Iliev A, Livneh A et al. The anti-DNA associated idiotype 8.12 is encoded by the VλII gene family and maps to the vicinity of L chain CDR1. J Immunol 1992; 149:3588-3595.
60. Lewis AP, Parry N, Peakman TC et al. Rescue and expression of human immunoglobulin genes to generate functional human monoclonal antibodies. Hum Antib Hybrid 1992; 3:146-152.
61. Paterson G, Wilson G, Kennedy PGE et al. Analysis of anti-GM1 ganglioside antibodies cloned from motor neuropathy patients demonstrates diverse V region gene usage with extensive somatic mutation. J Immunol 1995; 155:3049-3059.
62. Kabat EA, Wu TT. Identical V region amino acid sequences and segments of sequences in antibodies of different specificities: relative contributions of VH and VL genes, minigenes, and complementarity determining regions to binding of antibody-combining sites. J Immunol 1991; 147: 1709-1719.
63. Insel RA, Anderson Jr PW. Cross-reactivity with *Escherichia coli* K100 in the human serum anticapsular antibody response to *Haemophilus influenzae* type b. J Immunol 1982; 128:1267-1270.
64. Boswell CM, Irwin DC, Goodnight J et al. Strain-dependent restricted VH and VL usage by anti-bacterial levan monoclonal antibodies. J Immunol 1992; 148: 3864-3872.
65. Kabat EA, Nickerson KG, Liao J et al. A human monoclonal macroglobulin with specificity for α(2-8)-linked poly-N-acetyl neuramininc acid, the capsular polysaccharide of group B meningococci and *Escherichia coli* K1, which crossreacts with polynucleotides and denatured DNA. J Exp Med 1986; 164:642-654.
66. Cisar J, Kabat EA, Dorner et al. Binding properties of immunoglobulin combining sites specific for terminal or nonterminal antigenic determinants in dextran. J Exp Med 1975; 142:435-459.
67. Kabat EA. Antibody complementarity and antibody structure. J Immunol 1988; 141: S25-S36.
68. Padlan EA, Kabat EA. Model building study of the combining sites of two antibodies to α(1-6)dextran. Proc Natl Acad Sci USA 1988; 85:6885-6889.
69. Snyder JG, Dinh Q, Morrison SL et al. Structure and function of anti-fucosyllactosamine (Le^x) and galactosylgloboside antibodies. J Immunol 1994; 153: 1161-1169.
70. Nahm MH, Kim KH, Anderson PA et al. Functional capacities of clonal antibodies to *Haemophilus influenzae* type b polysaccharide. Infect Immun 1995; 63:2989-2994.

71. Lucas, AH, Granoff DM. A major cross-reactive idiotype associated with human antibodies to the *Haemophilus influenzae* b polysaccharide: expression in relation to age and immunoglobulin G subclass. J Clin Invest 1990; 85:1158-1166.
72. Lucas AH, Langley RJ, Granoff DM et al. An idiotypic marker associated with a germ-line encoded κ light chain variable region that predominates the vaccine-induced human antibody response to *Haemophilus influenzae* b polysaccharide. J Clin Invest 1991; 88:1811-1818.
73. Granoff D M, Shackelford PG, Holmes SJ et al. Variable region expression in the antibody responses of infants vaccinated with *Haemophilus influenzae* type b polysaccharide-protein conjugates: description of a new λ light chain-associated idiotype and the relation between idiotype expression, avidity, and vaccine formulation. J Clin Invest 1993; 91:788-796.
74. Lucas AH, Azmi FH, Mink CM et al. Age-dependent V region expression in the human antibody response to the *Haemophilus influenzae* type b polysaccharide. J Immunol 1993; 150:2056-2061.
75. Einhorn MS, Weinberg GA, Anderson EL et al. Immunogenicity in infants of *Haemophilus influenzae* tupe b polysaccharide in a conjugate vaccine with *Neisseria Meningitidis* outer-membrane protein. Lancet; 2: 299-302.
76. Decker MD, Edwards KM, Bradley R et al. Comparative trials in infants of four conjugate *Haemophilus influenzae* type b vaccines. J Pediatr 1992; 120:184-189.
77. Mageed A., Walker MR, Jefferis R. Restricted light chain subgroup expression of human rheumatoid factor paraproteins determined by monoclonal antibodies. Immunology 1986; 59:473-478.
78. Schroeder HW, Hillson JL, Perlmutter RM. Early restriction of the human antibody repertoire. Science 1987; 238:791-793.
79. Schroeder HW, Wang JY. Preferential utilization of conserved immunoglobulin heavy chain variable region gene segments during human fetal life. Proc Nat Acad Sci USA 1990; 87:6146-6150.
80. Cuisinier A-M, Gauthier L, Boubli L et al. Mechanisms that generate human immunoglobulin diversity operate from the 8th week of gestation in the fetal liver. Eur J Immunol 1993; 23:110-118.
81. Sanz I. Multiple mechanisms participate in the generation of diversity of human H chain CDR3 regions. J Immunol 1991; 147: 1720-1729.
82. Feeney AJ. Lack of N regions in fetal and neonatal mouse V-D-J junctional sequences. J Exp Med 1990; 172:1377-1390.
83. Kniskern PJ, Marburg S. Conjugation: Design, Chemistry, and Analysis. In: Ellis RW, Granoff DM, eds. Development and Clinical Uses of *Haemophilus* b Conjugate Vaccines, New York: Marcel Dekker, Inc., 1994; 37-69.
84. Schlesinger Y, Granoff DM, The Collaborative Vaccine Study Group. Avidity and bactericidal activity of antibody elicited by different *Haemophilus influenzae* type b conjugate vaccines. J Am Med Assoc 1992; 267:1489-1494.
85. Lucas AH, Granoff DM. Functional differences in iditypically defined IgG1 anti-polysaccharide antibodies elicited by vaccination with *Haemophilus influenzae* type b polysaccharide-protein conjugates. J Immunol 1995; 154:4195-4202.
86. Pascual V, Capra JD. Human immunoglobulin heavy-chain variable region genes: organization, polymorphism, and expression. Adv Immunol 1991; 49:1-74.
87. Susuki I, Pfister L, Glas A et al. Representation of rearranged VH gene segments in the human adult antibody repertoire. J Immunol 1995; 154:3902-3911.
88. Stewart AK, Huang C, Stollar BD et al. High-frequency representation of a single VH gene in the expressed human B cell repertoire. J Exp Med 1993; 177:409-418.
89. Cook GP, Tomlinson IM. The human immunoglobulin VH repertoire. Immunol Today 1995; 16:237-242.
90. Sasso EH, Buckner JH, Suzuki LA. Ethnic differences in polymorphism of an immunoglobulin VH3 gene. J Clin Invest 1995; 96:1591-1600.
91. Sasso EH, Van Dijk KW, Milner ECB.

Prevalence and polymorphism of human VH3 genes. J Immunol 1990; 145: 2751-2757.
92. Sasso EH, Silverman GJ, Mannik M. Human IgM molecules that bind staphylococcal protein A contain VHIII heavy chains. J Immunol 1989; 142:2778-2783.
93. Zouali M. B cell superantigens: implications for selection of the human antibody repertoire. Immunol Today 1995; 16:399-405.
94. Silverman GJ. Human antibody responses to bacterial antigens: studies of a model conventional antigen and a proposed model B cell superantigen. Intern Rev Immunol 1992; 9:55-76.
95. Chothia C, Lesk AM, Gherardi E et al. Structural repertoire of the human VH segments. J Mol Biol 1992; 227:799-817.
96. Kirkham PM, Mortari F, Newton JA et al. Immunoglobulin VH clan and family predicts variable domain structure and may influence antigen binding. EMBO J 1992; 11:603-609.
97. Clarke SH, Claflin J, Potter M et al. Polymorphism in anti-phosphocholine antibodies reflecting evolution of immunoglobulin families. J Exp Med 1983; 157:98-113.
98. Chen C, Bruderer U, Rittenberg MB. The developmental patterns of B cell precursors distinguishing between environmental and nonenvironmental forms of phosphocholine. Cell Immunol 1992; 143:378-388.
99. Claflin JL, Berry J. Genetics of the phosphocholine-specific antibody response to *Streptococcus pneumoniae*: germline but not mutated T15 antibodies are dominantly selected. J Immunol 1988; 141:4012-4019.
100. Kenny JJ, Moratz CM, Guelde G et al. Antigen binding and idiotype analysis of antibodies obtained after electroporation of heavy and light chain genes encoding phosphocholine specific antibodies: a model for T15-idiotype dominance. J Exp Med 1992; 176:1637-1643.
101. Feeney AJ, Thuerauf DJ. Sequence and fine specificity analysis of primary 511 anti-phosphorylcholine antibodies. J Immunol 1989; 143:4061-4068.
102. Foote J, Milstein C. Kinetic maturation of an immune response. Nature 1991; 352: 530-532.
103. Ching C, Roberts VA, Rittenberg MB. Generation and analysis of random point mutations in an antibody CDR2 sequence: many mutated antibodies lose their ability to bind antigen. J Exp Med 1992; 176: 855-866.
104. Kearney JF. Idiotypic networks. In: Paul WE, ed. Fundamental Immunology, third edition. New York:Raven Press Ltd, 1993; 887-902.
105. Bogen B, Weiss S. Processing and presentation of idiotypes to MHC-restricted T cells. Int Rev Immunol 1993; 10: 337-355.
106. Rademaekers A, Kölsch E. Regulation of an anti-polysaccharide immune response in BALB/c mice through a tight T and B lymphocyte idiotypic connection. Eur J Immunol 1995; 25:623-626.
107. Berek C, Milstein C. Mutation drift and repertoire shift in the maturation of the immune response. Immunol Rev 1987; 96:23-41.
108. Sikder SK, Borden P, Gruezo F, et al. Amino acid substitutions in VH CDR2 change the idiotype but not the antigen-binding of monoclonal antibodies to $\alpha(1\text{-}6)$ dextran. J Immunol 1989; 142:888-893.
109. Parhami-Seren B, Wysocki LJ, Margolies MN et al. Clustered H chain somatic mutations shared by anti-p-azophenylarsonate antibodies confer enhanced affinity and ablate the cross-reactive idiotype. J Immunol 1990; 145:2340-2346.
110. Källberg E, Gray D, Leanderson T. The effect of carrier and carrier priming on the kinetics and pattern of somatic mutation in the VκOx1 gene. Eur J Immunol 1995; 25:2349-2354.
111. Cohn M, Langman RE. The Protecton: the unit of humoral immunity selected by evolution. Immunol Rev 1990; 115:7-142.
112. Cohn M. Idiotype network views of immune regulation: for whom the bell tolls. In: Reichlin M, Capra JD, eds. Idiotypes. Orlando: Academic Press Inc., 1986:321-399.
113. Langman R. The Immune System. San Diego: Academic Pres Inc., 1989.
114. Schaible G, Rappold GA, Pargent W et al. The immunoglobulin κ locus: Polymor-

phism and haplotypes of caucasoid and non-caucasoid individuals. Hum Genet 1993; 91:261-267.

115. Pargent W, Schäble KF, Zachau HG. Polymorphism and haplotypes in the human immunoglobulin locus. Eur J Immunol 1991; 21:1829-1835.

116. Holmes SJ, Lucas AH, Osterholm MT et al. Immunoglobulin deficiency and idiotype expression in children developing *Haemophilus influenzae* type b disease after vaccination with conjugate vaccine. J Amer Med Assoc 1991; 266:1960-1965.

CHAPTER 10

THE HIV-1 GP120 SUPERANTIGEN: STRUCTURAL FEATURES AND ROLE IN VIRAL HOST-PATHOGEN INTERACTION

Lee Goodglick, Janet Townsley-Fuchs, Rick M. Fairhurst, Mehran Neshat, Denise Marcelo, Donald E. Mosier and Jonathan Braun

HIV INFECTION CAUSES DYSFUNCTION OF B CELLS AND HUMORAL IMMUNITY

Infection with human immunodeficiency virus type 1 (HIV-1) results in a multifaceted disturbance of the immune system. The pathophysiology of this infection centers on depletion of CD4 T cells and the consequent impaired cellular immunity. CD4 T cells are selectively deleted due to a series of events initiated by the binding of the human immunodeficiency virus (HIV) to the CD4 molecule via the viral envelope glycoprotein gp120.[1] The exact mechanism by which the virus leads to deletion of this population is unknown. However, several models have been proposed, such as direct cytotoxicity, gp120-induced polyclonal apoptosis, and oligoclonal superantigen-mediated deletion.[2-4]

The early stages of HIV infection are characterized by the in vivo polyclonal activation of B cells, reflected by hypergammaglobulinemia, elevated titers of autoantibodies and circulating immune complexes, lymphadenopathy due to B cell hyperplasia, and circulating B cells bearing activation markers.[5,6] In late stages of infection, an elevated occurrence of B cell lymphomas is an important clinical problem.[6,7]

When evaluated in tissue culture, B cells from HIV seropositive individuals are distinguished by their elevated frequency of spontaneously immunoglobulin (Ig) secreting cells consisting of both anti-HIV and polyclonal specificities,[8,9] and a striking cytokine secretory response to

Human B Cell Superantigens, edited by Moncef Zouali. © 1996 R.G. Landes Company.

gp120.[10,11] In B cells from normal individuals, HIV may directly stimulate proliferation and Ig secretion, related in part to a T cell-dependent response to the gp41 or gp160,[11-13] but notably not to gp120. Paradoxically, impairments in B cell function are superimposed on this hyperactive pattern, including poor response to neoantigens, particularly polysaccharides,[14] unresponsiveness to certain mitogens in vitro,[15] and the eventual depletion of absolute numbers of circulating B cells.[16] These abnormalities are not corrected by addition of normal T cells, suggesting that the defects are intrinsic to the B cell.[1]

The prevalent view has been that these B cell disorders are secondary to disturbed immunoregulation, an idea consistent with the striking cellular and cytokine immune abnormalities in HIV-infected individuals. However, our laboratory unexpectedly observed a clonal deficit which was selective for B cells bearing V_H3 genes in individuals with HIV infection.[17] This finding was inconsistent with the preceding view, since secondary immunoregulatory effects would not be expected to act in a clonally selective fashion. By analogy to the situation with CD4 T cells, we proposed that V_H3 B cell depletion involved direct binding of gp120 to a conserved domain of this Ig V gene family. V_H3 represents the largest V_H gene family with 30 or more members,[18] and the single most common family expressed at the population level throughout ontogeny (20-30%).[19,20] Consequently, dysfunction or deletion of this population could alone substantially account for the humoral immunodeficiency in this disease.

A series of studies have now validated this hypothesis, including demonstration of selective binding of gp120 to V_H3^+ Ig, gp120-induced activation of V_H3 B cells in vitro, and the predominance of gp120-specific B cells in the HIV-induced clonal expansion and eventual depletion of V_H3 B cells in clinical HIV infection.[21-25] These demonstrate the function and biologic significance of HIV-1 gp120 as a V_H3 superantigen (SAg), as previously reviewed (Fig. 10.1).[26-32] This article focuses on three areas. First, we will present what is now known about the structural features of V_H3 and gp120 required for their interaction, and how these compare to the interaction

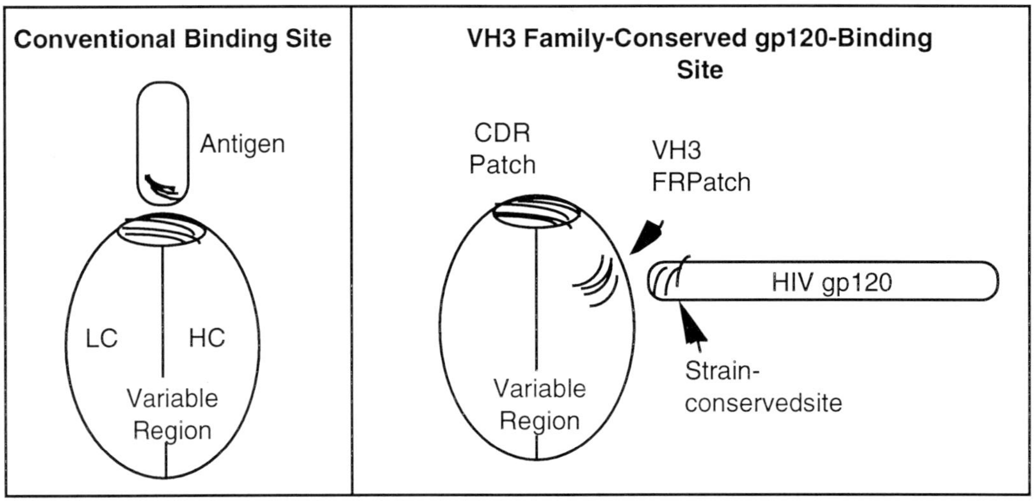

Fig. 10.1. Model of the V_H3-gp120 superantigen interaction. (Left) Conventional antigens bind to the antibody variable region through the CDR loops of the heavy and light chains. (Right) Superantigens such as gp120 are proposed to bind to an alternate site formed by strands of the FR1 and FR3 domains of the heavy chain only. The gp120 epitope is conserved among diverse strains, suggesting that this interaction is favorable for the virus life-cycle, and has been positively selected during HIV evolution.

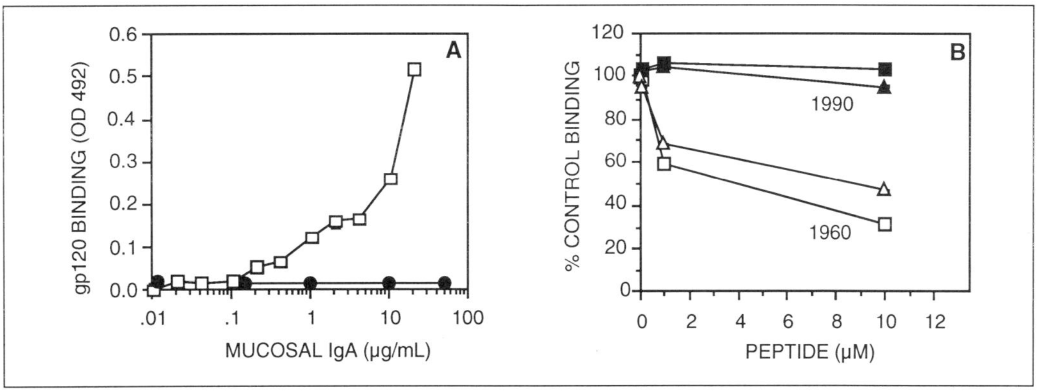

Fig. 10.2. Superantigen-specific binding of gp120 by secretory IgA. (A) ELISA wells coated with HIV-1 gp120 were reacted with indicated concentrations of purified colostral/secretory (square) or serum (circle) IgA, and detected with biotin-labeled anti IgA and streptavidin-poly HRP. (B). Colostral IgA (square) or serum IgM (triangle) were preincubated with 20mer peptides at the indicated concentrations either bearing (1960 peptide; open symbols) or lacking (1990; closed symbols) the C2 decamer motif; the mixtures were then tested for gp120 binding as in (A).

between V_H3 and other SAgs. Second, we will review emerging information on the biologic factors controlling the abundance of this group of V_H3 antibodies. Finally, we will present our current understanding of the role of the V_H3-gp120 interaction in HIV immunopathogenesis, particularly with respect to HIV transmission.

SELECTIVE BINDING OF HIV-1 GP120 BY V_H3 IG

In healthy individuals, serum IgM displays detectable binding activity to HIV-1 gp120.[21-23] Purified serum IgG also binds gp120, although with ~10- fold lower activity[21,23] (also, Townsley-Fuchs et al, "HIV-1 gp120 superantigen-binding serum antibodies. A host factor in homosexual HIV-1 transmission," 1996, submitted for publication). Serum IgA lacks detectable binding activity (testing up to 50 μg/mL IgA). In contrast, activity is observed with colostral (secretory) IgA at concentrations comparable to serum IgG (Fig. 10.2). A panel of monoclonal antibodies have also been established which display or lack this binding activity (Table 10.1). Some features of this panel should be noted. First, binding activity is not a uniform feature of antibodies, but instead is restricted to antibodies of the V_H3 gene family. Thus, binding activity is enriched 5-10 fold in polyclonal antibodies fractionated for reactivity with the V_H3-binding domain of *S. aureus* protein A (SpA).[21] Similar findings have been observed for serum IgG and secretory IgA (Townsley-Fuchs, *op. cit.*; R. Fairhurst and M. Neshat, unpublished). Where suitable analysis has been possible, active monoclonal antibodies have been identified as V_H3 gene family members. Second, binding is not restricted to particular light chain isotypes, indicating that a variety of light chain gene products are permissive for this binding activity. Third, binding activity is not dependent on the entire heavy chain; in fact, a pair of gp120-binding antibodies have been identified (NANUC-1, -2) as recombinant Fab proteins.[33,34] Thus, binding does not require multimeric antibody structure, although this does not rule out a possible role for the C_H1 constant region domain.

There are two technical points which should be noted. First, reliable detection by ELISA is best achieved by an amplification system: wells are coated with gp120 in PBS (to minimize "plate-binding"; see below, polyreactivity), reacted with test antibody, and detected by biotin-labeled anti-Ig, streptavidin conjugated to poly-(horseradish peroxidase) complexes, and colometric substrate.[23] Avidity of binding has been analyzed by competition measurements with soluble gp120[21-23] and by surface plasmon resonance (Neshat, Goodglick, and Braun, unpublished). Antibodies typically show binding in the range of K_D ~1 μM, although certain monoclonal antibodies display higher avidity (< 0.01 μM) (Table 10.2).[21] Second, inhibition of binding is produced by typical components of tissue culture media interfere with detection (fetal calf serum, albumin), and minor contaminants in bacterially expressed proteins. Assays are best performed using Tween 20 (0.5%) as a blocking agent, and test monoclonal and recombinant proteins require careful purification prior to binding analysis (see below, polyreactivity).

HIV gp120 binds a substantial fraction (~6%) of the B cells in HIV-uninfected individuals.[21] Binding requires membrane Ig and is CD4 independent. Two-color flow cytometry with anti-V_H antibodies reveals that this B cell subset expresses V_H3 gene products. Thus, over 70% were accounted for using the avail-

Table 10.1. HIV-1 gp120 binding activity of selected antibodies

Antibody	Isotype	V_H Family* or V_H gene	Antigen§	SpA	gp120
RSJ	IgM		WM	+++	+++
HEA	IgM	VH3-30	WM	+++	+++
VNG	IgM		WM	++	++
VIN	IgM	VH3-23	WM	-	+
TAAO	IgA,G¶	mouse VH3	DNS	+	+++
NANUC-1	rFab	VH3-30	pANCA	-	++
NANUC-2	rFab	VH3-30	histone H-1	-	++
SMI	IgM	V_H1	rheum. factor	-	-
ALV	IgM		WM	-	-
BEN	IgM		WM	-	-
TSU7	IgA, G¶	mouse V_H1	dextran	-	-
P313	rFab	V_H1	tetanus tox.	-	-

Monoclonal antibodies were characterized for binding to HIV-1 gp120 or modified SpA.[2-3,33]
*Families identified by anti-idiotopes (HEA, VIN) or direct sequencing(TAAO, TSU7, NANUC-1, NANUC-2, P313).
§WM, Waldenstrom's macroglobulinemia; DNS, dansyl hapten;
Comparative binding is tabulated by antibody concentration giving ELISA absorbance of 0.4: +++, < 0.1 μg/mL; ++ < 1 μg/mL, +, < 5 μg/mL.
¶Transfectoma antibodies engineered with IgG or IgA constant region domains.[34]

Table 10.2. Binding avidity of gp120-binding monoclonal antibodies to selected antigens

	Apparent Dissociation Contant (Kd in nmol/l)			
	RSJ	HEA	VNG	VIN
gp120	210	2	430	10
Thyroglobulin	40	110	310	290
Actin	> 2,000	> 2,000	250	47
Fc IgG	> 2,000	> 2,000	nd	164
Tetanus toxoid	> 2,000	> 2,000	778	149
CD4	> 2,000	> 2,000	> 2,000	163

Competitive ELISA was used to measure binding avidity for the indicated antigens. Note that antibodies react with thyroglobulin, but range from no (RSJ, HEA) to broad (VNG, VIN) polyreactivity.

able anti-V_H3 reagents (16/6, B6, and BK2; specific for VH3-23, VH3-30, and VH3-15, respectively). In contrast, B cells expressing other common V gene idiotopes were at the limit of detection among gp120-binding B cells. It is notable that only approximately 25% of V_H3^+ B cells were gp120-binding. Since this heterogeneity was not related to the levels of membrane Ig, it indicates that sequence differences in V_H and V_L may be permissive or nonpermissive for gp120-Ig interaction.

RELATIONSHIP OF V_H3 BINDING TO GP120, SPA, AND POLYREACTIVITY

There are three reasons to believe that the SpA and gp120 interact with distinct V_H3 sequences: (a) Several monoclonal antibodies are now known to be discordant in binding to SpA and gp120 (Table 10.1). (b) While fractionation of polyclonal antibody with SpA immunoaffinity columns enriches for gp120-binding Ig, it also reveals that only 50% of total gp120-binding activity displays detectable avidity for SpA (Townsley-Fuchs et al, *op. cit.*). (c) The frequencies of gp120- and SpA-binding in total B cells are approximately ~6% and ~25%, respectively (i.e., ~25% and ~75% of V_H3 B cells).[21,35] One explanation for this discordance is the variability in SAg-binding avidity. With respect to SpA, binding heterogeneity among different V_H3 recombinant Fabs has been related to sequence polymorphisms of V_H3 family-specific residues.[36] It is likely that the same holds true for gp120 interaction. Nonetheless, since gp120- and SpA-binding vary independently, it would appear that key contact residues for binding of these two ligands to the V_H3 IG are distinct. Competition studies offer a distinct approach for evaluating the relationship of SpA and gp120 binding to V_H3. Curiously, this has not been technically feasible, because by both ELISA and immunoprecipitation analysis, SpA and gp120 directly bind each other (L. Goodglick, unpublished). The basis for this surprising interaction deserves further analysis.

A second issue is the subset of antibodies with detectable binding activity to a diversity of antigens.[37-42] Such "polyreactive" antibodies represent ~5% of normal adult serum IgM or IgM-secretory precursor cells, but only ~0.05% of IgG or IgA. The frequency are nearly all of the B1 subpopulation, is higher in children, and is increased in mature isotypes of individuals with various autoimmune diseases. The frequency of V_H3 use in these antibodies is moderately elevated (~50% V_H3). Originally, these antibodies were perceived as indiscriminately "sticky", but more recent quantitative studies with monoclonal antibodies have revealed distinct patterns of antigen recognition and avidity. Nearly all react with the Fc fragment of IgG (K_D = 12-60 μM), although this may be in part due to the typical use of this antigen as the screening agent to select polyreactive B cell clones. In contrast, binding to other antigens is usually restricted to only a minority of "polyreactive" antibodies. For example, avidity for actin among 12 monoclonals was minimal in 4 ($K_D \geq$ 1000 μM), and moderate for the 6 (K_D = 0.7-9 μM). Similarly, only ~30% of such antibodies from a large EBV panel detectably bound thyroglobulin, and these did so with moderate avidity (K_D = 0.2-0.6 μM).[40]

Some information is now available on the shared structures of these antibodies which confer these antigen-binding patterns. Domain-swapping studies mainly implicate the heavy chain CDR3, although there may be additional contributions of heavy (polyreactive) or light chain (anti-Fc) V gene motifs.[42-48] An interesting exception is natural anti-thyroglobulin antibodies, which are restricted to the V_H3-23 gene and often distinct from "polyreactivity".[38-40,42]

Binding of polyreactive antibodies depends on conventional complementarity-determining region (CDR) interactions (including critical CDR3) and V_L-encoded sequences, and is usually of low avidity (K_D > 10 mM). In contrast, SAgs depend on apparently framework (FR)-type V_H sequences, and are often of high-avidity

(K_D < 0.1 μM). These findings indicate that superantigenicity and polyreactivity are structurally and functionally distinct, and may be independently expressed by individual antibodies. Also, thyroglobulin might prove to be part of an emerging family of endogenous SAgs, now represented by the hepatic Fv protein and the I/i carbohydrate.[30,49]

DEFINING THE INTERACTION DOMAINS

V_H3

In studies of evolutionary shared framework sequences defining Ig heavy chain families and clans, Schroeder and his colleagues noted the particular conservation of surface-exposed regions, and their potential role in a novel form of antigen-binding outside the classic CDR loop region.[50] In the case of SpA, necessary binding segments of V_H3 include FR1, FR3, and the V_H3-invariant portion of CDR2.[51,52] Comparison of sequence-defined antibodies among gp120 binders and nonbinders is shown in Figure 10.3. The gp120-binding V_H3 antibodies are homologous (compared to the nonbinding V_H1 antibodies) in the FR1 and FR3 V_H3 region, particularly in the surface-exposed beta sheets.[50,53] No similarities in heavy chain V_κ family or CDR motifs were observed among the group of antibodies (not shown). Similarly, domain swap experiments using the NANUC-2 antibody thus far implicate FR1, FR3, and CDR2; different CDR3 segments are permissive (Neshat, Goodglick, Braun, unpublished). The I/i carbohydrate antigen is avidly bound by many antibodies using the VH4-34 gene, and this binding is mediated by FR1 in concert with suitable CDR3 segments.[54] This latter study raises the possibility that FR1 facilitates proper conformation of the CDR3 loop and does not resolve whether FR1 contributes contact residues to ligand binding. The same reservation is appropriately expressed for the existing data on SpA interaction by V_H3. Hence, the structural premise of a framework patch of contact residues for V_H SAgs will probably require more direct analysis of ligand-V_H interaction, such as reporter group analysis[55] or X-ray crystallography.

gp120

The envelope glycoprotein of HIV-1 is composed of a noncovalently linked heterodimer, consisting of gp120 and the transmembrane gp41 protein.[56,57] These are derived from a single gp160 precursor by proteolysis during Golgi processing, and incorporated into the budding virion after trafficking to common plasma membrane sites. HIV gp120 is a heavy glycosylated, 411 amino acid protein composed of five conserved regions (C1-C5) and five variable regions (V1-V5) distinguished by pronounced strain-specific mutation and variation. CD4 is the primary cell-surface receptor for gp120, interacting with a discontinuous gp120 domain which includes amino acid residues in the C3 and C4 regions. Regions of gp120 and gp41 are necessary for the process of virus cell fusion and cellular tropism, including V3, the predominant antibody neutralizing domain.[55]

HIV gp120 from a number of strains display binding activity for V_H3 Ig, indicating that the interaction is more likely to involve constant region vs. variable region domains.[21] A large panel of gp160 peptides were used to identify the epitope responsible for the SAg activity of gp120.[23] Peptides were tested in a competition binding assay which measured the inhibition of V_H3 Ig binding to HIV-1_{SF2} gp120. Comparison of the active peptides from overlapping and distinct regions of gp120, and evaluation of a mutant peptide series, revealed a minimal decamer motif: Lys-n-Asn/Ile-x-x-n-x-Gln/Ser-p-Val (n, nonpolar; p, polar, x, unrestricted). It is interesting that different V_H3 antibodies displayed distinct fine specificities for the decamer sequence. This observation may indicate that fixed motif sequences interact with the most conserved amino acids in the V_H3 binding domain, while other residues (e.g., positions 2, 6, 9) contact

Framework 1

	====	====	====	====	==4.1==	====	====	====								====	====	====	====	==4.2==	====	====	====							
VH3-30 >	gln	val	gln	leu	val	glu	ser	gly	gly	gly	val	val	gln	pro	gly	arg	ser	leu	arg	leu	ser	cys	ala	ala	ser	gly	phe	thr	phe	ser
TAAO >	glu	...	lys	...	glu	...	...	...	...	...	leu	...	...	...	...	gly	...	met	lys	...	...	...	...	thr	...	...	...	...	...	...
NANUC1 >				...	glu	gln	...	...	...	...	...	...	...	...	...	lys	...	...	...	...	...	...	...	...	...	...	...	...	...	arg
NANUC2 >				...	glu	...	...	...	...	...	...	...	...	...	...	lys	...	...	...	...	...	...	...	...	...	...	...	...	...	arg
SMI >	...	...	...	...	...	gln	...	...	ala	glu	...	lys	lys	...	...	ser	...	val	lys	val	...	...	lys	...	...	...	gly	...	...	...
P313 >				...	glu	gln	...	...	ala	glu	...	lys	lys	...	...	ser	...	val	lys	val	...	...	arg	...	...	...	gly	...	...	asn
TSU7 >	...	...	...	...	gln	gln	...	...	ala	glu	leu	met	lys	...	...	ala	...	val	lys	ile	...	...	lys	...	thr	...	tyr	...	...	...
									vh3																		vh3			
									xxx									xxx												
									SpA										SpA								SpA			

Framework 3

	====	====	====	==4-4==	====	====	====	====				====	====	====	==4-3==	====	====	====													
VH3-30 >	arg	phe	thr	ile	ser	arg	asp	asn	ser	lys	asn	thr	leu	tyr	leu	gln	met	asn	ser	leu	arg	ala	glu	asp	thr	ala	val	tyr	tyr	cys	ala
TAAO >	...	...	...	...	...	...	...	asp	...	...	arg	arg	val	...	...	...	...	...	thr	...	...	...	...	...	...	gly	ile	...	...	...	thr
NANUC1 >	...	...	...	...	...	...	...	lys	...	...	...	...	...	...	...	...	...	...	...	...	...	...	...	...	...	...	...	...	...	...	...
NANUC2 >	...	...	phe	...	...	...	...	...	...	...	...	...	...	...	...	...	leu	...	...	...	...	...	...	...	...	...	...	...	...	...	...
SMI >	...	val	...	...	thr	ala	...	lys	...	thr	ser	...	...	...	met	glu	leu	ser	...	...	...	ser	...	...	...	...	...	...	...	...	...
P313 >	...	val	...	...	thr	ala	...	glu	...	thr	gly	...	ala	...	met	glu	leu	ser	...	...	...	ser	glu	...	...	...	ile	...	...	...	...
TSU7 >	lys	ala	...	phe	thr	ala	...	thr	...	ser	...	...	ala	...	met	...	leu	ser	...	...	thr	ser	...	...	ser	...	...	...	...	...	...
		vh3		vh3		vh3											vh3												vh3		
		xxx															xxx														
		SpA						SpA					SpA																		

Fig. 10.3. Framework region sequences of V_H3 gp120-binding and V_H1 non-binding antibodies. Binders include TAAO, NANUC-1, NANUC-2. Non-binders include TSU7, SMI, and P313. The beta strands are indicated using the Padlan nomenclature[68]. Notations: xxx, important for CDR conformation;[47,53] vh3, invariant residues unique to human vh3 and mouse vh3c;[50] SpA, sequences present in SpA binders and unique to V_H3.[51-52]

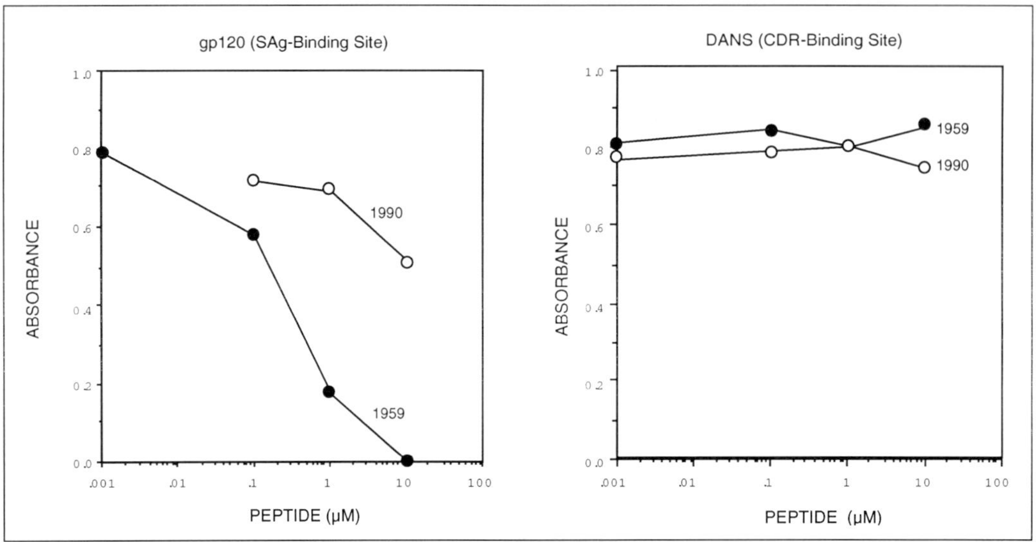

Fig. 10.4. Superantigen peptide 1959 competes for gp120 but not hapten binding. TAAO-IgA (0.1 μg/mL) was equilibrated overnight with peptides at the indicated concentrations, then reacted with ELISA wells coated either with gp120 (left) or DANS-BSA (right). 1959, gp120 C2 domain peptide bearing the decamer superantigen sequence; 1990, negative control gp120 C3 domain peptide.

divergent V_H3 residues in the domain. The C3 decamer peptide (KWNDTLRQIV) may be the optimal available sequence, because it shows the greatest specificity for V_H3 binding under conditions which minimize detection of polyreactive V_H3 activity.

It remains uncertain whether this peptide motif represents the sequence displayed by gp120 for V_H3 interaction. The motif recurs in the C2, C3, and C4 regions of gp120; among them, the relevant C4 segment is documented to be surface-exposed, based on its role in binding to CD4 and certain monoclonal antibodies. No suitable reagents have been available to test whether or not this is the case for the other candidate segments. It also should be appreciated that these peptide competitors are not likely to adopt a free solution conformation analogous to one assumed in the native gp120 protein and may even interact with V_H3 as serendipitous mimetic ligands. Site directed mutagenesis of these candidate sites is thus necessary to establish which if any are involved in V_H3 interaction.

One use of these peptides is to compare the location of gp120 binding with respect to the conventional antigen binding site. We selected TAAO for detailed study, because it was isolated as a conventional murine hybridoma specific for the DANS hapten (dimethylamino-napthalene-sulphonate). Since the "CDR" binding site of this antibody has a defined ligand, this allowed us to compare binding at the anti-DANS (CDR) versus gp120 (SAg-binding) sites. As shown in Figure 10.4, gp120 binding was efficiently competed with the superantigenic decamer peptide (1960, C2 domain), but not by an irrelevant gp120 peptide (1990, C3 domain). In contrast, DANS binding was unaffected by either peptide. Reciprocally, DANS-binding activity was competed with soluble DANS-BSA, but not gp120 or BSA alone (not shown). These findings provide additional evidence that the putative FR patch (gp120 binding site) is functionally and physically distinct from CDR patch (classic antigen-binding site).

It is also notable that these peptides do not inhibit V_H3-SpA interaction. This might be taken as evidence that the peptides interact with V_H3 in a site distinct from that recognized by SpA. However, technical factors, such as the higher avidity of SpA vs. gp120 binding of V_H3 Ig, might account for this observation.

IMMUNOBIOLOGY OF THE GP120-V_H3 INTERACTION: GP120-BINDING AS A STABLE POLYMORPHIC TRAIT

Since HIV gp120 is a membrane Ig ligand for a significant fraction of B cells, it should produce the antigen receptor signaling required for the normal program of B cell activation. Evidence for this prediction was first obtained in vitro, when it was observed that gp120 replaced anti-Ig in the Ig secretory activation of V_H3 B cells (IgG secretion with IL-4/anti-CD40). Specificity for V_H3 B cell activation was reflected in the preferential response of D12 (V_H3) idiotope vs. IV.6 (a $V_\kappa III$ idiotope with low V_H3 family use).[21] Similarly, during the early stages of natural HIV infection, the abundance of gp120 and T cell help would be expected to selectively increase the abundance of B cells and serum Ig from the V_H3 subset. This prediction was confirmed in a cross-sectional clinical study of subjects with HIV infection.[22] Thus, B cells expressing the D12 V_H3 idiotope were increased in frequency 3-fold in HIV seropositive versus seronegative groups. This was selective for the D12 population, since total B cell numbers were identical in the two groups. A 4-fold increase in levels of serum anti-gp120 D12 IgM was also observed. This change was again selective for V_H3, since the prevalence of D12 anti-gp120 dropped later in disease, concordant with the decline in D12 B cells, and discordant with the persistently high titers of anti-gp120 in this population. Similar results were reported by Zouali and colleagues using V_H family-specific quantitative PCR.[30]

Could this stimulatory effect of HIV infection be a factor in the remarkable rate of B cell lymphoproliferation also associated with HIV infection? At present, no large study of Ig V gene use in HIV-associated lymphoma has been reported, although evidence from one group indicates that V_H3 representation may be deficient (T Kipps, personal communication). If so, one explanation might be preferential depletion of V_H3 B cells later in HIV infection, which may affect the pool of V_H3 B cells available for neoplastic outgrowth.[17] In addition, other immunologic abnormalities and opportunistic infection with transforming viruses (e.g., Epstein-Barr virus, or EBV) are likely to predominate as factors in HIV lymphomagenesis.[26,27]

Ig V_H3 predominance has been observed in sequence analysis of gp120-reactive B cell monoclonals and phage-display selectants derived from individuals with natural HIV infection.[24,25] However, these observations do not permit assessment of this selective V_H3 gene. Since only a minority of V_H3 antibodies express this gp120-binding activity, further analysis of this issue requires delineation of those B cells expressing the hallmarks of gp120 superantigen-binding (sensitivity to decamer inhibition, and sequence features of the pertinent V_H3 family subset).

We have attempted to model the effect of HIV infection in SCID-hu-PBL mice.[58] In this system, certain HIV-1 strains (e.g., SF162) are pathogenic, resulting in depletion of the engrafted human CD4 T lymphocytes, while others are nonpathogenic (e.g., SF33). These differences reflect specific tropic or cytopathic properties of the viral strains, since they are not correlated with viral load. Our question was whether this system might model either V_H3 B cell activation or depletion during HIV infection. The results of two such experiments are shown in Table 10.3. SF162 infection severely reduced all serum Ig activities, indicating a global effect on B cell activity (perhaps related to the depletion of helper T cell function). In contrast, SF33 preserved serum Ig activities, and one experiment reflected a selective increase in anti-gp120 (vs. total) IgM.

Where do these gp120-binding V_H3 antibodies come from? A recent study has revealed that the abundance of the gp120-binding V_H3 family subset in serum IgM and IgG of HIV in nonimmune individuals is a polymorphic trait (Townsley-Fuchs et al, *op. cit.*). Among a group of 75 individuals, anti-gp120 activity for both IgM

Table 10.3. Effect of HIV-1 infection on V_H3 serum IgM production in SCID-hu-PBL mice

Group	Total IgM (μg/ml)	anti-gp120 IgM (units/ml)	anti-SpA IgM (units/ml)*
Expt. 1			
Mock	285 + 85	43 + 7	330 + 65
SF33	340 + 120	20 + 5	350 + 95
SF162	50 + 10	7 + 3	40 + 5
Expt. 2			
Mock	100 + 40	1.0 + 0.3	nd
SF33	220 + 80	4.0 + 2.0	nd
SF162	50 + 15	< 0.1	nd

SCID mice were reconstituted with 5 x 10^6 blood lymphocytes and inoculated with 100 tissue culture infectious doses of HIV-1 virus as described in ref. 58. Three weeks after infection (corresponding to the period of CD4 T cell depletion in SF162), blood samples were collected and assayed for the indicated antibody activities (total IgM, "V_H3" IgM [modified SpA-binding], and anti-gp120 IgM). Serum Ig activities were preserved by SF33, but were severely reduced by SF162. No consistent selective effect of infection was observed on V_H3 or anti-gp120 IgM, compared to the response of total IgM. (*) One unit is calculated by regression analysis of absorbance produced by 10 μg/ml of a mixed donor preparation of purified serum IgM (Ref. 22).

and IgG ranged 40-fold, and was uncorrelated with total isotype levels. Moreover, this trait was stable when monitored in 16 individuals followed for 4 months or longer. This observation may be related to the stable predominance of B cell clonality due to the combined action of genetic traits and the equilibrium achieved after antigen-driven clonal competition.[18,20,47,59] In fact, this polymorphism is most simply explained by the positive selection of the natural V_H3 "anti-gp120" repertoire by a crossreactive antigen. An appealing structural class of such antigens are capsular polysaccharides, because of the highly restricted V family and gene use typically observed for B cell responses to these molecules. An elegant precedent is the remarkable predominance of V_H3-23 and V_H3-15 gene usage in the human response to *H. influenzae* capsular polysaccharide (bearing the phosphoribosyl phosphate repeating unit).[47,60,61]

ROLE OF NATURAL V_H3 ANTI-GP120 ANTIBODIES IN RESISTANCE TO HIV INFECTION

The gp120 subunit of the envelope glycoprotein is the major target for neutralizing antibodies to HIV. These antibodies fall into two categories, specific either for the V3 loop or conformational determinants affecting CD4 binding, and are typically strain-specific.[62] Conversely, anti-HIV antibodies under certain circumstances enhance infection by HIV in vitro, in most cases by a complement-dependent mechanism.[63] The gp120 epitope specificities of enhancing antibodies were diverse, since most anti-peptide antisera were enhancing (excluding only those recognizing the V3 loop). It is likely that targeting of virus by this mechanism to macrophages and follicular dendritic cells (FDCs) is important for propagation of the infection in vivo.[64,65] Finally, the apparently narrow repertoire of the anti-HIV antibody response is perceived as an obstacle to effective natural or vaccine-elicited anti-viral immunity. The mechanism of this repertoire restriction is uncertain, but has been attributed to processes such as antigenic sin and molecular mimicry.

These mechanisms also pertain to the subset of naturally-occurring subset of gp120-binding antibodies. In particular, we have been curious to determine whether these preexisting antibodies influence the success of transmission in an individual first encountering HIV. In principle, such antibodies may produce their effect by opsonizing virus and promoting its destruction by cellular and noncellular mechanisms. It is also notable that nonimmune serum fixes complement to gp120 and HIV-1 virions by the classical pathway, presumably through action of this class of antibodies.[66,67]

We have addressed this question through an epidemiologic project of 240 subjects selected from the NIH Multicenter AIDS Cohort Study (Townsley-Fuchs et al, *op. cit.*). Initially seronegative MACS subjects were grouped by statistical criteria into those who were highly resistant or susceptible to infection, based on their levels of high risk behavior, and duration of time to seroconversion. Archival pre-seroconversion sera (> 2 years prior to infection) were tested for IgM and IgG binding activity for two putative V_H3 SAgs (gp120 and modified SpA) and a conventional antigen (tetanus toxoid). It should be noted that the stable polymorphism observed for anti-gp120 V_H3 levels among individuals is a critical element permitting this experimental design.

We observed that preimmune gp120-binding IgG was decreased in susceptible men by 40% and 30%, compared to resistant and control groups, respectively. This finding was specific, since significant differences were not observed for IgG levels in these populations to modified SpA or tetanus toxoid. Analysis of risk-group quartiles indicated that increasing levels of these antibodies conferred an odds-ratio of 5.46 for resistance to infection. Since no other biologic host factors have been defined to play a role in HIV transmission, this finding presents the first example of such a protective host factor.

DISCUSSION

This review has related the current state of knowledge about the interaction of HIV-1 gp120 with V_H3^+ Igs. Structurally, gp120 appears to interact with V_H3 in the same region utilized by SpA (FR1, CDR2, FR3), although sequence heterogeneity among different V_H3 antibodies influence the avidity of the interaction. A decamer peptide motif has been identified which mimics the epitope of gp120 involved in V_H3 binding. This reagent has proved useful in distinguishing "superantigen" from other modes of antibody-antigen interactions. HIV gp120 can serve as a membrane Ig ligand for V_H3 B cell activation in vitro, and some B cell changes in HIV infection indicate that a similar ligand-specific selection of V_H3 B cells may occur in vivo. Confirmation of an infection-associated B cell SAg effect is warranted, and will especially benefit from development of a suitable model animal systems.

The most striking biologic correlate of V_H3-gp120 interaction is its apparent role in resistance to HIV transmission. We envision that the virus is opsonized by such antibodies and delivered to a variety of cell types suboptimal or unsuitable for viral propagation in the new host (Fig. 10.5). If the size of the viral inoculum is near the threshold for successful transmission, then even a moderate reduction in virus delivery to suitable target cells may have a significant impact on the rate of transmission. Accordingly, individuals with low levels of these antibodies would be at greater risk for successful viral transmission, as observed experimentally.

The model highlights several gaps in our knowledge. What Ig compartment plays the protective role: Lumenal IgA? Interstitial IgG or IgM in mucosal or lymphoid tissue? What is the mechanism of protection: Complement destruction of virus? Redirection of virus to non-T cells? One favorable property of the V_H3-gp120 interaction is that the gp120 sequence involved in V_H3 binding is conserved among strains, and thus could confer broad protection: Is there an effective or safe way to augment these antibody levels? Can they be elicited in the correct anatomic compartment? Progress on these issues will determine whether this mechanism plays a significant pathogenic role in HIV transmission, and whether it could be a target of preventative therapy. Such information

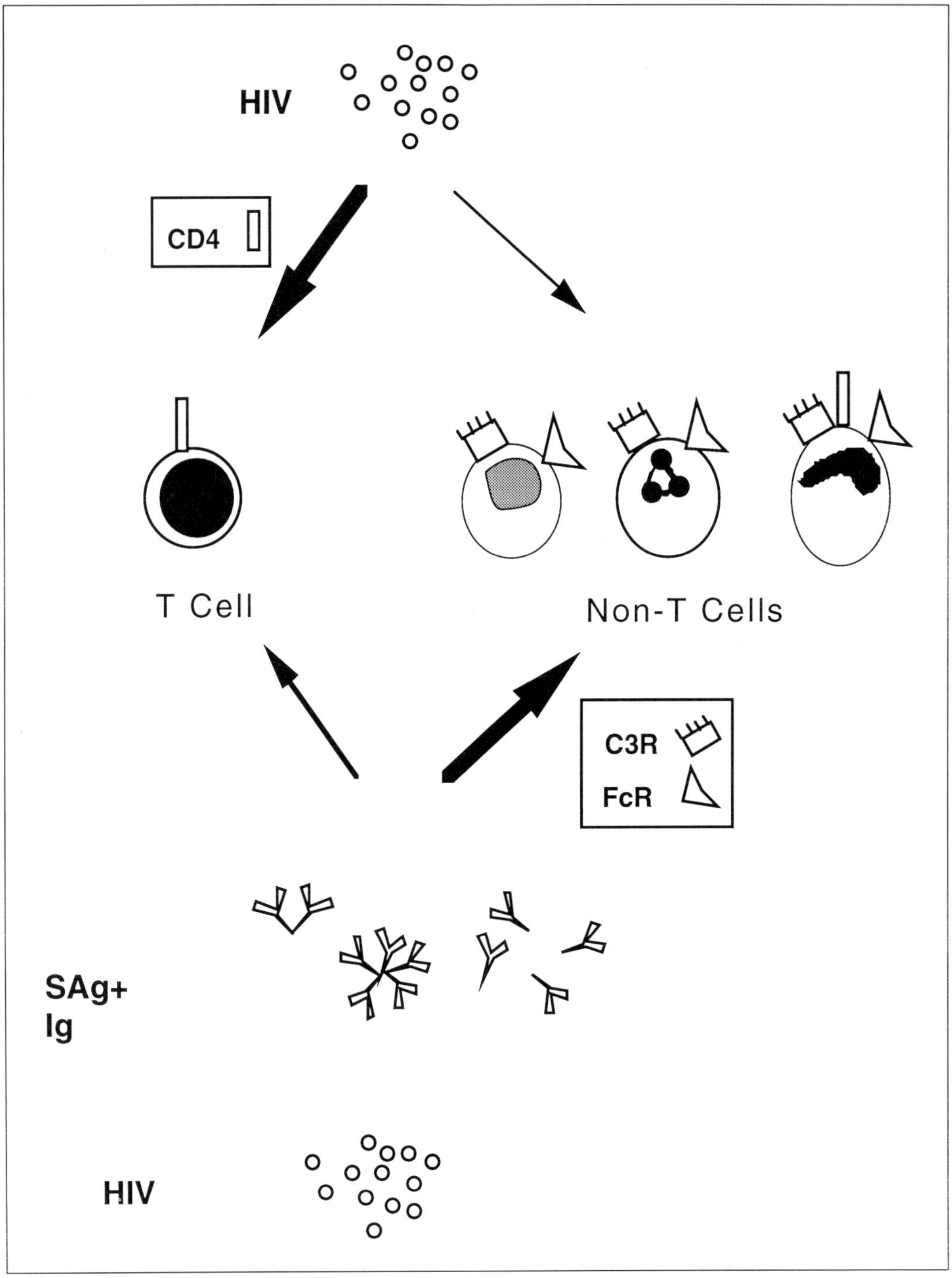

Fig. 10.5. Model of the effect of V_H3 anti-gp120 on transmission of HIV infection.

is also likely to shed light on other potential roles of SAg binding in host-pathogen interaction.

Acknowledgments

We are grateful to our colleagues for their role in phases of this work: Karin Reimann, and Drs. Linda Berberian, Roger Detels, Janis Giorgi, Thomas Kipps, Otoniel Martinez-Maza, Sherie Morrison, Nora Sun, and Yadira Valles-Ayoub. We thank our colleagues for reagents: Drs. James Berenson, Mary Territo, Carlos Barbas III, Andrew Saxon, Mark Eggena, Marshall Posner, and Susan Zolla-Pazner. Peptides and anti-gp120 antibodies were obtained through the AIDS Research and Reference Reagent Program, NIH. HIV-1 gp120 was a generous gift of Dr. Kathelyn Steimer, Chiron Corporation. This work was supported by NIH CA12800, AI38545, the University-wide AIDS Research Program, the Margaret E. Early Trust, and the Jonsson Comprehensive Cancer Center.

References

1. Sheppard HW, Ascher MS. The natural history and pathogenesis of HIV infection. Annu Rev Microbiol 1992; 46:533-64.
2. Imberti L, Sottini A, Bettinardi A et al. Selective depletion in HIV infection of T cells that bear specific T cell receptor Vβ sequences. Science 1991; 254:860-2.
3. Groux H, Torpier G, Monte D et al. Activation-induced death by apoptosis in $CD4^+$ T cells from human immunodeficiency virus-infected asymptomatic individuals. J Exp Med 1991; 175:331-40.
4. Siliciano RF, Lawton T, Knall C et al. Analysis of host-virus interactions in AIDS with anti-gp120 T cell clones: effect of HIV sequence variation and a mechanism for $CD4^+$ cell depletion. Cell 1988; 54:561-75.
5. Said JW. AIDS-related lymphadenopathies. Seminars in Diagnostic Pathology 1988; 5:365-75.
6. Martinez-Maza O, Crabb E, Mitsuyasu RT et al. Infection with the human immunodeficiency virus (HIV) is associated with an in vivo increase in B lymphocyte activation and immaturity. J Immunol 1987; 138:3720-4.
7. Levine AM. Acquired immunodeficiency syndrome-related lymphoma. Blood 1992; 80:8-20.
8. Amadori A, Zamarchi R, Ciminale V et al. HIV-1-specific B cell activation: A major constituent of spontaneous B cell activation during HIV-1 infection. J Immunol 1989; 143:2146-52.
9. Shirai A, Cosentino M, Leitman-Klinman SF et al. Human immunodeficiency virus infection induces both polyclonal and virus-specific B cell activation. J Clin Invest 1992; 89:561-66.
10. Reickmann P, Poli G, Fox CH et al. Recombinant gp120 specifically enhances tumor necrosis factor-alpha production and Ig secretion in B lymphocytes from HIV-infected individuals but not from seronegative donors. J Immunol 1991; 147:2922-77.
11. Chirmule N, Kalyanaraman VS, Lederman S et al. HIV-gp160-induced T cell-dependent B cell differentiation: Role of T cell-B cell activation molecule and IL-6. J Immunol 1993; 150:2478-86.
12. Nair MPN, Pottahil R, Heimer EP et al. Immunoregulatory activities of human immunodeficiency virus (HIV) proteins: effect of HIV recombinant and synthetic peptides on immunoglobulin synthesis and proliferative responses by normal lymphocytes. Proc Natl Acad Sci USA 1988; 85:6498-501.
13. Yarchoan R, Redfield R, Broder S. Mechanisms of B cell activation in patients with acquired immunodeficiency syndrome and related disorders. J Clin Invest 1986; 78:439-48.
14. Ballet J, Sulcebe G, Couderc L et al. Impaired anti-pneumococcal antibody response in patients with AIDS-related persistent generalized lymphadenopathy. Clin Exp Immunol 1987; 68:479-87.
15. Terpstra FG, Al BJM, Roos MTL et al. Longitudinal study of leukocyte functions in homosexual men seroconverted for HIV: rapid and persistent loss of B cell function after HIV infection. Eur J Immunol 1989; 19:667-73.
16. Reddy MM, Goetz RG, Gorman JM et al. Human immunodeficiency virus type 1 infection of homosexual men is accompanied

by a decrease in circulating B cells. J AIDS 1991; 4:428-34.

17. Berberian L, Valles-Ayoub Y, Sun N et al. A VH clonal deficit in human immunodeficiency virus-positive individuals reflects a B cell maturational arrest. Blood 1991; 78:175-9.
18. Matsuda F, Shin EK, Nagaoka H, et al. Structure and physical map of 64 variable segments in the 3' 0.8-megabase region of the human immunoglobulin heavy-chain locus. Nature Genetics 1993; 3:88-94.
19. Guigou V, Cuisinier A, Tonnelle C et al. Human immunoglobulin VH and VK repertoire revealed by in situ hybridization. Mol Immunol 1990; 27:935-40.
20. Stewart AK, Huang C, Stollar BD et al. High-frequency representation of a single VH gene in the expressed human B cell repertoire. J Exp Med 1993; 177:409-18.
21. Berberian LS, Goodglick LA, Kipps TA et al. VH3 Ig Gene Products: Natural Ligands for HIV gp120. Science 1993; 261:1588-91.
22. Berberian LS, Shukla J, Jefferis R et al. Effect of HIV infection on VH3 (D12 idiotope) B cells in vivo. J AIDS 1994; 7:641-6.
23. Goodglick L, Zevit N, Neshat MS et al. Mapping the Ig superantigen-binding site of HIV-1 gp120. J Immunol 1995; 155: 5151-9.
24. Barbas CFI, Collet TA, Amberg W et al. Molecular profile of an antibody response to HIV-1 as probed by combinatorial libraries. J Mol Biol 1993; 230:812-23.
25. David D, Goossens D, Desgranges C et al. Molecular characterization of human monoclonal antibodies specific for several HIV proteins: Analysis of the VH3 family expression. Immunol Lett 1995; 47:107-12.
26. Monroe JG, Silberstein LE. HIV-mediated B lymphocyte activation and lymphomagenesis. J Clin Immunol 1995; 15:61-8.
27. Andris JS, Capra JD. The molecular structure of human antibodies specific for the human immunodeficiency virus. J Clin Immunol 1995; 15:17-26.
28. Kohler H, Muller S, Nara PL. Deceptive imprinting in the immune response against HIV-1. Immunol Today 1994; 15:475-8.
29. Goodglick LA, Braun J. Revenge of the microbes: Superantigens of the T of B cell lineage. Am J Pathol 1994; 144:623-36.
30. Zouali M. B cell superantigens: Implications for selection of the human antibody repertoire. Immunol Today 1995; 16:399-405.
31. Goodglick L, Aldrovandi G, Zack JA et al. HIV-1 gp120, an immunoglobulin superantigen. In:Tomonari, K., ed. Viral Superantigens. Boca Raton: CRC Press, 1996: in press.
32. Pantaleo G, Fauci A. Tracking HIV during disease progression. Curr Opinion Immunol 1994; 6:600-5.
33. Eggena ME, Vidrich A, Targan SR et al. Phage display cloning and characterization of an immunogenetic marker (pANCA) in ulcerative colitis. J Immunol 1996; in press.
34. Smith RI, Coloma MJ, Morrison SL. Addition of a mu-tailpiece to IgG results in polymeric antibodies with enhanced effector functions including complement-mediated cytolysis by IgG4. J Immunol 1995; 154:2226-36.
35. Silverman GJ, Sasano M, Wormsley SB. Age-associated changes in binding of human B lymphocytes to a VH3-restricted unconventional bacterial antigen. J Immunol 1993; 151:5840-55.
36. Sasano M, Burton DR, Silverman GJ. Molecular selection of human antibodies with an unconventional bacterial B cell antigen. J Immunol 1993; 151:5822-39.
37. Lydyard PM, Quartey-Papafio RP, Bröker BM et al. The antibody repertoire of early human B cells. III. Expression of cross-reactive idiotopes characteristic of certain rheumatoid factors and identifying VkappaIII, VHI, and VHIII gene family products. Scand J Immunol 1990; 32:709-16.
38. Kasaian MT, Ikematsu H, Casali P. Identification and analysis of a novel human surface $CD5^-$ B lymphocyte subset producing natural antibodies. J Immunol 1992; 148:2690-702.
39. Harindranath N, Goldfarb IS, Ikematsu H et al. Complete sequence of the genes encoding the VH and VL regions of low- and high-affinity monoclonal IgM and IgA1 rheumatoid factors produced by $CD5^+$ B cells from a rheumatoid arthritis patient. Int Immunol 1992; 3:865-75.

40. Casali P, Notkins AL. Probing the human B cell repertoire with EBV: Polyreactive antibodies and CD5+ B lymphocytes. Annu Rev Immunol 1989; 7:513-35.
41. Newkirk MM, Rauch J, Mageed RA et al. Restricted immunoglobulin variable region gene usage by hybridoma rheumatoid factors from patients with systemic lupus erythematosus and rheumatoid arthritis. Mol Immunol 1993; 30:255-63.
42. Sanz I, Casali P, Thomas JW et al. Nucleotide sequences of eight human natural autoantibody VH regions reveals apparent restricted use of VH families. J Immunol 1989; 142:4054-61.
43. Martin T, Duffy SF, Carson DA et al. Evidence for somatic selection of natural autoantibodies. J Exp Med 1992; 175:983-91
44. Ichiyoshi Y, Casali P. Analysis of the structural correlates for antibody polyreactivity by multiple reassortments of chimeric human immunoglobulin heavy and light chain V segments. J Exp Med 1994; 180:885-95.
45. Crouzier R, Martin T, Pasquali J. Heavy chain variable region, light chain variable region, and heavy chain CDR3 influences on the mono- and polyreactivity and on the affinity of human monoclonal rheumatoid factors. J Immunol 1995; 154:4526-35.
46. Adib-Conquy M, Gilbert M, Christodoulou C, Avrameas S. Reactivity and structure of a mouse anti-F(ab')2 IgM. Comparison of its variable region sequences with those of a structurally close polyreactive natural IgM. Mol Immunol 1994; 31:555-62.
47. Vargas-Madrazo E, Lara-Ochoa F, Almagro JC. Canonical structure repertoire of the antigen-binding site of immunoglobulins suggests strong geometrical restrictions associated to the mechanism of immune recognition. J Mol Biol 1995; 254:497-504.
48. Cheung SC, Takeda S, Notkins AL. Both VH and VL chains of polyreactive IgM antibody are required for polyreactivity: Expression of Fab in Escherichia coli. Clin Exp Immunol 1995; 101:383-86.
49. Silverman GJ, Roben P, Bouvet J et al. Superantigen properties of a human sialoprotein involved in gut-associated immunity. J Clin Invest 1995; 96:417-26.
50. Kirkham PM, Mortari F, Newton JA et al. Immunoglobulin VH clan and family identity predicts variable domain structure and may influence antigen binding. EMBO J 1992; 11:603-9.
51. Randen I, Potter KN, Li Y et al. Complementarity-determining region 2 is implicated in the binding of staphylococcal protein A to human immunoglobulin VHIII variable regions. Eur J Immunol 1993; 23:2682-6.
52. Hillson JL, Karr NS, Oppliger IR et al. The structural basis of germline-encoded VH3 immunoglobulin binding to staphylococcal protein A. J Exp Med 1993; 178:331-6.
53. Saul FA, Poljak RJ. Structural patterns at residue positions 9, 18, 67 and 82 in the VH framework regions of human and murine immunoglobulins. J Mol Biol 1993; 230:15-20.
54. Li YC, Spellerberg MB, Stevenson FK et al. The II binding specificity of human VH4-34 (VH4-21) encoded antibodies is determined by both VH framework region 1 and complementarity determining region 3. J Mol Biol 1996; 256:577-89.
55. Hubbell WL, Altenbach C. Investigation of structure and dynamics in membrane proteins using site-directed spin labeling. Curr Opinion Struct Biol 1994; 4:566-73..
56. Levy JA. Pathogenesis of human immunodeficiency virus infection. Microbiol. Rev 1993; 57:183-245.
57. Moore JP, Sattentau QJ, Wyatt R et al. Mapping the topology of the human immunodeficiency virus surface glycoprotein gp120 with a panel of monoclonal antibodies. J Virol 1994; 68:469-84.
58. Mosier DE, Gulizia RJ, MacIsaac PD. Rapid loss of CD4+ T cells in human-PBL-SCID mice by noncytopathic HIV isolates. Science 1993; 260:689-92.
59. Fish S, Zenowich E, Fleming M et al. Molecular analysis of original antigenic sin. I. Clonal selection, somatic mutation, and isotype switching during a memory B cell response. J Exp Med 1989; 170: 1191-1209.
60. Bona C. Molecular characteristics of antipolysaccharide antibodies. Springer Semin Immunopathol 1993; 15:103-18.
61. Adderson EE, Shackelford PG, Quinn A et al. Restricted immunoglobulin VH us-

age and VDJ combinations in the human response to Haemophilus influenzae type b capsular polysaccharide. Nucleotide sequences of monospecific anti-Haemophilus antibodies and polyspecific antibodies cross-reacting with self antigens. J Clin Invest 1993; 91:2734-43.
62. Zolla-Pazner S, Gorny MK. Passive immunization for the prevention and treatment of HIV infection. AIDS 1992; 6:1235-47.
63. Burke DS. Human HIV vaccine trials: Does antibody-dependent enhancement pose a genuine risk? Perspect Biol Med 1992; 35:511-30.
64. Spiegel H, Herbst H, Niedobitek G et al. Follicular dendritic cells are a major reservoir for human immunodeficiency virus type 1 in lymphoid tissues facilitating infection of $CD4^+$ T-helper cells. Am J Pathol 1992; 140:15-22.
65. Pantaleo G, Graziosi C, Demarest JF et al. HIV infection is active and progressive in lymphoid tissue during the clinically latent stage of disease. Nature 1993; 362:355-8.
66. Saarloos M, Lint TF, Spear GT. Efficacy of HIV-specific and 'antibody-independent' mechanisms for complement activation by HIV-infected cells. Clin Exp Immunol 1995; 99:189-95.
67. Süsal C, Kirschfink M, Kröpelin M, et al. Complement activation by recombinant HIV-1 glycoprotein gp120. J Immunol 1994; 152:6028-34.
68. Padlan EA. Anatomy of the antibody molecule. Molec Immunol 1994; 31:169-217.

CHAPTER 11

Superantigens and the Versatility of HIV-Mediated B Cell Interactions

Saoussen Karray, Laure Juompan and Moncef Zouali

The immune system has the potential to generate a large repertoire of recognition elements able to interact with the enormous number of environmental antigens and to distinguish self from non-self. This unique discriminating property is mediated by the variable (V) regions of the T cell (TcR) and B cell (BcR) receptors. The V regions of the BcR are composed of three heavy chain (H) genes, {variable (V_H), diversity (D_H) and joining (J_H)}, and of two V light chain (L) genes, V_L and J_L.[1] Generation of a functional immunoglobulin (Ig) molecule is the result of combinatorial assembly whereby these gene segments tissue- and site-specifically rearrange in a temporally ordered fashion during B cell development. For example, D_H-J_H joining occurs at the pre-B cell stage and is followed by V_H-D_HJ_H assembly.[2] In humans, pre-B cells become detectable at about eight weeks of fetal life and assembly of V_L and J_L gene segments occurs at the pre-B to B cell transitional stage and results in the synthesis of a complete Ig molecule that will be displayed on the surface of the B lymphocyte.[3] This VDJ joining plays a key role in diversifying the Ig repertoire, particularly at the level of the third complementarity-determining region (CDR). The diversity of the CDR3, which is critical for antigen binding, relies on use of a relatively limited number of D_H genes that are prone to somatic mutations, on addition of N nucleotides by terminal deoxytransferase, and on insertion of P nucleotides at the ends of V_H, D_H and J_H genes. In contrast to the multiple mechanisms of CDR3 diversity, only somatic mutation is involved in generating CDR1 and CDR2 diversity.

In conventional antigen binding, the antibody paratope is formed by the combination of the six CDRs, three from the heavy chain and three from the light chain. There is, however, an alternate mode of BcR and

TcR interactions with a group of antigens, termed superantigens (SAg), which, in principle, does not require contributions from the CDRs. In contrast to conventional antigens which exhibit a clonal specificity towards B cells, SAg interact primarily with the V_H portion of the Ig molecule and trigger all B cells bearing the appropriate V_H, regardless of the other J_H, D_H, J_L and V_L segments. As there are a limited number of V_H genes, this property results in stimulation of a large proportion of the repertoire.[4] Here, we discuss the implications of B cell SAg interactions with regard to evolutionary organization of the mammalian immune system. We also summarize data on the pathological consequences of SAg-like properties of gp120 of the human immunodeficiency virus (HIV). Since B cell SAg interact with the products of a particular human V_H gene-family, it is useful to first highlight the essential features of the human V_H genes at both the germline and somatic levels.

INTERSPERSION, POLYMORPHISM AND SHUFFLING OF HUMAN V_H GENES

Studies of the V_H locus of different species have revealed that the organization of V_H segments is not evolutionarily conserved. The human gene complex contains approximately 100 V_H segments located on the telomeric portion of the long arm of chromosome 14 with an average of 22 kb per functional V_H gene. Based on nucleotide sequence homology, V_H genes can be classified into seven families, V_H1 to V_H7, with members of each family sharing at least 80% homology.[5,6] Unlike the human V_H locus organization, all V_H segments of the rabbit seem to be members of one highly conserved gene-family,[7] and, in birds, a unique functional gene is diversified by segmental gene conversion with a pool of pseudogenes.[8] In addition to this family-categorization, nucleotide conservation of the first (FR1) and third (FR3) framework regions allows further classification of V_H families into three clans. Clan I includes the V_H1, V_H5 and V_H7 families; clan II encompasses the V_H2, V_H4 and V_H6 families; and clan III contains the V_H3 family.[9] With over 20 V_H3 gene segments, this latter family makes the largest contribution to the functional repertoire, followed by the V_H1 and the V_H4 families.[10,11] In contrast to the murine V_H locus[12] where members of the 14 known families are clustered on chromosome 12, members of human V_H gene families are interspersed throughout the entire locus and even on other chromosomes, including chromosomes 15 and 16. This chromosomal dispersion is not unique to V_H genes. For example, although the approximately 30 functional human D_H gene segments are located between the single V_H6 gene and the six functional J_H segments, a number of human D_H gene segments[13] are also dispersed outside the functional chromosome 14.

The human V_H locus is highly polymorphic with insertions and deletions of multiple V_H segments. For example, the 3-23 gene is duplicated and resides on two distinct loci, both of which are polymorphic with ethnic differences at each,[14] and the 3-30.3 gene results from insertion of a 50 kb between the 3-30 and 4-31 V_H genes. In addition to duplication and deletion, there is evidence for translocation of V_H-containing DNA fragments[15,16] which is reminiscent of what is seen in the human V_κ locus. However, although both the V_H and V_κ loci appear to have evolved by frequent duplication and reorganization, their genomic organizations are quite different. In this respect, the V_H locus was studied recently by mapping DNA fragments hybridized to nonrepetitive intergenic probes, which enables tracing V_H duplication and translocation. By determining the content and the distribution of two repetitive sequences [short interspersed elements (*Alu* repeats) and long interspersed elements (L1 repeats)], these studies showed that the locus underwent recent duplication and dynamic reshuffling of DNA containing V_H segments, and the divergence time of the duplicated V_H segments was estimated to be 30 to 38, 22 to 40, and 55 million years for V3-9/V3-20/V3-43, V3-7/V3-21/V3-48 and V3-13/V3-47P V_H gene segments, respectively.[17] Obviously, these polymorphisms could affect the available repertoire. For example, a vaccine preparation against *Haemophilus influenzae* type b (Hib) induces different immune responses among individuals, and this functional difference could be due to V_H gene polymorphisms.[18,19] In this respect, it would be useful to develop assays to screen for expression of the polymorphic V regions of the anti-Hib antibody repertoire in vaccine recipients.

PHYLOGENETIC CONSERVATION OF V_H3-LIKE GENES

In addition to dominating the antibody repertoire, the V_H3 gene family exhibits a unique evolutionary characteristic. When the evolution of Ig gene families is considered, studies of the human and murine species, which are descendent from lines that diverged some 70 million years ago, revealed that the human V_H3 gene-family is phylogenetically related to the J558 mouse family which is the largest in the murine species.[9] More recently, an analysis of cartilaginous fishes, which are the most distantly related species to humans (they diverged from the line that lead to humans and mice some 450 million years ago) to have an immune system, revealed that the human V_H3 gene-family exhibits the highest sequence homology to V_H families from the horned shark (*Heterodontus francisci*), the little skate (*Raja erinacea*) and the nurse shark (*Ginglymostoma cirratum*).[20] Therefore the V_H3 gene family arose in the earliest stage of the immune system and has been conserved throughout evolution, even though the germline organization of the V_H loci is different in mammals and in cartilaginous fishes.[21]

OVER-EXPRESSION OF V_H3 GENE MEMBERS

Not only is the V_H3 gene family the most abundant, but, in addition, some of its members are overutilized in the somatic repertoire. If V_H gene use were totally random, one would predict that the utilization of each V_H gene family would depend on its size and that members of a given family might be expressed at an equal frequency. It appears, however, that certain individual V_H genes are used more frequently than others, even at early stages of ontogeny. For example, analysis of V_H-D_H-J_H rearrangements during fetal life revealed that the J_H3 and the D_HQ52 gene segments are preferentially rearranged compared to rearrangements of the adult.[22,23] Similar studies of V_H3 gene segments isolated from adult B cells showed that the 3-23 V_H gene, also called V_H26, is frequently used.[24,25] From such studies, it seems clear that the expression of V_H genes is independent of their chromosomal location. For instance, some of the V_H3 genes that are frequently expressed in early ontogeny are located at a distal position to the J_H locus, while the J_H-proximal V_H5 gene member is not expressed in the fetal repertoire. It is likely therefore that a number of factors govern selection of individual V_H genes, including their number in the genome. For example, duplication of some genes in some haplotypes may result in their overexpression.

ANTIBODIES TO PATHOGENS USE PREDOMINANTLY V_H3 GENES

Until recently, studies of human antibody V regions were essentially restricted to the fetal B cell repertoire, to autoantibodies and to malignant B cells, leaving the normal adult immune repertoire less explored. As there is a restricted usage of V_H genes during early development and in the adult preimmune repertoire, characterization of the V genes expressed in response to pathogens is important to understand maturation and diversification of the repertoire. Only recently attention was turned to analysis of the secondary immune response to pathogens, including viruses of the herpes family (Herpes simplex virus and Varicella-zoster virus), the surface antigens of Hepatitis B virus, the rabies vaccine, *Haemophilus influenzae* type b and *Bordetella pertussis*. From several studies, it appears that different antibodies to the same pathogen can use different putative V_H germline genes. Conversely, the same putative germline gene can be used by antibodies to different pathogens. This overlap may suggest that the potentially functional V_H gene repertoire is smaller than the structural repertoire. As seen in the total adult repertoire where some genes are overexpressed, there are also examples of individual gene segments or gene families being preferentially utilized in response to certain pathogens. Not unexpectedly, the V_H genes expressed by antibodies to pathogens exhibit somatic mutations in their CDRs and FRs and have high replacement/silent mutation (R/S) ratios typical of secondary immune responses with amino acid changes that represent a footprint of an antigen-driven process. The families expressed in the antibody repertoire to pathogens are those found in the unselected adult B cell repertoire, with the V_H3 gene family dominating the repertoire, and some members being more frequently utilized. The V_H1 and the V_H4 families are equally expressed, and the V_H5 gene family is rarely encountered.[18,26-29] Here, it is of note that some V_H genes initially isolated from tumor cells were also found in response to foreign antigens,[30] including a somatically mutated V_H6 gene segment of an antibody to *Bordetella pertussis*,[29] and a V_H5 gene family member expressed by a monoclonal anti-idiotypic antibody to rabies vaccine.[26]

Thus, the V_H gene pool utilized by antibodies to exogenous antigens overlaps with that of fetal B cells, autoantibodies and malignant B cells. Remarkably, the V_H3 gene-family dominates these repertoires, suggesting that V_H3-like elements have been positively selected during evolution in response to motifs shared by common pathogens. In sharp contrast with what was observed with human immune responses to infectious agents, the repertoire developed in response to HIV does not conform to this V_H3 dominance. Before discussing this biased repertoire, it is necessary to first summarize the alteration of B cell functions seen during HIV infection.

B CELL ABNORMALITIES IN HIV INFECTION

Although B cells are not directly infected by HIV, functional abnormalities of B cells and of humoral responses are common in HIV-infected patients. They include hypergammaglobulinemia, enhanced serum levels of IgG, IgA, IgE and IgM in children, the presence of circulating immune complexes and autoantibodies, and in vitro spontaneous IgG production by circulating lymphocytes.[31,32] The occurrence of oligoclonal Igs ranging from 10 to 45% of those examined has also been reported in HIV-1^+ subjects.[33] In addition, B cell proliferation and Ig production induced in vitro by polyclonal activators, as well as primary responses in vivo, are impaired soon after HIV infection in most patients.[34] The mechanisms causing hyperactivation of the B cell compartment in HIV-1-infected patients have not yet been clarified. Initially, B cell hyperactivation was attributed to frequent infection by B cell activators, such as Epstein-Barr virus (EBV) and cytomegalovirus.[32] Then, the direct B cell-activating role of HIV components was adduced[32] and several viral proteins, as well as the inactivated HIV-1 virus itself, can directly stimulate B cells to proliferate and differentiate into Ig-producing cells.[35] Conversely, some specific HIV-1 glycoproteins may decrease responsiveness of B cells to polyclonal stimulators.[36] This spectrum of B cell abnormalities raises the question of whether HIV alters the mechanisms of selection of the antibody repertoire.

PROBING THE ANTI-HIV ANTIBODY REPERTOIRE BY COMBINATORIAL LIBRARIES

Human anti-HIV monoclonal antibodies can be produced through the combinatorial library technology which is based on the use of an antigen to select antibodies of a desired specificity from a library generated on the surface of a bacteriophage. Parenthetically, in addition to providing a tool to probe antibody diversity to HIV, this approach may allow identification of neutralizing epitopes that could be useful in vaccine design and preparation of reagents for passive immunotherapy. The first phage display library was prepared from the bone marrow of a 31-year-old homosexual male who had been HIV-1-seropositive for six years, but had no symptoms.[37] The library was screened against gp120 of the HIV-$_{LAI}$ strain which is very rare in the USA, and a panel of 36 anti-gp120 Fabs has been derived. Most of them react with a conformational epitope on the CD4 binding site of gp120 from the LAI, SF2 and MN isolates, and some of them are neutralizing in vitro. Their affinity for gp120 was in the order of 10^8 M^{-1}. Sequence analysis of 33 Fabs revealed that the H chains could be organized into seven groups.[38] Each group contained members with identical V_H-D_H-J_H regions, implying common genealogical clonal origins. In addition to this recurrent use, identical or related H chains were found paired with very different L chains. It seems therefore possible that the H chain dictates the antibody specificity. Surprisingly, a significant number of these anti-gp120 antibodies utilize V_H3 genes, thus contrasting with the V_H gene family profile seen with anti-gp120 antibodies obtained by EBV transformation and/or somatic cell fusion (see below). It is therefore important to consider the relevance of these library-derived antibodies to the in vivo immune response. It is thought that human hybridomas result from fusion of activated, but not terminally differentiated B cell populations, and that Epstein-Barr virus immortalizes resting B cells. In phage libraries, the starting material is mRNA, which derives essentially from activated and differentiated B cells. Therefore, this approach essentially probes the repertoire of plasma cell populations. More importantly it does not reveal faithfully the H-L pairings that occur in B cells in vivo. Many of these combinations may not exist in vivo, but rather arise fortuitously during library construction from the random recombination of H and L chains during shuffling of the phage libraries. Therefore only one chain, H or L, could be involved in antigen binding in vivo. Furthermore, it is even possible that neither chain is involved in binding and that only the random combinations bind antigen in vitro. It is, for example, intriguing that in one group of the antibodies generated, the CDR3 region was conserved against a background of considerable variation in the V_H gene segment, a pattern not seen in V_H sequences of antibodies obtained from hybridoma or EBV-transformed anti-HIV B cell clones. Also intriguing is the extensive promiscuity reported for these sequences wherein one or a few H chains are paired with very different L chains. Such a H chain promiscuity has also been described in several reports using combinatorial libraries to other antigens. Other factors may skew the representation of the antibody response as studied by the combinatorial approach, including unequal PCR priming, the presence of restriction sites in certain antibody genes, or the preferential expression of certain antibodies on the phage surface. For example, at least 5% of the total repertoire is lost because of the presence of internal cloning sites. We therefore conclude that, while the combinatorial library technology is useful to generate antibodies for passive immunotherapy, it does not provide a valuable approach to probe the diversity of the antibody repertoire to HIV.

SKEWED V_H GENE-FAMILY UTILIZATION IN MONOCLONAL ANTIBODIES TO HIV

Using EBV-transformed B cell clones and somatic cell hybridomas, the V_H gene repertoire of monoclonal antibodies to HIV antigens was studied in several laboratories.[29,39-46] The D_H gene segments used were found to be rather long, with evidence for D_H-D_H joining, D_H inversions and/or N segment addition.[47] In some cases, the D_H gene segments appear to result from the fusion of an inverted D_H segment to a second D_H segment. P nucleotide additions at the V_H to D_H junctions were also observed in a number of cases. As with other human antibodies, however, complete homology cannot be easily found with known germ-line D_H segments. J_H gene segment utilization also appears to be random (Table 11.1). Comparison of the V_H region sequences of these antibodies to germ-line and fetal V_H sequences revealed a significant load of somatic point mutations, with a high R/S mutation ratio in the CDRs. This high R/S ratio is strongly indicative of positive selection with antigen.[48] However, in some cases the nucleotide changes

Table 11.1. Molecular characteristics of anti-HIV-1 human monoclonal antibodies secreted by B cell clones and hybridomas

Antibody	Target antigen	Epitope	V_H gene: V_H family	V_H gene: Closest germline relative (% Homology)	D_H gene	J_H gene	Ref.
71-31, (γ1)	p24	UKN	V_H1	UKN	DM2	J_H4	29
MD2F4, (γ1/κ)	p25	AA 144-152	V_H1	1-69, (95.2)	DXP5	J_H6	45
GSD2B5B10, (γ1/κ)	p25	UKN	V_H1	1-69, (96.7)	DXP5/DXP'1	J_H3b	45
CE10G11G2, (γ1/λ)	p34	UKN	V_H1	1-2, (92.8)	DIR1	J_H4b	45
K14, (γ1/λ)	gp41	UKN	V_H3	3-23, (89.9)	UKN	J_H4	43
No. 86, (γ1/κ)	gp41	AA586-620	V_H1	1-69, (89.7)	D21/0.5	J_H4	42
120-16, (γ2)	gp41	AA 644-663	V_H4	4-61, (87.2)	UKN	J_H2	29
98-6, (γ2)	gp41	AA 644-663	V_H4	4-39, (85.2)	UKN	J_H4	29
F240, (γ1)	gp41	AA 592-606	V_H3	3-11, (81)	UKN	UKN	46
3D6, (γ1/κ)	gp41	UKN	V_H3	3-9, (97)	UKN	UKN	88
NG3B7, (γ1/κ)	gp41	UKN	V_H3	3-23, (94.83)	DK1/DIR1	J_H3b	45
DZ33, (γ1/λ)	gp41	AA 827-843	V_H3	3-30, (95.5)	DLR2/DIR1	J_H4b	45
DaB2B3, (γ1/κ)	gp41	UKN	V_H1	1-46, (85.5)	DIR2	J_H3b	45
C31, (γ1/κ)	gp120	Conformational	V_H2	2-26, (96.6)	DIR1/DL3	J_H5b	45
T48.16-G8, (γ/κ)	gp120	Conformational	V_H4	4-59, (96.9)	DXP5	J_H3b	45
F172, (γ/λ)	gp120	AA 604-625	V_H4	4-39, (85.5)	DXP'1/D21.9	J_H3	45
15e, (γ1)	gp120	CD4BS*	V_H4	4-39, (93.8)	DXP1	J_H6	44
21h, (γ1)	gp120	CD4BS*	V_H3	3-11, (94.3)	DLR4	J_H5	44
gp13, (γ1/κ)	gp120	CD4BS*	V_H5	V_H32, (94.2)	DXP1	J_H6	43
gp44, (γ1/λ)	gp120	CD4BS*	V_H1	1-46, (94.9)	UKN	J_H4	43
gp68, (γ1/κ)	gp120	CD4BS*	V_H1	1-69, (87.8)	UKN	J_H4	43
MN215, (γ1/λ)	gp120	V3 loop	V_H3	3-21, (96.3)	UKN	J_H4	43
No.13, (γ1/λ)	gp120	UKN	V_H1	1-69, (88.6)	UKN	J_H4	42
S1-1, (γ1/λ)	gp120	CD4BS*	V_H1	1-69, (89.4)	UKN	J_H4	42
HBW4, (γ1/λ)	gp120	UKN	V_H2	S12-2, (95.8)	UKN	J_H5	42
F105, (γ1/κ)	gp120	CD4BS*	V_H4	4-59, (94.8)	DLR4	J_H5	41
268-D, (γ1)	gp120	V3 loop	V_H4	4-59, (88.5)	UKN	J_H3	29
257-D, (γ1)	gp120	V3 loop	V_H5	5-51, (95.5)	UKN	J_H4	29
F285, (γ1)	gp160	UKN	V_H1	1-69, (87)	UKN	UKN	46

(*): CD4 binding site

D_H genes in an inverted orientation are underlined

UKN: Unknown

were clustered within the FRs. This mutation pattern suggests that this region might play a role in antigen binding.[26,40] In general, the V_H genes utilized appear to have accumulated mutations at a higher rate than did the expressed V_L. A higher number of mutations in the V_H than in the V_L regions has been previously been observed in mouse and human antibodies of other specificities.[49] Also, mutations accumulate in some genes more frequently than in others. It is possible that different mutational rates may be exerted on different genes, or that changes in some V genes may lead to antigen-binding loss mutants more frequently than in others. What is, however, striking in human antibodies to gp120 is the underrepresentation of V_H3 family genes. As discussed above, this family has been reported to be the most frequently expressed subgroup of human V_H genes in antibodies to various antigens.[22,24,25,50,51] Remarkably, in contrast to the V_H gene-family skewing, human monoclonal antibodies derived from HIV-infected individuals do not exhibit any obvious V_L family-restriction.[52]

This V_H3 gene-family underexpression is also demonstrable by serological studies of polyclonal antibodies from HIV-infected subjects.[53] In molecular studies, the PBL of AIDS patients were also found to have reduced expression of V_H3 family-genes and this deficiency was noted in the lymph node and spleen of some of these patients.[54] A strong reduction of B cells expressing the D12 idiotope, a marker of V_H3 gene products, was also detectable in AIDS individuals. However, this reduction was preceded by a three-fold elevation in $D12^+$ B cells in HIV seropositive subjects compared to negative controls. The same differences were also seen in the level of circulating anti-gp120 $D12^+$ antibodies.[55] Other studies analyzing IgM, IgD and IgG mRNA of $CD19^+$ B cells of HIV-infected subjects have shown a marked under-expression of Igs expressing the V_H3 gene-family by IgM^+, IgG^+ and IgM^+IgD^+ naive B cells. This underexpression is associated with a low $CD4^+$ count.[56] Beside the V_H3 gene-family-specific B cell deletion, some observations suggested that the V_H clonal deficit in HIV infected individuals may be due to a B cell maturational arrest at the germinal center stage.[54] Indeed, destruction of germinal centers in lymph nodes, and more particularly of follicular dendritic cells, is observed early in infection.[57-59] In addition, histological abnormalities of B cell zones in the germinal centers of lymph nodes has also been reported.[60,61] Such alterations of the germinal center, which is important in immunological memory, could result in an altered immune response to HIV.

LACK OF CONTINUED DIVERSIFICATION OF THE ANTI-HIV ANTIBODY RESPONSE

An alternative approach to probe antibody diversity is to investigate the spectrotype of the antibody response. Several reports showed that the anti-gp120 antibody spectrotype in the serum of early stage HIV-infected patients has a restricted heterogeneity. The spectrotype of anti-HIV antibodies is oligoclonal, has a restricted heterogeneity and fails to expand during the course of the disease,[62,63] which may suggest that during HIV infection, the number of B cell clones originally recruited is limited and does not expand despite persistent exposure to gp120 epitopes. Thus, paradoxically, despite the continuous viral replication and exposure of gp120 to the immune system, there is a lack of continued diversification of the anti-gp120 antibody response. Several hypotheses might account for this repertoire bias.

B CELL SUPERANTIGENS AND REPERTOIRE BIAS IN HIV INFECTION

It is of interest to speculate on the mechanism(s) underlying these B cell abnormalities. HIV shows remarkable genetic and biologic diversity, and certain virus isolates are believed to be more pathogenic than others. How HIV destroys the immune system and causes disease remains an intriguing question. During HIV infection, there is a marked depletion of B cells. Since it is unlikely that B cells are directly killed by the virus, other mechanisms must be responsible for this B cell deficit, and HIV must be killing uninfected cells indirectly. Several non-mutually exclusive mechanisms may be proposed. First, it is possible that the loss of B cells may be linked to the fact that HIV destroys the bone marrow where naive B cells are produced. Second, because HIV progressively destroys the architecture of the lymph node, it may be that homing of the B cells becomes altered, hence an accelerated death. Third, since certain gp120 determinants mimic autologous human antigens,[64] it is conceivable that this mimicry lowers the number of HIV epitopes that may be the target of immune recognition, and, subsequently, hampers diversification of the antibody response. Fourth, 55% of gp120 molecular mass is contributed by carbohydrates and this high glycosylation extent may interfere with presentation by antigen-presenting cells or with presentation of the processed peptides as well. It could also confer resistance to protease activity and influence antigen recognition by antibody. Fifth, it is also known that the HIV genome, and particularly *env* genes, exhibit a high degree of heterogeneity.[65,66] This variability results in the presence of multiple variants of gp120, even within a single individual, and in divergence in approximately 50% of the amino acids expressed in the hypervariable loops of the envelope proteins. This property may also serve to restrict the antibody response and only a few epitopes will be recognized with little cross-reactivity between different isolates. Sixth, an alternative explanation may involve regulatory sequences associated with specific Ig V-region genes that could be modulated by different factors, such as cytokines. Since an abnormal cytokine profile, including IL-6, is observed during HIV infection,[67,68] it is possible that such a modification influences B cell development. This possibility is supported by the observation that in common immunodeficiency syndrome, which is also characterized by a germinal center maturational arrest of B cells, a substantial elevated IL-6 production has been reported.[69,70] Finally, another pathway might be related to the B cell SAg properties of gp120 (Figs. 11.1 and 11.2). We favor the view that the deletion of V_H3^+ cells is triggered by a binding event mediated by gp120 which is consequently responsible for the clonal restriction, since the antibody repertoire will be deprived of a significant proportion of its members V_H3 genes represent at least 50% of the overall repertoire. Since B cell SAgs bind the V_H portion of the Ig molecule, they can trigger all B cells bearing the appropriate V_H regardless of the other J_H, D, J_L and V_L segments.[4] It is possible that such an inappropriate B cell activation via gp120 binding to V_H3^+ B cells renders the B cell anergic, and unable to respond to further exogenous stimuli. More dramatically, when these cells encounter antigen, they may become prone to apoptosis. This possibility is supported by the observation that there is an accelerated B cell apoptosis in the lymph nodes of HIV-infected subjects [71] and by the demonstration that there is a progressive loss of V_H3^+ B cells.[55] The under expression of the Ig V_H3 gene family in AIDS patients, and its over-expression in HIV seropositive individuals are also reminiscent of an activation by a SAg followed by a clonal deletion of the activated cell subset.[4] Since this pattern is typical of the consequences of the interaction of T cells with SAgs, it is useful to discuss the potential role of T cell SAgs during HIV infection.

SUPERANTIGENS FOR T CELLS DURING HIV INFECTION

The discovery of superantigens for murine and human T cells,[72] provided a potential explanation for the severe $CD4^+$ T cell deletion seen during HIV infection. Initially, a semi-quantitative PCR analysis of TcR variable genes demonstrated a re-

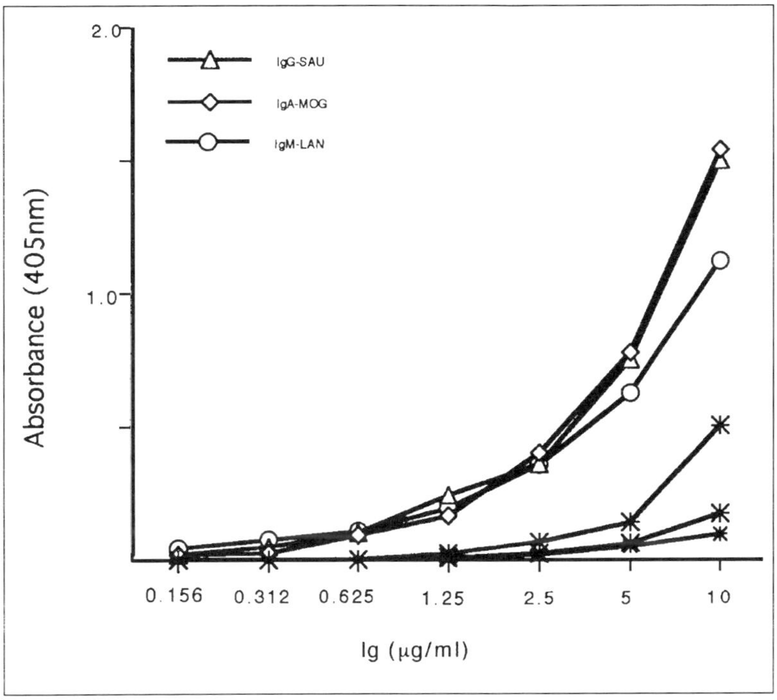

Fig. 11.1. Superantigen binding of gp160 to human Igs of various isotypes. ELISA wells were coated overnight at 4°C with 50 ng/well of recombinant gp160 from the MN isolate. After washing and saturation with 0.1% bovine serum albumin, human monoclonal Igs were incubated for 90 min at 37°C. After washing, binding was revealed with alkaline phosphatase-labeled anti-human Ig conjugates (1/1000 diluted). Three Ig (IgA, IgG and IgM) that gave negative binding are indicated by stars.

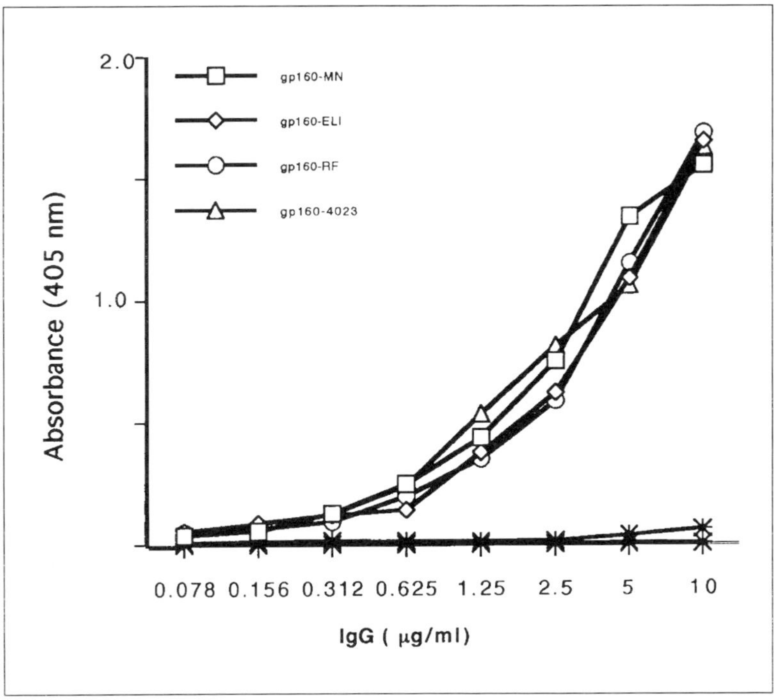

Fig. 11.2. Superantigen binding of a human monoclonal IgG1κ to gp160 from various HIV isolates. ELISA wells were coated overnight at 4°C with 50 ng/well of recombinant gp160s from the isolates indicated. After washing and saturation with 0.1% bovine serum albumin, human monoclonal Igs were incubated for 90 min at 37°C. After washing, binding was revealed with alkaline phosphatase-labeled anti-human IgG conjugates (1/1000 diluted). An IgG that gave negative binding with the four gp160s is indicated by stars.

stricted pattern of Vβ genes expressed with an under-representation of Vβ17 genes in AIDS patients compared to normal individuals.[73] This selective Vβ deletion, as measured by a PCR assay of mRNA, in AIDS patients generated much excitement. Subsequently, a number of investigations were initiated to identify the putative SAg. Here, it is of note that the HIV genome, particularly the *env* gene, is known to undergo extensive variation throughout its viral cycle. If HIV produces a SAg encoded by a variable part of its genome and if this SAg is responsible for the $CD4^+$ T cell depletion seen in HIV patients, one would expect a variable degree of loss of $CD4^+$ T cells bearing the target Vβ gene products. However, the use of Vβ-specific monoclonal antibodies revealed an absence of Vβ-specific T cell deletion and no common "whole" of a specific T cell subset in the repertoire of HIV-1 subjects at the various clinical stages of the disease.[74-76] These observations suggest that if a SAg activity is present during HIV infection, it would rather be related to an ubiquitous infectious agent that might be associated with the frequent opportunistic infections seen during the late stages of the disease. In fact, recent work provides evidence that a SAg secreted by cytomegalovirus-infected monocytes enhances HIV replication in $V\beta12^+$ T cells.[77] More specifically, studies using monoclonal antibodies to TcRs have shown that, while there is an absence of selective Vβ T cell depletion in HIV patients, $V\beta12^+$ cells become a preferential target for HIV replication after having been activated by an HIV-associated SAg presented by non-T cells.[75,78,79]

On the other hand, it is known that T cell subsets triggered by SAgs may not be completely deleted, but may be rather anergized for a variable time-period. For example, the superantigen toxic shock syndrome toxin-1 (TSST-1) of staphylococci is thought to be responsible for toxic shock syndrome. In these patients, there is an acute rise in the percentage of T cells expressing Vβ2 genes. During later stages of the disease, the percentage of $V\beta2^+$ T cells drops back to normal levels and T cell deletion is not apparent.[80] It is therefore possible that, during HIV infection, some $V\beta^+$ T cell subsets are targeted by a putative SAg without being deleted. It is also remarkable that the skewing of the viral burden to the Vβ12 subset does not correlate with a clinical stage of the disease. Since this $V\beta12^+$ target subset is not deleted in AIDS patients, it was suggested that it may, in fact, represent a viral reservoir from which HIV gradually disseminates to infect other cells and tissues. Accordingly, this Vβ12 subset may function as a viral reservoir in a majority of patients, and, by comparison with positively selected CD4 T cells, it was estimated that the majority of the HIV-1 viral burden in the peripheral blood of one patient is contained within the Vβ12 subset, even though this subset represents only less than 2% of all T cells.[77] It is possible that infection of an adult host with HIV-1 in vivo might also initially target Vβ12 cells, because HIV-1 is often skewed to the Vβ12 subset. These findings suggest that the Vβ selective element may be a SAg that could derive from an ubiquitous integrated virus. Since HIV-1 activates transcription of *Herpes* virus genes, such as cytomegalovirus, it could lead to expression of an otherwise silent gene, the production of which may depend on HIV-1 infection. In summary, HIV-1 replicates more efficiently in T cells expressing TcR using certain Vβ genes, such as Vβ12, a Vβ specificity that is consistent with an HIV-1 SAg. In peripheral cells, the targeted Vβ subsets are not deleted and it is possible that these subsets represent a viral reservoir in vivo. This SAg-like activity appears to promote Vβ-slective HIV-1 replication in vitro and in vivo in patients infected with HIV-1. In addition to these studies, other experiments found that gp160 exhibits gp160-like properties for T cells.[81,82] Clearly, additional work is required to elucidate the role of T cell SAg in HIV infection.

THE POWER OF MICROBIAL ADAPTATION

It must be emphasized that gp120 in not the only known SAg for B cells. Historically, protein A (SpA) was the first SAg to be discovered.[83] It is a cell-wall-associated protein of the Gram-positive pathogenic bacterium *Staphylococcus aureus*. It makes up nearly 7% of the cell wall of this strain and is present in approximately 95% of all pathogenic strains, with five repeated domains protruding from the cell surface. Biological responses to SpA include activation of the complement system, hypersensitivity reactions, cell-mediated cytotoxicity, interferon production, activation of polyclonal antibody synthesis and stimulation of lymphocytes.[84] It was initially thought that SpA plays an important role in immunopathology owing to its specific interaction with the Fc portion of Ig from many mammalian species with each of the five domains binding the Ig molecule. This protein has also been tested in the treatment of cancer and immune complex disorders.[85] However, more recent data show that SpA also binds to the Fab of Ig in a V_H3 gene family-specific manner.[83] An example of this binding is shown in Figure 11.3. This SAg-like interaction is suspected to play a role in the virulence of *S. Aureus*. In addition to SpA, protein G also binds the Fab portion,[86] but it is unknown whether this interaction is V_H gene-family specific. Several bacterial proteins with affinity for the constant region of IgG have been identified and characterized. Protein A of *S. aureus* and protein G of group C and G streptococci are the best known. Many strains of *Streptococcus pyogenes*, the most important streptococcal species in clinical medicine, also have M proteins which exhibit IgG-binding activity and are regarded as major virulence determinants due to their anti-phagocytic activity. Among these M-like proteins, protein H of *S. pyogenes* has been well studied.

It is interesting that proteins A, G and H have evolved convergently.[87] Despite a lack of sequence homology in their binding regions they all interact with the same region of IgG. That a number of species of pathogenic bacteria have proteins on their surface which bind to IgG suggests that Ig-binding proteins participate in essential microbial functions, adding selective advantages to the bacteria. That a bacterial surface protein, SpA, has developed separate binding sites for the Fc and Fab domains, the two important motifs in the Ig, emphasizes the power of microbial adaptation. The observation that a bacterial surface protein, SpA, and a viral envelope protein, gp120, exhibit a similar specificity for V_H3 gene-family products deserves consideration. It is thought that the relationship between host and pathogens represents a delicate balance between multiple molecular events, and pathogenicity and virulence are highly polygenic properties. The emergence of a closely related binding site in a bacterial and a viral protein further underlines the complexity of the molecular interactions underlying the relationship between infecting microorganisms and their human host. Studying the evolution of protein-binding regions is interesting not only from a general biological point of view, but also to understand how these SAg proteins may play a role in enhancing microbial virulence. For the prevention, the diagnosis and the treatment of infectious diseases, it is therefore critical to better understand the SAg-mediated host-parasite interactions.

ACKNOWLEDGMENTS

We thank Drs. J.-P. Bouvet, P. Lambin, M.-P. Kieny and J.-L. Preudhomme for generous gift of reagents. This work was supported by grants from the Institut Pasteur and the Fondation pour la Recherche Médicale (FRM, SIDACTION). SK is an investigator of the Centre National de la Recherche Scientifique (CNRS), LJ is a post-doctoral fellow of the FRM, and MZ is an investigator of the Institut National de la Recherche et de la Santé Médicale (INSERM).

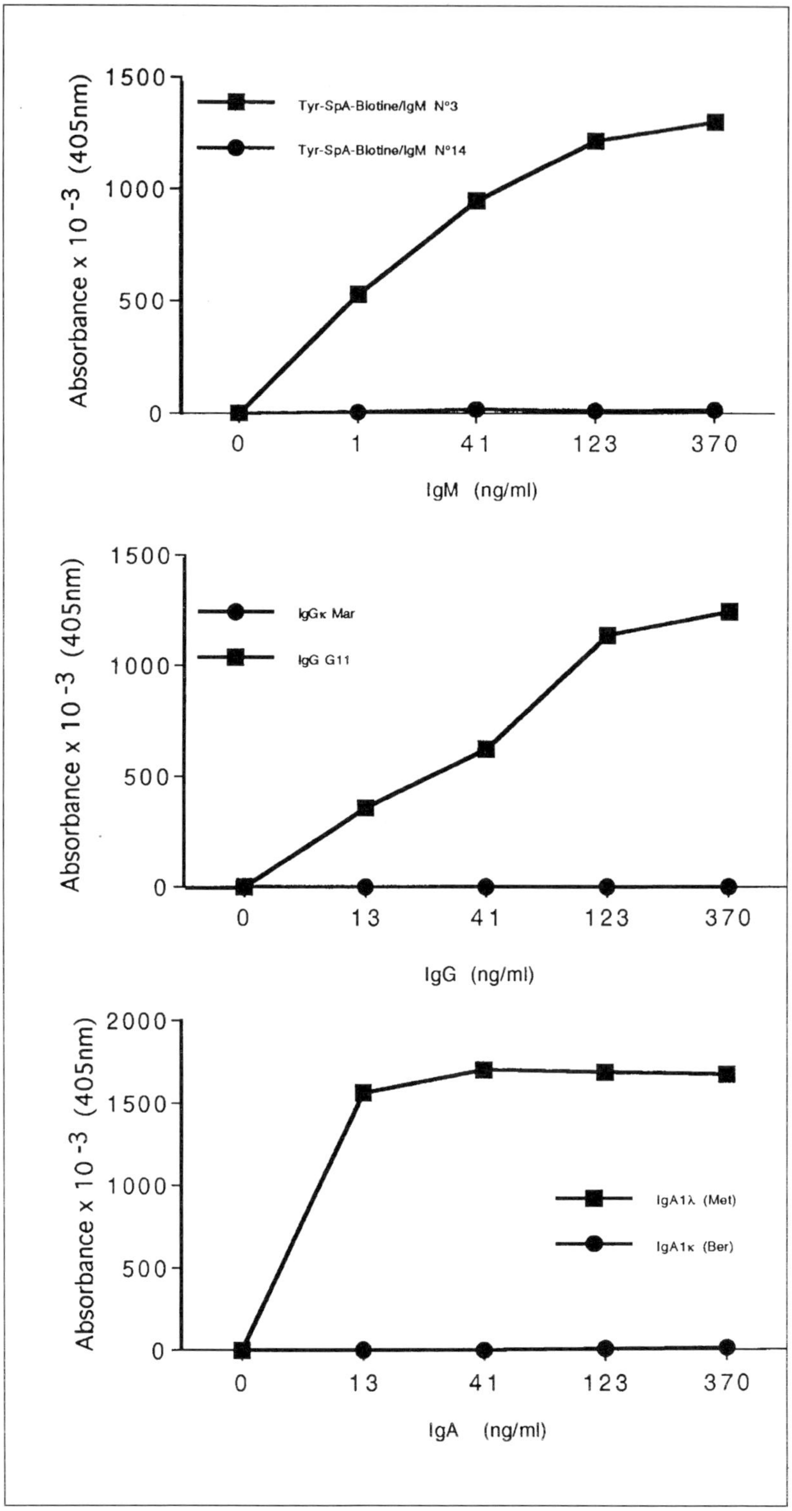

Fig. 11.3. Binding of biotinylated Tyr-SpA to human Igs. SpA was treated with Iodine Chloride to destroy the Fc-binding site (Tyr-SpA) and ELISA wells were coated overnight at 4°C with 500 ng/well of anti-human Ig. After washing and saturation with 0.1% bovine serum albumin, human monoclonal Igs were incubated for 90 min at 37°C. After incubation with biotinylated Tyr-SPA, binding was revealed with an alkaline phosphatase-labeled extravidine conjugate (1/70000 diluted).

References

1. Tonegawa S. Somatic generation of antibody diversity. Nature 1983; 302:575-81.
2. Alt FW, Blackwell TK, De Pinho RA et al. Regulation of genome rearrangement events during lymphocyte differentiation. Immunol Rev 1986; 89:5-30.
3. Rolink A, Melchers F. Molecular and cellular origins of B lymphocyte diversity. Cell 1991; 66:1081-94.
4. Zouali M. B cell superantigens: Implications for selection of the human antibody repertoire. Immunol. Today 1995; 16:399-405.
5. Matsuda F, Shin EK, Nagaoka H et al. Structure and physical map of 64 variable segments in the 3' 0.8-megabase region of the human immunoglobulin heavy-chain locus. Nature Genet 1993; 3:88-94.
6. Cook GP, Tomlinson IM, Walter G et al. A map of the human immunoglobulin VH locus completed by analysis of the telomeric region of chromosome 14q. Nature Genet 1994; 7:162-8.
7. Currier SJ, Gallarda JL, Knight KL. Partial molecular genetic map of the rabbit VH chromosomal region. J Immunol 1988; 140:1651-9.
8. Weill JC, Reynaud CA. The chicken B cell compartment. Science 1987; 238:1094-8.
9. Kirkham PM, Mortari F, Newton JA et al. Immunoglobulin VH clan and family identity predicts variable domain structure and may influence antigen binding. EMBO J 1992; 11:603-9.
10. Guigou V, Cuisinier AM, Tonnelle C et al. Human immunoglobulin VH and VK repertoire revealed by in situ hybridization. Mol Immunol 1990; 27:935-40.
11. Zouali M, Theze J. Probing VH gene-family utilization in human peripheral B cells by in situ hybridization. J Immunol 1991; 146:2855-64.
12. Kofler R, Geley S, Kofler H et al. Mouse variable-region gene families: complexity, polymorphism and use in non-autoimmune responses. Immunol Rev 1992; 128:5-21.
13. Zouali M. Unravelling antibody genes. Nature Genet 1994; 7:118-20.
14. Sasso EH, Buckner JH, Suzuki LA. Ethnic differences of polymorphism of an immunoglobulin VH3 gene. J Clin Invest 1995; 96:1591-600.
15. Chen PP, Yang PM. A segment of human Vh gene locus is duplicated. Scand J Immunol 1990; 31:593-9.
16. Sasso EH, Willems van Dijk K, Bull A et al. VH genes in tandem array comprise a repeated germline motif. J Immunol 1992; 149:1230-6.
17. Matsumura R, Matsuda F, Nagaoka H et al. Structural analysis of the human VH locus using nonrepetitive intergenic probes and repetitive sequence probes. Evidence for recent reshuffling. J Immunol 1994; 152:660-6.
18. Lucas AH, Azmi FH, Mink CM et al. Age-dependent V region expression in the human antibody response to the Haemophilus influenzae type b polysaccharide. J Immunol 1993; 150:2056-61.
19. Adderson EE, Shackelford PG, Insel RA et al. Immunoglobulin light chain variable region gene sequences for human antibodies to Haemophilus influenzae type b capsular polysaccharide are dominated by a limited number of V kappa and V lambda segments and VJ combinations. J Clin Invest 1992; 89:729-38.
20. Barre S, Greenberg AS, Flajnik MF et al. Structural conservation of hypervariable regions in immunoglobulins evolution. Nature Struct Biol 1994; 1:915-20.
21. Litman GW, Rast JP, Shamblott MJ et al. Phylogenetic diversification of immunoglobulin genes and the antibody repertoire. Mol Biol Evol 1993; 10:60-72.
22. Schroeder H Jr., Wang JY. Preferential utilization of conserved immunoglobulin heavy chain variable gene segments during human fetal life. Proc Natl Acad Sci U S A 1990; 87:6146-50.
23. Hillson JL, Oppliger IR, Sasso EH et al. Emerging human B cell repertoire. Influence of developmental stage and interindividual variation. J Immunol 1992; 149:3741-52.

24. Stewart AK, Huang C, Stollar BD et al. High-frequency representation of a single VH gene in the expressed human B cell repertoire. J Exp Med 1993; 177:409-418.
25. Demaison C, David D, Letourneur F et al. Analysis of human VH repertoire expression in peripheral CD19+ B cells. Immunogenetics 1995; 42:342-352.
26. van der Heijden RW, Bunschoten H, Pascual V et al. Nucleotide sequence of a human monoclonal anti-idiotypic antibody specific for a rabies virus-neutralizing monoclonal idiotypic antibody reveals extensive somatic variability suggestive of an antigen-driven immune response. J Immunol 1990; 144:2835-9.
27. Andris JS, Ehrlich PH, Ostberg L et al. Probing the human antibody repertoire to exogenous antigens. Characterization of the H and L chain V region gene segments from anti-hepatitis B virus antibodies. J Immunol 1992; 149:4053-9.
28. Ikematsu H, Harindranath N, Ueki Y et al. Clonal analysis of a human antibody response. II. Sequences of the VH genes of human IgM, IgG, and IgA to rabies virus reveal preferential utilization of VHIII segments and somatic hypermutation. J Immunol 1993; 150:1325-37.
29. Andris JS, Brodeur BR, Capra JD. Molecular characterization of human antibodies to bacterial antigens: utilization of the less frequently expressed VH2 and VH6 heavy chain variable region gene families. Mol Immunol 1993; 30:1601-16.
30. Berman JE, Mellis SJ, Pollock R et al. Content and organization of the human Ig VH locus: definition of three new VH families and linkage to the Ig CH locus. Embo J 1988; 7:727-38.
31. Biagiotti R, Giudizi MG, Almerigogna F et al. Abnormalities of in vitro immunoglobulin production in apparently healthy haemophiliacs: relationship with alterations of T cell subsets and with HTLV-III seropositivity. Clin Exp Immunol 1986; 63:354-8.
32. Fauci AS, Schnittman SM, Poli G et al. NIH conference. Immunopathogenic mechanisms in human immunodeficiency virus (HIV) infection. Ann Intern Med 1991; 114: 678-93.
33. Crapper RM, Deam DR, Mackay IR. Paraproteinemias in homosexual men with HIV infection. Lack of association with abnormal clinical or immunologic findings. Am J Clin Pathol 1987; 88:348-51.
34. Miedema F, Petit AJ, Terpstra FG et al. Immunological abnormalities in human immunodeficiency virus (HIV)-infected asymptomatic homosexual men. HIV affects the immune system before CD4+ T helper cell depletion occurs. J Clin Invest 1988; 82:1908-14.
35. Pahwa S, Pahwa R, Saxinger C et al. Influence of the human T lymphotropic virus/lymphadenopathy-associated virus on functions of human lymphocytes: evidence for immunosuppressive effects and polyclonal B cell activation by banded viral preparations. Proc Natl Acad Sci U S A 1985; 82:8198-202.
36. Amadori A, Faulkner-Valle GP, De Rossi A et al. HIV-mediated immunodepression: in vitro inhibition of T lymphocyte proliferative response by ultraviolet-inactivated virus. Clin Immunol Immunopathol 1988; 46:37-54.
37. Burton DR, Barbas C3, Persson MA et al. A large array of human monoclonal antibodies to type 1 human immunodeficiency virus from combinatorial libraries of asymptomatic seropositive individuals. Proc Natl Acad Sci U S A 1991; 88:10134-7.
38. Barbas C3, Collet TA, Amberg W et al. Molecular profile of an antibody response to HIV-1 as probed by combinatorial libraries. J Mol Biol 1993; 230:812-23.
39. Felgenhauer M, Kohl J, Ruker F. Nucleotide sequences of the cDNAs encoding the V-regions of H- and L-chains of a human monoclonal antibody specific to HIV-1 gp41. Nucleic Acids Res 1990; 18:4927.
40. Andris JS, Johnson S, Zolla-Pazner S et al. Molecular characterization of five human anti-human immunodeficiency virus type 1 antibody heavy chains reveals extensive somatic mutation typical of an antigen-driven immune response. Proc Natl Acad Sci U S A 1991; 88:7783-7.

41. Marasco WA, Bagley J, Zani C et al. Characterization of the cDNA of a broadly reactive neutralizing human anti-gp120 monoclonal antibody. J Clin Invest 1992; 90:1467-78.
42. Moran MJ, Andris JS, Matsumato Y et al. Variable region genes of anti-HIV human monoclonal antibodies: nonrestricted use of the V gene repertoire and extensive somatic mutation. Mol Immunol 1993; 30:1543-51.
43. van der Donk EM, Schutten M, Osterhaus AD et al. Molecular characterization of variable heavy and light chain regions of five HIV type 1-specific human monoclonal antibodies. AIDS Res Hum Retroviruses 1994; 10:1639-49.
44. Bagley J, Dillon PJ, Rosen C et al. Structural characterization of broadly neutralizing human monoclonal antibodies against the CD4 binding site of HIV-1 gp120. Mol Immunol 1994; 31:1149-60.
45. David D, Goossens D, Desgranges C et al. Molecular characterization of human monoclonal antibodies specific for several HIV proteins: analysis of the VH3 family. Immunol Letters 1995; 47:107-12.
46. Wisnewski A, Cavacini L, Posner M. Human antibody variable region gene usage in HIV-1 infection. J AIDS 1996; 11:31-8.
47. Desiderio SV, Yancopoulos GD, Paskind M et al. Insertion of N regions into heavy-chain genes is correlated with expression of terminal deoxytransferase in B cells. Nature 1984; 311:752-5.
48. Shlomchik M, Mascelli M, Shan H et al. Anti-DNA antibodies from autoimmune mice arise by clonal expansion and somatic mutation. J Exp Med 1990; 171:265-92.
49. Bensimon C, Chastagner P, Zouali M. Human lupus anti-DNA autoantibodies undergo essentially primary V kappa gene rearrangements. EMBO J 1994; 13: 2951-62.
50. Zouali M. Development of human antibody variable genes in systemic autoimmunity. Immunol Rev 1992; 128:73-99.
51. Demaison C, Chastagner P, Theze J et al. Somatic diversification in the heavy chain variable region genes expressed by human autoantibodies bearing a lupus-associated nephritogenic anti-DNA idiotype. Proc Natl Acad Sci U S A 1994; 91:514-8.
52. David D, Zouali M. Variable region light chain genes encoding human antibodies to HIV-1. Mol Immunol 1995; 32:77-88.
53. Muller S, Wang H, Silverman GJ et al. B cell abnormalities in AIDS: stable and clonally-restricted antibody response in HIV-1 infection. Scand J Immunol 1993; 38:327-34.
54. Berberian L, Valles-Ayoub Y, Sun N et al. A VH clonal deficit in human immunodeficiency virus-positive individuals reflects a B cell maturational arrest. Blood 1991; 78:175-9.
55. Berberian L, Shukla J, Jefferis R et al. Effects of HIV infection on VH3 (D12 idiotope) B cells in vivo. J AIDS 1994; 7:641-6.
56. David D, Demaison C, Bani L et al. Selective variations in vivo of VH3 and VH1 gene family expression in peripheral B cell IgM, IgD and IgG during HIV infection. Eur J Immunol 1995; 25:1524-1528.
57. Koopman G, Pals ST. Cellular interactions in the germinal center: role of adhesion receptors and significance for the pathogenesis of AIDS and malignant lymphoma. Immunol Rev 1992; 126:21-45.
58. Tenner-Racz K. Human immunodeficiency virus associated changes in germinal centers of lymph nodes and relevance to impaired B cell function. Lymphology 1988; 21: 36-43.
59. Frost SD, McLean AR. Germinal centre destruction as a major pathway of HIV pathogenesis. J AIDS 1994; 7:236-44.
60. Tenner-Racz K, Racz P, Dietrich M et al. Monoclonal antibodies to human immunodeficiency virus: their relation to the patterns of lymph node changes in persistent generalized lymphadenopathy and AIDS. AIDS 1987; 1:95-104.
61. Martinez-Maza O, Crabb E, Mitsuyasu RT et al. Infection with the human immunodeficiency virus (HIV) is associated with an in vivo increase in B lymphocyte activation and immaturity. J Immunol 1987; 138:3720-4.
62. Grimaldi LM, Roos RP, Devare SG et al. Restricted heterogeneity of antibody to

gp120 and p24 in AIDS. J Immunol 1988; 141:114-7.
63. D'Amelio R, Biselli R, Nisini R et al. Spectrotype of anti-gp120 antibodies remains stable during the course of HIV disease. J AIDS 1992; 5:930-5.
64. Neurath AR, Strick N, Li YY et al. Improbability of harmful autoimmune responses resulting from immunization with HIV-1 envelope glycoproteins. AIDS Res Hum Retroviruses 1993; 9:1195-208.
65. Hahn BH, Shaw GM, Taylor ME et al. Genetic variation in HTLV-III/LAV over time in patients with AIDS or at risk for AIDS. Science 1986; 232:1548-53.
66. Wain-Hobson S, Sonigo P, Danos O et al. Nucleotide sequence of the AIDS virus, LAV. Cell 1985; 40:9-17.
67. Clerici M, Shearer GM. The Th1-Th2 hypothesis of HIV infection: new insights. Immunol Today 1994; 15:575-81.
68. Hagiwara E, Sacks T, Leitman-Klinman SF et al. Effect of HIV infection on the Frequency of Cytokine-Secreting cells in Human Peripheral Blood. AIDS Res and Human Retroviruses 1996; 12:127-32.
69. Breen EC, Rezai AR, Nakajima K et al. Infection with HIV is associated with elevated IL-6 levels and production. J Immunol 1990; 144:480-4.
70. Adelman DC, Matsuda T, Hirano T et al. Elevated serum interleukin-6 associated with a failure in B cell differentiation in common variable immunodeficiency. J Allergy Clin Immunol 1990; 86:512-21.
71. Muro-Cacho CA, Pantaleo G, Fauci AS. Analysis of apoptosis in lymph nodes of HIV-infected persons. Intensity of apoptosis correlates with the general state of activation of the lymphoid tissue and not with stage of disease or viral burden. J Immunol 1995; 154:5555-66.
72. White J, Herman A, Pullen AM et al. The V beta-specific superantigen staphylococcal enterotoxin B: stimulation of mature T cells and clonal deletion in neonatal mice. Cell 1989; 56:27-35.
73. Imberti L, Sottini A, Bettinardi A et al. Selective depletion in HIV infection of T cells that bear specific T cell receptor V beta sequences. Science 1991; 254:860-2.
74. Laurence J, Hodtsev AS, Posnett DN. Superantigen implicated in dependence of HIV-1 replication in T cells on TCR V beta expression. Nature 1992; 358:255-9.
75. Posnett DN, Kabak S, Hodtsev AS et al. T cell antigen receptor V beta subsets are not preferentially deleted in AIDS. AIDS 1993; 7:625-31.
76. Boyer V, Smith LR, Ferre F et al. T cell receptor V beta repertoire in HIV-infection individuals: lack of evidence for selective V beta deletion. Clin Exp Immunol 1993; 92:437-41.
77. Dobrescu D, Ursea B, Pope M et al. Enhanced HIV-1 replication in V beta 12 T cells due to human cytomegalovirus in monocytes: evidence for a putative herpesvirus superantigen. Cell 1995; 82:753-63.
78. Laurence J, Hodtsev AS, Posnett DN. Superantigens in infectious diseases, including AIDS. Ann N Y Acad Sci 1993; 685:746-55.
79. Dobrescu D, Kabak S, Mehta K et al. Human immunodeficiency virus 1 reservoir in $CD4^+$ T cells is restricted to certain V beta subsets. Proc Natl Acad Sci U S A 1995; 92:5563-7.
80. Choi Y, Lafferty JA, Clements JR et al. Selective expansion of T cells expressing V beta 2 in toxic shock syndrome. J Exp Med 1990; 172:981-4.
81. Akolkar PN, Chirmule N, Gulwani-Akolkar B et al. V beta-specific activation of T cells by the HIV glycoprotein gp 160. Scand J Immunol 1995; 41:487-98.
82. Akolkar PN, Gulwani-Akolkar B, Chirmule N et al. The HIV Glycoprotein gp160 has Superantigen-like Properties. Clin Immunol Immunopathol 1995; 76:255-65.
83. Sasso EH, Silverman GJ, Mannik M. Human IgM molecules that bind staphylococcal protein A contain VHIII H chains. J Immunol 1989; 142:2778-83.
84. Langone JJ. Protein A of Staphylococcus aureus and related immunoglobulin receptors produced by streptococci and pneumonococci. Adv Immunol 1982; 32:157-252.
85. Bansal SC, Bansal BR, Thomas HL et al. Ex vivo removal of serum IgG in a patient with colon carcinoma: some biochemical, immunological and histological observations. Can-

cer 1978; 42:1-18.

86. Derrick JP, Wigley DB. Crystal structure of a streptococcal protein G domain bound to an Fab fragment. Nature 1992; 359: 752-4.
87. Frick IM, Akesson P, Cooney J et al. Protein H—a surface protein of Streptococcus pyogenes with separate binding sites for IgG and albumin. Mol Microbiol 1994; 12: 143-51.
88. Felgenhauer M, Kohl J, Ruker F. Nucleotide sequences of the cDNAs encoding the V-regions of H- and L-chains of a human monoclonal antibody specific to HIV-1 gp41. Nucleic Acids Res 1990; 18:4927.

CHAPTER 12

Protein Fv (Fv Fragment Binding Protein): A Mucosal Human Superantigen Reacting with Normal Immunoglobulins

Jean-Pierre Bouvet, René Pirès and Canh P. Quan

Fv fragment-binding protein (protein Fv: pFv) is a gut-associated molecule, described in 1990 by our group.[1] It can bind human and animal immunoglobulins (Igs), irrespective of preliminary immunization. The molecule was first discovered in stools of patients suffering from viral hepatitis C. In these patients, pFv is under a free form, leading to interferences with enzyme-linked immunosorbent assays (ELISA) used to detect viral antigens. This phenomenon was first shown not to be virus-specific. Subsequently, it was found to be due to a molecule of the normal human digestive lumen exhibiting biological properties of major interest. Here we present the main structural and functional properties of this molecule, which seems to be an important factor of humoral digestive immunity and which binds the variable (V) domain V_H of the nonimmune Ig heavy (H) chain. This binding is closely related to that of the superantigenic protein A (SpA) of *Staphylococcus aureus*.

DETECTION OF PFV IN PATIENTS WITH HEPATITIS

The easiest assay to detect pFv under its free form, derives from the sandwich ELISA by which it was discovered. This assay was at first designed to detect unknown viral antigens released from the liver in the intestine lumen of patients suffering from viral hepatitis C. Fecal extracts were incubated with antibody-coated wells, and the captured antigens revealed by the same peroxidase-labeled antibody (Fig. 12.1). The preparation suspected to contain antibodies to the test antigens consisted of serum IgG from convalescent hepatitis patients or from squirrel mon-

Human B Cell Superantigens, edited by Moncef Zouali.

keys inoculated with viral hepatitis C. The positivity of this assay correlated with both clinical and biological findings since 50% of these patients were positive as compared with a very low percentage of normal subjects. However, an immune specificity control, which consisted of preimmune serum IgG from six month-old babies or from noninoculated squirrel monkeys, showed that the assay was not antibody-specific since it gave positive results with control IgG. These findings led us to postulate that an Ig-binding molecule was present in the gut of these patients (Fig. 12.1). We then ruled out the possibility of a trivial artifact and confirmed our hypothesis by a series of experiments, including absorption with insolubilized IgG and competitive inhibitions with soluble unlabeled IgG.[1]

The pFv assay is currently standardized as follows. ELISA plates are coated with 100 μL per well of phosphate buffered saline (PBS) containing 2.5 μg/mL of normal polyclonal human IgG or of their F(ab')2 fragments. After a one-hour incubation at 37°C, the wells are washed with a PBS solution containing 1% (vol/vol) of Tween-20 (PBS-Tween) and then saturated by incubation overnight at 4°C with a PBS solution containing 2% (wt/vol) skim milk powder and sodium azide. The plates can then be stored for 3 or 4 days at 4°C. After extensive washing with PBS-Tween, dilutions of the sample in a PBS solution

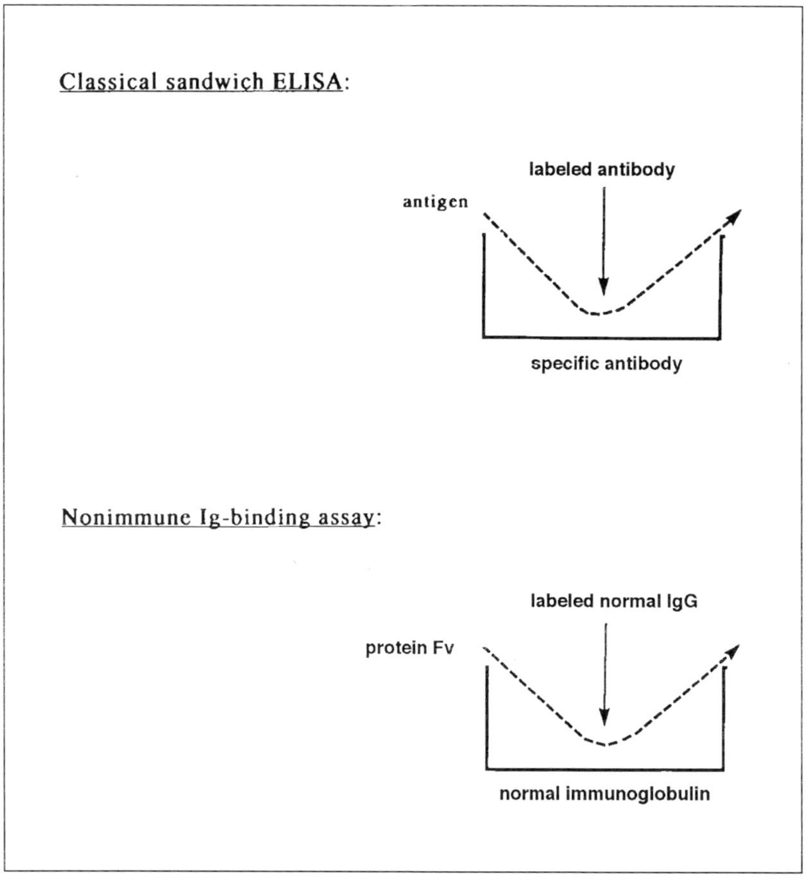

Fig. 12.1. Comparison between a classical sandwich ELISA and the nonimmune Ig-binding assay. In classical ELISAs, antigens are usually captured by antibody-coated wells and then revealed by a second antibody labeled with an enzyme. In contrast, in our nonimmune assay, the wells are coated with nonspecific Igs which are recognized by Ig-binding molecules (Fc- or Fab-specific). During a second step, the plurivalent pFv is revealed by capture of nonspecific Igs labeled with an enzyme.

containing 1.16 mM of sodium deoxycholate—this physiological detergent providing the best solubility for pFv—are incubated at 37°C for one hour, allowing the nonimmune binding of pFv, followed by an extensive washing with PBS-Tween. The multivalent pFv, bound to the Ig-coated plate, is then revealed by incubation at 37°C for one hour with peroxidase-labeled normal IgG diluted in PBS-milk, followed by an extensive washing with PBS. The peroxidase activity is detected with *o*-phenylenediamine and the optical density read at 492 nm after addition of 4N sulfuric acid. This assay differs from classical ELISAs since it does not involve an antigen-binding, reaction but an unconventional nonimmune binding.

MOLECULAR CHARACTERISTICS OF PFV

Even with high pFv activity samples, no Ig binding was found in eluates from gel permeation columns, irrespective of the pore size and of the carbohydrate or the acrylamide nature of the gel. This phenomenon was explained by the presence of trace amounts of calibrating IgG, adsorbed in the gel and in the column filters. Therefore we used fresh gels and calibrated the columns with markers containing no Fab. In addition, the yield of recovery of pFv after elution was highly increased by using deoxycholate-containing buffers. Under these non-dissociating conditions, the apparent molecular mass was 175 kDa. When investigated by either preparative[1] or analytical[2] SDS-PAGE, this size dropped to 82-85 kDa, indicating that the molecule associates two noncovalently linked subunits of the same size. Reduction of the disulfide bridges by treatment with dithiotreitol did not modify these values showing that each subunit contains one polypeptide chain. Whether these chains are different or identical has not yet been determined, but a homodimeric structure is currently assigned to pFv.

Preparative isoelectrofocusing in granulated gels[1] or in solution[3] showed the isoelectric charge to be very acidic (pi: 4.2), a property suggesting the presence of sialic residues. Indeed, treatment of pFv with neuraminidase led to a significant decrease of its binding activity.[1,3] Similarly, the use of various enzymes allowed investigation of the molecular nature of pFv.[1,3] Pronase and pepsin abolished the activity evidencing that the molecule is a protein. In contrast, treatments with trypsin and with chymo–trypsin did not modify the size and activity of pFv, suggesting the presence of a large protective carbohydrate moiety. This conclusion may account for the persistence of this protein in the digestive lumen. Finally, the lack of cleavage by DNAse, RNAse and lipases ruled out the presence of the corresponding substrates in pFv.

BINDING SPECIFICITY OF PFV

When incubated with animal Igs, pFv reacts with molecules from an extremely large number of species.[4] These include animals phylogenetically distant from humans such as the sturgeon: the genetic distance between these two species exceeds 400 x 10^6 years (Table 12.1). Similarly, Igs from more evolved fishes (goldfish, trout, carp), amphibians (axolotl, claw toad), reptile (python) and birds (quail, chicken) are also recognized. In mammals, Igs from monkeys (rhesus, squirrel monkey, cynomolgus), carnivorous (dog, cat), rodents (rat, mouse), lagomorphs (rabbit) and from one ungulates species (pig) are reactive. In contrast, Igs from other ungulates (cow, horse, sheep, goat) do not react significantly with pFv. This lack of reactivity with Igs from most ungulates seems to correlate with their strict herbivorous diet (whereas the pig is omnivorous), and is associated with an apparently interfering Ig structure selectively denatured by a 4M guanidine-HCl dissociative treatment.[4]

The specificity for human Igs was further investigated with myeloma proteins and was found to be independent of their H chain isotype: (IgG, IgA, IgM, IgD and IgE) and subclass ($\gamma1$, $\gamma2$, $\gamma3$, $\gamma4$, $\alpha1$ and $\alpha2$), their H chain allotype (Gm1 and Gm4), and their light (L) chain isotype (κ and λ).[1,5] These results suggested a specificity for the V_H domain, which is common to all classes. Indeed, by using isolated chains or fragments (Table 12.2), we showed that only V_H-containing molecules were able to bind pFv, provided that their preparation had not required cleavage of the intradomain disulfide bridge of V_H.[6] F(ab')2, Fab, and Fv fragments were found to be reactive, as well as the dimeric H chains from IgA2m(1) which can be isolated without cleavage of disulfide bridges. In contrast, Fc fragments, Fb fragments and dimeric L chains were unreactive. Finally, the H chains prepared by the usual

Table 12.1. Protein Fv binding to immunoglobulins of various nonprimate species

Species	Class	Order	Phylogenetic* distanceto humans	Diet**	pFv binding
Dog	*Mammalia*	*Carnivora*	110	Carnivorous	++
Cat	*Mammalia*	*Carnivora*	110	Carnivorous	+++
Mouse	*Mammalia*	*Rodentia*	110	Other	++
Rat	*Mammalia*	*Rodentia*	110	Other	+++
Rabbit	*Mammalia*	*Lagomorpha*	110	Other	++
Horse	*Mammalia*	*Perrissodactyla*	110	Herbivorous	±
Cow	*Mammalia*	*Artiodactyla*	110	Herbivorous	±
Sheep	*Mammalia*	*Artiodactyla*	110	Herbivorous	-
Goat	*Mammalia*	*Artiodactyla*	110	Herbivorous	-
Pig	*Mammalia*	*Artiodactyla*	110	Other	+++
Hen	*Aves*	*Galliformes*	270	Other	+++
Quail	*Aves*	*Galliformes*	270	Other	++
Python	*Reptilia*	*Squamata*	270	Carnivorous	+++
Claw Toad	*Amphibia*	*Anura*	380	Carnivorous	+++
Axolotl	*Amphibia*	*Urodela*	380	Carnivorous	+
Carp	*Osteichthyes*	*Ostariophysi*	380	Other	++
Goldfish	*Osteichthyes*	*Ostariophysi*	380	Other	++
Trout	*Osteichthyes*	*Salmoniformes*	380	Carnivorous	+
Sturgeon	*Osteichthyes*	*Chondrostei*	400	Other	+++
Shark (Dogfish)	*Chondrichthyes*	*Elasmobranchii*	420	Carnivorous	-

* Million years since divergence from the human phylum.
** Carnivorous, herbivorous or other (including omnivorous)

Table 12.2. V_H domain specificity of pFv, as investigated by its binding to Ig fragments

Fragment	Constitutive domains*	pFv binding
F(ab')2	**V_H**, V_L, C_H1, C_L, h	+
Fab	**V_H**, V_L, C_H1, C_L	+
Fc	h, C_H2, C_H3	-
(H)2**	**V_H**, C_H1, C_H2, C_H3	+
(L)2***	V_L, C_L	-
Fb	C_H1, C_L	-
Fv	**V_H**, V_L	+

* V_H and V_L: variable domains of the heavy (H) and light (L) chains; C_H and CL: constant domains of the H and L chains; h: hinge region of the H chain.
** H chain dimers were prepared from urea-dissociated IgA2m(1).
*** L chain dimers were from Bence Jones proteins or were prepared from urea-dissociated IgA2m(1).

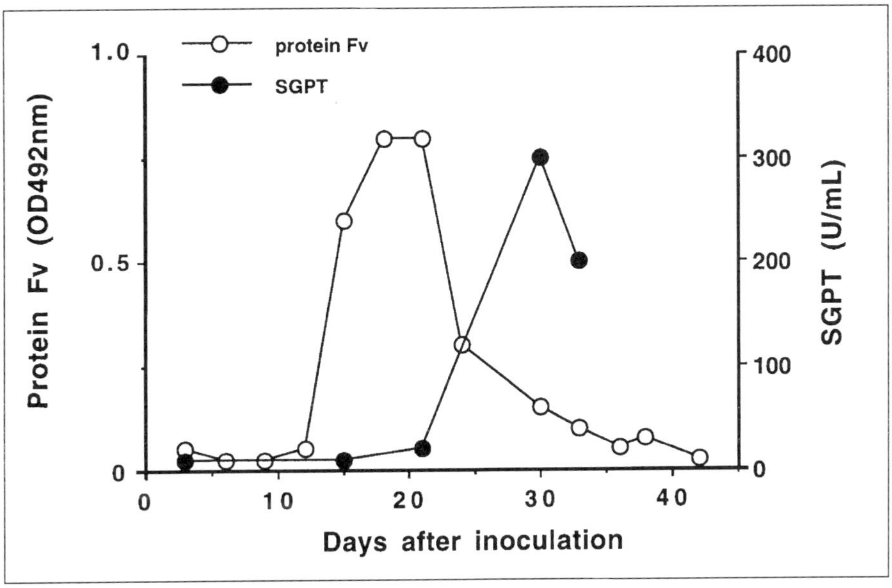

Fig. 12.2. Transient appearance of free protein Fv in the stools of a rhesus monkey injected with a human non-A, non-B, non-C, non-E hepatitis virus, preceding the elevation of the serum glutamic-pyruvic transaminase (SGPT).

reduction-dissociation procedure did not react.

The structure recognized by pFv in the V_H domain is not located within the antigen-binding site since antigen-antibody and pFv-Ig interactions do not interfere significantly.[6] Simultaneous dissociation and reduction irreversibly denatured the V_H structure, whereas each of these treatments carried out alone was not denaturing. These data demonstrate that the Ig structure involves a discontinuous sequence protected from dissociation by its proximity to the intrachain disulfide bridge. Moreover, comparison of human and animal V_H sequences confirms that accessible areas of the framework regions (FR) FR1 and FR3 are both close to this bridge and highly conserved throughout evolution. In a recent paper, Silverman et al[2] have shown that essentially all IgM antibodies that use V_H3 domains can bind pFv, but that a limited range of lengths of the third complementarity-determining region (CDR3) is associated with optimal binding affinity. The similarity of this binding with that of the alternative pathway of SpA suggests that pFv recognizes a structure involving FR1 and FR3 in a lateral pocket of the V_H domain.[7,8]

PRESENCE IN NORMAL SUBJECTS AND IN OTHER ANIMAL SPECIES

In initial experiments, pFv was rarely detected in stool extracts from normal subjects. We therefore hypothesized that the negative results were due to an unusual binding of pFv to intestinal secretory IgA (SIgA), inhibiting detection by the Ig-binding assay. To denature irreversibly both bound and unbound SIgA, stool extracts from normal subjects were treated with guanidine and dithiotreitol. This treatment revealed hidden pFv molecules in the stools of most normal subjects.[3] Gel permeation analysis showed that pFv-SIgA complexes can reach very large sizes. Complexes of as large as 3,000 kDa included primarily F(ab')2α fragments of SIgA, forming polymeric antibody structures that we compared to "immune fortresses".

In two studies, the presence of pFv was evidenced in monkeys from different species (squirrel monkey, cynomolgus, rhesus) during experimental viral hepatitis,[9,10] in which the release of free pFv accompanies, or just precedes, the rise of transaminases (Fig. 12.2). Investigation of laboratory animals shows the presence in rats of a gut-associated molecule with a similar specificity and molecular form (manuscript in preparation).

VALENCY AND STRUCTURE OF PFV

The smallest size observed with the spontaneous F(ab')2α-pFv complexes exhibiting approximately 800 kDa suggested that these structures are formed by one molecule of pFv (175 kDa) saturated with six molecules of 100-kDa F(ab')2 fragments. To determine whether the two V_H domains of each F(ab')2 molecule were involved in the binding, free pFv was saturated in vitro with a large excess of F(ab')2, and the size of the complexes was determined by gel permeation.[3] The results confirmed that one molecule of pFv cannot bind more than six F(ab')2 molecules, whatever the large excess of these fragments. A direct method using Fab fragments to measure valency was not possible since pFv affinity for these monomers is much lower than for dimeric Ig fragments.

Its unusual resistance to proteolytic cleavage suggests that pFv is not linear, but that it rather exhibits a globular structure. The two-dimensional diagram presented in Figure 12.3 corresponds to a pFv complex formed under a large excess of F(ab')2 fragments. The constant (C) C_L and C_H1 domains are not shown since their representation requires a three-dimensional diagram. It is likely that the F(ab')2 arms lead to staple-like or to chair-like shapes similar to those described for immune complexes.[11] It is also possible that these arms point towards six different directions.

ATTEMPTS TO PURIFY PFV

Purification of pFv by usual methods, such as gel permeation, ion-exchange chromatography, hydrophobic interactions, pre-

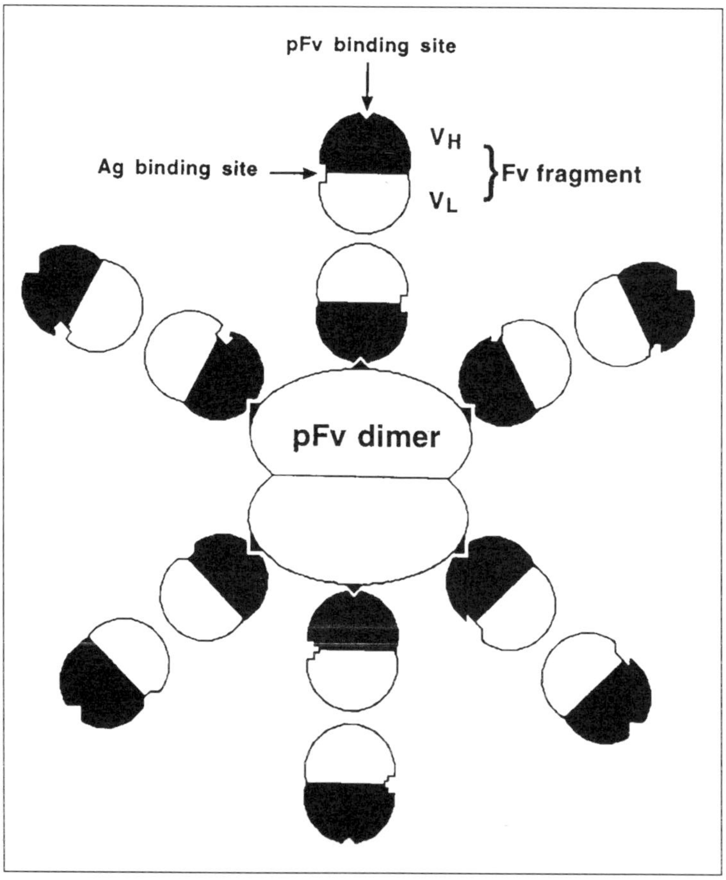

Fig. 12.3. Schematic two-dimensional representation of a pFv complex under a large excess of F(ab')2 fragments. The 175 kDa pFv is a non-covalent homodimer of an acidic sialoglycoprotein. The six functional valencies of the dimer can bind the V_H domain of Igs throughout a conserved structure located outside the antigen-binding site to form an "immune fortress-like" polymer. The C_H1 and C_L domains are not represented. At equivalence, the size of the polymer can be much larger and subsequently poorly soluble because of the presence of more than one pFv molecule in each complex.

parative isofocusing and electrophoresis were unsatisfactory both due to a low concentration of the molecule, as compared to that of impurities, and to its poor solubility. Even affinity chromatography by incubation with IgG covalently bound to SpA-Sepharose beads was unsuccessful. Despite the fact that pFv was fully absorbed, elution did not occur unless the V_H structure was irreversibly denatured by reduction-dissociation. Unfortunately, this method also released L chains and other fragments, and pFv was lost during the successive separation steps. Purification by immunoabsorption with antibodies to denatured pFv could not be achieved since this molecule is poorly immunogenic and does not allow generation of monoclonal or polyclonal reagents.

SEMI-QUANTITATIVE MEASUREMENT OF PFV

The concentration of pFv can be estimated by measuring the amount of labeled IgG binding to pFv after successive incubations of the test sample with F(ab')2-precoated wells. During incubation, one to five (mean = 3) of the six valencies of pFv are occupied by the coated F(ab')2 molecules, complete saturation being avoided by using a low coating concentration. Conversely, the pFv/labeled IgG molar ratio ranges from five to one, with a reasonable mean value of three. In this assay the labeled IgG is functionally monovalent since it is added in a very large excess. The supernatants of each well are successively incubated three times under the same conditions and the wells are revealed simultaneously. A correspondence curve is established using the same plate by measuring the peroxidase activity of dilutions of the labeled IgG, which allows conversion of optical densities (OD492nm) into ponderal values of bound IgG. The results of each well are summed and the amount of pFv can finally be calculated according to the following formula:

$$\text{pFv (ng)} = \left(\frac{\text{captured IgG (ng)}}{3}\right) = \left(\frac{\text{pFv molecular mass}}{\text{IgG molecular mass}}\right)$$

The values obtained with three different preparations of high activity confirmed the minute concentrations of pFv, reaching only 100 ng/mL for the most concentrated extract investigated.

TISSUE ORIGIN OF pFv

In our initial studies, several findings strongly suggested that pFv was produced by the liver. Indeed, a large amount of this molecule was detected in the sole patients suffering from liver diseases,[12] and a similar Fab-binding activity was found in liver extracts. Moreover, incubation of liver microscopical slices with peroxidase-labeled F(ab')2 showed a selective binding to hepatocytes (unpublished results). However, attempts to detect free or combined pFv in human bile have remained unsuccessful, a conclusion challenging our first interpretation. Nevertheless, the protein is certainly synthesized by the body and not by the digestive flora since it is sialylated, a phenomenon never observed with bacterial proteins. Moreover, its presence has been detected in fetal rats (manuscript in preparation).

"IMMUNE FORTRESSES" IN THE DIGESTIVE LUMEN

The capacity of pFv to bind Igs without impairing the antigen-antibody reaction must potentiate antibody functions in the gut. One of the major roles of gut antibodies is to augment the conveyance of pathogens with the mucus stream.[13] This clearance is increased by agglutination, which requires polymeric IgA. It has been shown in vitro that pFv induces, or increases, the agglutinating activity of antibodies both on erythrocytes,[14] bacteria[3] and viruses.[3] In vivo, the frequent bacterium-associated proteolytic degradation of SIgA is balanced by formation of macromolecular complexes with pFv,[3] which maintain the agglutinating properties of these antibodies. It is therefore likely that these immune fortresses actually correspond to "super-antibody" structures, which may induce polyspecific agglutinations of pathogens.

COMPLEMENT ACTIVATION AND SUPERALLERGEN PROPERTIES OF PFV

Activation of the complement cascade by the direct (classical) pathway is normally induced by binding of the antibodies to the corresponding antigens. Similarly, pFv binding to IgG1 or to IgM, but not to IgG4 and or to F(ab')2 fragments, activates complement by the same mechanism, irrespective of antibody specificities.[14] This function might be of importance as a pathogenic cofactor in the inflamed gut where both serum components and lumenal molecules can diffuse throughout the injured mucosa.

As for other isotypes, the V_H domain of IgE can bind pFv. Incubation of this molecule with human mast cells or basophils, sensitized with monoclonal or polyclonal IgE via binding to the Fcε receptor, stimulates both the release of preformed mediators (histamine, tryptase) and the de novo synthesis of leukotriene C4 and of prostaglandin D_2.[5] This activation occurs through the same pathway as that of allergens, but is independent of the antibody activity. It is likely that under normal conditions, pFv could desensitize gut mast cells by a low-dose and continuous contact, preventing hypersensitivity reactions triggered by true allergens.

RELATIONSHIP WITH B CELL SUPERANTIGENS

We presently have no direct evidence of the role of pFv in immune regulation. However, a large body of evidence indicates a close relationship with SpA in terms of specificity for the V_H domain (submitted for publication). Both molecules recognize V_H3 gene family products and are mutual inhibitors of V_H-mediated Ig binding, pFv displaying a much higher affinity than SpA. It is therefore likely that this molecule is either an endogenous SpA-like activator of B cells or, in contrast, a specific inhibitor of SpA-induced B cell activation. Preliminary results showing that pFv can suppress the pokeweed mitogen-induced proliferation of human B cells (Fig. 12.4) are in favor of such an inhibitory function. Anyhow, pFv is actually a superantigen at the Ig level.

CONCLUDING REMARKS

To summarize, pFv seems to be a key factor in mucosal immunity since it leads to the formation of large nonimmune complexes of SIgA or fragments (immune fortresses) in the colonic lumen. Besides its co-agglutinating properties, this molecule displays potentially important functions: it is a complement activator, a super aller-

Fig. 12.4. (Opposite page) Inhibition of pokeweed mitogen-induced activation of normal human peripheral B lymphocytes by dilutions of protein Fv. Mononuclear cells were isolated from heparinized human blood by a Ficoll-Hypaque gradient and stimulated by pokeweed mitogen (PWM). The cells were cultured in triplicate at a concentration of 2 x 10^5 per 0.2 mL in RPMI 1640 supplemented with 10% fetal calf serum, glutamine and antibiotics. PWM was used at a final concentration of 1 µg/mL. On day 0, dilutions of pFv were added to each well, and proliferations were analyzed on day 5 after an 18-hour incubation with ^{3}H-thymidine. Control cultures without pFv or PWM established the degree of inhibition. The percentage of inhibition was calculated according to the following formula:

$$\%\ inhibition = \left(\frac{cpm_{control} - cpm_{test}}{cpm_{control}}\right) \times 100$$

where $cpm_{control} = cpm_{PWM} - cpm_{medium}$, and $cpm_{test} = cpm_{(pFv+PWM)} - cpm_{pFv}$.
In a representative experiment, $cpm_{PWM} = 61{,}292 \pm 1{,}134$, $cpm_{medium} = 27{,}327 \pm 773$, $cpm_{(pFv+PWM)} = 988 \pm 169$, and $cpm_{pFv} = 966 \pm 64$. The specificity control is provided by the same pFv preparation depleted from pFv by incubation with IgG-Sepharose. Note that the pFv preparation contains some co-stimulating material as revealed by the negative values of the inhibition test carried out after absorption.

gen and a V_H3-specific superantigen. The main future directions of research in the field of pFv will be the determination of its tissue origin and the establishment of its molecular structure. Molecular cloning and expression leading to the production of large amounts of recombinant material, will further extend the knowledge of the biological activities of this important molecule.

Acknowledgments

This work was supported by grants from the Institut Pasteur. JP Bouvet and CP Quan are INSERM and CNRS investigators, respectively. We are indebted to Professor J Pillot (Institut Pasteur), who kindly gave us results presented in Figure 12.2, to Dr S Iscaki (Institut Pasteur) for wise discussions of the manuscript, and to Professor J Charlemagne (Faculty of Sciences, University of Paris) for discussion of Table 12.1.

References

1. Bouvet JP, Pirès R, Lunel-Fabiani F et al. Protein F: a novel F(ab)-binding factor, present in normal liver, and largely released in the digestive tract during hepatitis. J Immunol 1990; 145: 1176-1180.
2. Silverman GJ, Roben P, Bouvet JP, Sasano M. Superantigen properties of a human sialoprotein involved in gut-associated immunity. J Clin Invest 1995; 96: 417-426.
3. Bouvet JP, Pirès R, Iscaki S, Pillot J. Nonimmune macromolecular complexes of Ig in human gut lumen: possible enhancement of antibody functions. J Immunol 1993; 151: 2562-2571.
4. Bouvet JP, Pirès R, Charlemagne J et al. Non-immune binding of human protein Fv to immunoglobulins from various mammalian and non-mammalian species. Scand J Immunol 1991; 34: 491-496.
5. Patella V. Bouvet JP, Marone G. Protein Fv produced during viral hepatitis is a novel activator of human basophils and mast cells.

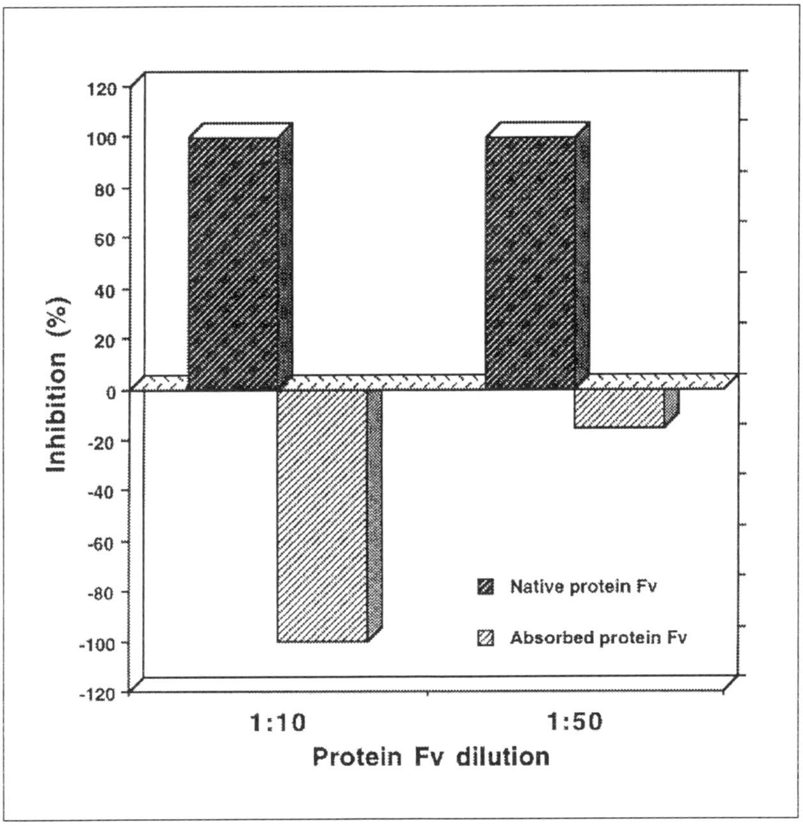

J Immunol 1993; 151: 5685-5698.
6. Bouvet JP, Pirès R, Quan C et al. Non-immune VH-binding specificity of human protein Fv. Scand J Immunol 1991; 33: 381-386.
7. Hillson JL, Karr NS, Oppliger IR et al. The structural basis of germline-encoded V_H3 immunoglobulin binding to staphylococcal protein A. J Exp Med 1993; 178: 331-336.
8. Sasano M, Burton DR, Silverman GJ. Molecular selection of human antibodies with an unconventional bacterial B cell antigen. J Immunol 1993; 151: 5822-5839.
9. Sharma MD, Maillard P, Vrati S et al. Serial passage of West-European sporadic non-A non-B hepatitis in rhesus monkeys by inoculation with fecal extracts. J Med Virol 1990; 30: 36-41.
10. Diallo A, Lazizi Y, Le Guenno B, Pillot J. Hepatitis-E-virus-associated antigen: improved detection in stools by protein Fv removal. Res Virol 1991; 142: 449-459.
11. Feinstein A, Moon EA, Richardson NE. The three-dimensional conformation of γM and γA globulin molecules. Ann NY Acad Sci 1971; 190: 104-121.
12. Bouvet JP. Role of a liver F(ab')2-binding molecule in mucosal immunity. In: Tsuchiya M, Yodoi J, Hibi T, Miura S, eds. Current Topics in Mucosal Immunology 1993. Amsterdam: Excerpta Medica. 1994; 169-174.
13. Sanderson IR, Walker A. Mucosal barrier. In: Ogra PL, Mestecky J, Lamm ME, Strober W, McGhee JR, Bienenstock J, eds. Handbook of Mucosal Immunology. San Diego: Academic Press, 1994: 41-51.
14. Ruffet E, Pirès R, Bouvet JP. Activation of the classical pathway Fv (Fv fragment-binding protein). Scand J Immunol 1994; 40: 359-362.

CHAPTER 13

Immunoglobulin Nucleotide Binding Site: A Possible Superantigen Receptor

Heinz Kohler, Gabriela Pavlinkova and Boyd Haley

INTRODUCTION

For many years the antigen binding site on immunoglobulins has been considered the only site in the variable region of antibodies.[1] Unlike conventional receptor-ligand relationships (i.e., hormones or cytokines), the antibody binding site consists of a large collection of different structures for a myriad of different ligands, called antigens. Thus, the antigen binding site can only be described biochemically in general terms as a subdomain within the variable immunoglobulin (Ig) domains. The characteristic feature of the antigen binding site is its assemblage of the six so-called complementary determining regions, or CDR, which participate in the formation of the site. Depending on the structure of the antigen, the site is either a flat or curved surface, or a variably deep pocket or grove. Furthermore, the six CDRs contribute differently and selectively in the formation of the site.

In addition to the antigen binding site, recently discovered unconventional or alternative binding sites reside also in the variable domains. The present volume contains detailed description of these sites. The intriguing aspect of the variable antibody structure is the dual role as a highly polymorphic receptor structure for the vast repertoire of antigens and at the same time as a receptor for a handful of nonantigen ligands. The antibody molecule accomplishes this dual function by keeping antigen contacting regions as independent subdomains separated from nonantigen receptor structures. The basis for this separation comes in part from the independent genetic elements encoding of the third CDR in both chains and the ability of the V genes to maintain regions with high mutation rates in the first and second CDRs. Non-CRD regions are con-

Human B Cell Superantigens, edited by Moncef Zouali. © 1996 R.G. Landes Company.

sidered to provide the structural framework of the variable Ig domains, hence the term framework region. Ligand binding to both sites, the antigen and the nonconventional binding site, have profound physiological consequences meditated by the Ig B cell receptor. Because of the similarities with the so-called T cell superantigens, these B cell ligands have received the same connotation.

Unlike antigen binding sites, the unconventional binding site structures are not clonally expressed on B cells. Thus, the response to B cell triggering via unconventional sites binding involves variable sizes of B cell subsets, hence the term B cell superantigen.

All known ligands for the unconventional sites are proteins (see this volume). Binding to these sites typically does not interfere with antigen binding. Furthermore, these proteins are derived from bacteria, viruses or cellular products. They are biologically active molecules involved in specific cellular or pathogenic mechanisms.

Here we will discuss a recently discovered binding site on antibodies which meets several criteria of an unconventional immunoglobulin binding site.

THE DISCOVERY OF A NUCLEOTIDE BINDING SITE IN ANTIBODIES

Nucleotides such as GTP and ATP play an important regulatory and triggering role for many enzymes and proteins. The involvement of nucleotides in antibodies has not been described or suggested, although other members of the immunoglobulin superfamily have binding sites for nucleotides. For example the BiP chaperone for Ig chains requires ATP for the release of nascent light and heavy chains.[2] Thus, it was surprising to observe incorporation of a photo-reactive ATP probe into Ig chains as part of an immunoprecipitated ATPase. We decided to study this Ig photolabeling in more detail.[3] The key question in our mind concerned the preservation of antibody function, in particular the capacity to bind the antigen. The second issue which surfaced was whether this photoinsertion is restricted to an unique affinity site or whether the Ig molecule is randomly labeled at several sites. ATP photoprobes are known to react with many serum proteins such as albumin; therefore it was not at all obvious whether the photoinsertion observed with antibodies would be site-specific and different from the nonspecific labeling of serum albumin.

Monoclonal mouse antibodies, specific for lymphoma idiotypes on mouse and human B cell lymphoma cell lines, were used to assess the site specificity and the preservation of antigen binding site upon photolysis with 8-azido-ATP.

The S1C5 monoclonal antibody recognizes sIgM on 38C13 murine lymphoma[4] and the monoclonal 5D10 is idiotype specific for the DHL-4 human lymphoma cell line.[5] Both antibodies were photolysed with increasing concentration of 8-azido-ATP and incorporation of label was analyzed by SDS-PAGE under reducing conditions. Both, heavy and light chains, showed incorporation of the radiolabel (data not shown). Subsequently a large number of monoclonal and polyclonal antibodies were reacted with the radioactive photoprobe and screened for incorporation by autoradiography. An example of affinity labeling of several antibodies is shown in Figure 13.1. So far all antibodies studied could be labeled with the ATP photoprobe; however, we noticed differences in the amount of incorporated label into light and heavy chains. Some antibodies carried more label on the heavy chain and less on the light chain than others. Since these differences were not related to Ig class or species of origin, we concluded that the variable degree of incorporation into the Ig chains might be due to sequence differences in the variable domain and that the site of incorporation would be in the variable domains of the Ig chains. This would also suggest that incorporation into a variable domain structure could affect the antigen binding site.

Photolabeled antibodies were tested in RIA and cell binding for binding to their corresponding antigens and found, to our surprise and relief, to bind. To demonstrate the specificity in the binding of affinity labeled antibody to target cell, cold antibody was used as inhibitor of cell binding. In Figure 13.2 the inhibition of binding of ^{32}P-photolabeled S1C5 to 38C13 tumor cells by unlabeled S1C5 is shown.

CHARACTERIZATION OF THE ATP-BINDING SITE

Titration of the photoreaction on several antibodies produced a plateau at 150-250 μMol concentration of photolabel. This saturation effect indicated that the photolabel inserts into a unique site and that random insertion would not occur at

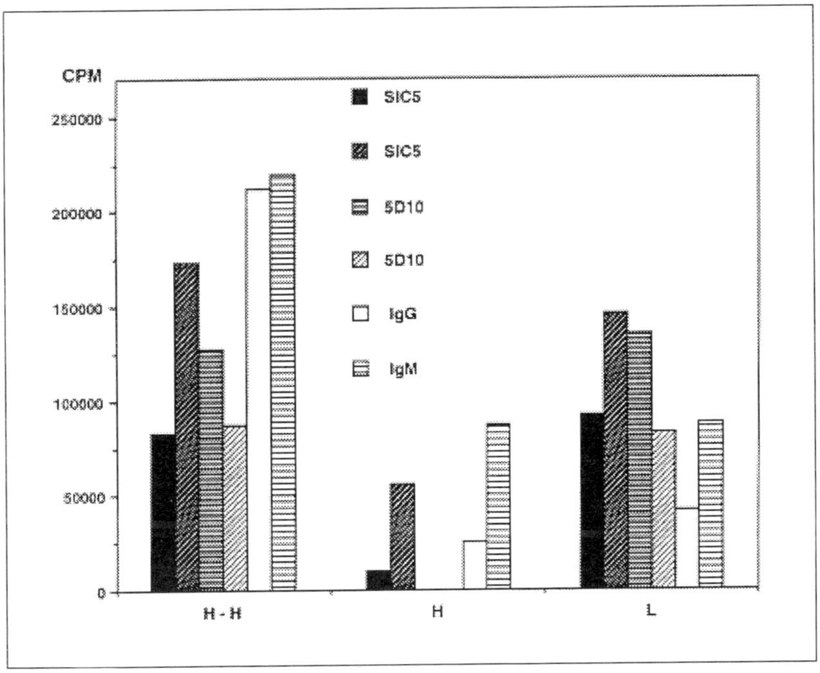

Fig. 13.1. Photoinsertion of γ^{32}P azido-ATP into several mouse immunoglobulins. Monoclonal mouse antibodies S1C5, 8019, 5D10, and mouse ployclonal IgM and IgG were photo-affinity labeled as described.[9] Labeled antibodies were separated on SDS-PAGE; radioactivity associated with protein bands is expressed in cpm. H-H denotes heavy chain dimers, H free heavy chain and L light chain.

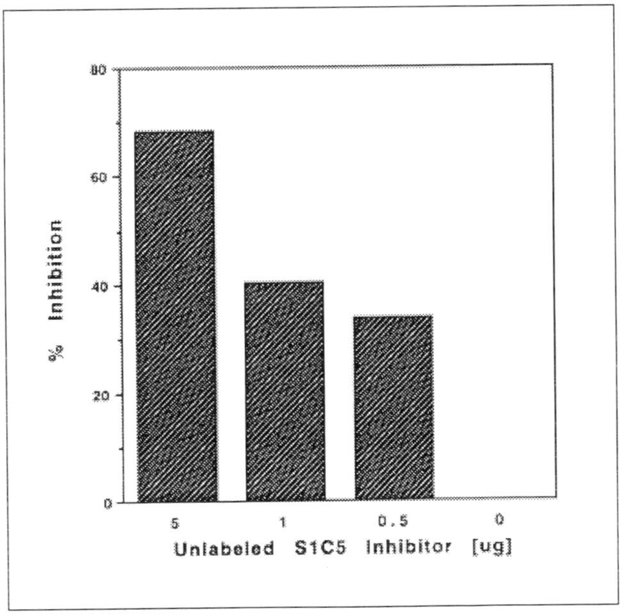

Fig. 13.2. Inhibition of binding of affinity radiolabeled SIC5 to insolubilized 38C13 tumor cells by unlabeled S1C5. Monoclonal S1C5, specific for the idiotype of the mouse 38C13 B cell lymphoma, was labeled with γ^{32}P azido-ATP as in Fig. 13.1. Labeled S1C5 was added to 38C13 tumor cells in the presence of increasing amounts of unlabeled S1C5 for 2 hours at 4C^{0}. After washing the amount of bound radioactivity was determined and expressed as percent inhibition of binding in absence of unlabeled S1C5.

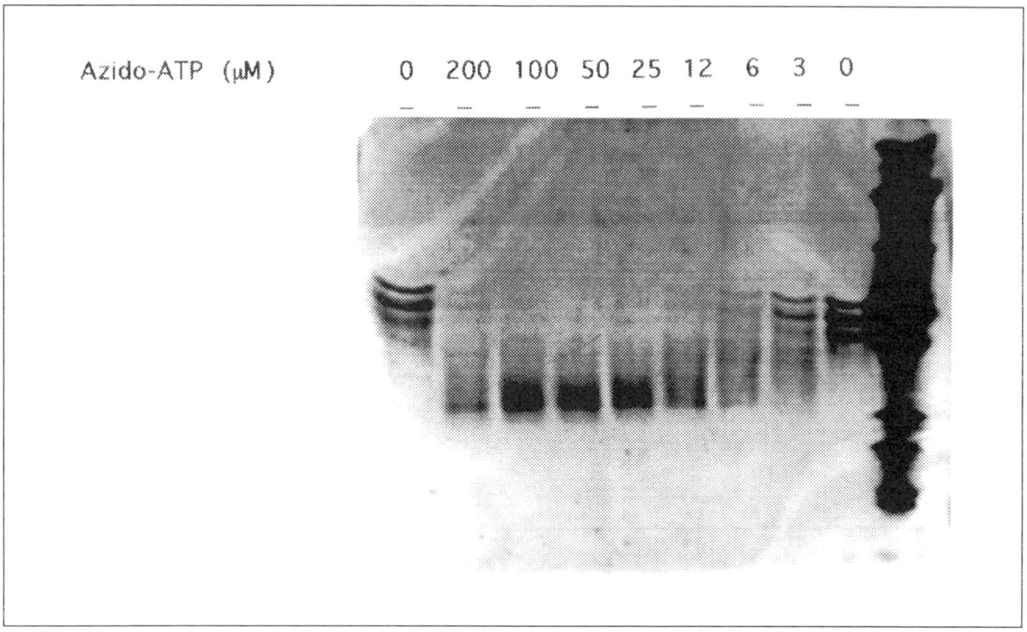

Fig. 13.3. Isoelectric focusing of S1C5 antibody. S1C5 was photo affinity labeled with increasing concentrations of 8-azido-ATP. Labeled S15 was applied to isoelectric focusing gels, pH range 3-9, and stained with Commassie blue.

the saturating concentration of photolabel. In Figure 13.3 the isolectric focusing patterns of a photo-affinity labeled monoclonal antibody using increasing concentrations of the probe are shown. The typical native three banding pattern of the monoclonal antibody converts with increasing concentrations of label to a single species with more acid isoelectric point.

Furthermore, protection experiments using nucleotides and aromatic amino acids implied K_D values for the photolabel in the range of 50-100 μM. Collectively these findings hinted strongly at the existence of an high affinity site on antibodies for heterocyclic ring compounds. The search for structural location of such a site followed protocols established for the determination of hapten binding sites[6] on antibodies or ATP sites on ATPases.[7] From the onset of our studies it was obvious that this site is not a typical ATP binding site, but might rather represent a hydrophobic pocket on the antibody molecule surface with the potential for aromatic ring base stacking.

At the same time Marianne Schiffer from the National Laboratory at Argonne became interested in our labeling experiments and initiated a search for a hydrophobic pocket on existing antibody Fab structures. She scanned the surface of Fab structures[8] for crevices which could accommodate the structure of ATP seen earlier in an ATP binding crystal. She could fit the ATP structure into a site located between the H-L interface away from the CDRs of the antigen contacting surface. By this time we had isolated a pair of labeled peptides from two monoclonal photoinserted antibodies, S1C5 and 8019. These peptides were derived from a tryptic digest of the intact molecules and were separated on a metal chelating column and HPLC. We had earlier cloned the V-genes and determined their DNA sequence in collaboration with Soshona Levy at Stanford and Ed Blalock at University of Alabama. The sequence of the labeled peptides could be easily placed into the V domains of H and L chains for both antibodies. Interestingly, the peptides included sections from

CDR and framework sequences. Each peptide contained aromatic residues, tyrosine and tryptophan, which can provide base stacking forces. Most importantly, both peptides from the H and L chains, made up the hydrophobic pocket in the H-L interface, into which Marianne Schiffer had fitted the ATP. The computer modeled insertion of ATP showed base stacking of the purine ring with a tryptophan residue at position H103 of the heavy chain. This tryptophan is one of the few invariant residues in the variable domain. Furthermore, the ATP makes also contact with a fairly conserved tyrosin residue in the light chain at position 36. There are additional residues in the pocket which are sufficiently close to the azido group of the photolabel to form a covalent bond after light exposure. Since these residues are part of the hypervariable CDR regions it is expected that this microenvironment differs in different antibodies and that therefore the extend of incorporation into light and heavy chains is different in different antibodies. Such different H/L photoincorporation has actually been seen in our labeling experiments. Collectively, photolabeling experiments, protein chemical analysis and computer modeling synergistically produced a molecular description of a novel affinity site on antibodies for nucleotides. The biological role of such a site, however remains a mystery. Nevertheless, it is highly tempting to assume that this site might have the function of a receptor site for a ligand which could function as a superantigen.

THE UTILITY OF THE SITE FOR CHEMICAL ANTIBODY ENGINEERING

The discovery of an affinity site on antibodies for photoreactive probes offers a new methodology to couple to anti-tumor antibodies therapeutically active and radio-image producing compounds. Currently applied coupling methods attach randomly active compounds to the antibody surface thereby altering or blocking the sensitive antibody binding site. The new method takes advantage of a naturally existing site which has high affinity for chemical ring structures, such as ATP and adenosine. The phosphate group and the ribose of both compounds can be used for attaching molecules of biological interest.

To demonstrate the feasibility of using photoreactive nucleotides or nucleosides we used the biotin-avidin system which is widely used to measure antigen-antibody binding. Biotin was conjugated to azido-ATP via a phosphate ester linkage and to the oxidized ribose of azido-adenosine via aldehyde condensation reaction. Both azido-biotin reagents were photolysed to antibodies using standard reaction conditions. Saturation of photolabeling with both compounds was similar. Monoclonal and polyclonal photo-affinity biotinlylated antibodies were tested in ELISA and FACS and found to give read-outs comparable to conventionally biotinylated antibodies. Furthermore, we assumed that the affinity and relative specificity of the nucleotide-photoprobes could afford direct photo-affinity biotinylation of antibodies in serum or in culture supernatant from hybridoma cells lines. Sera from HIV-1 infected individuals and control normal sera were biotinylated without prior purification and used in ELISA (Fig. 13.4). The ELISA results demonstrated that antibodies against HIV-1 antigens can be detected without using secondary antibody.

CONCLUSION

A general affinity site on immunoglobulins of different classes and species was discovered using a nucleotide photoprobe.[9] Insertion of ATP or adenosine compounds does not interfere with antigen binding as tested with a large panel of monoclonal and polyclonal antibodies. The site is formed by invariant residues in the Fv domains of H and light chains and is easily accessible from the surface of the Ig structure. Since the site has high affinity for nucleotides containing purine bases it is suggested that biological functions are associated with this site. Preliminary data with catalytic antibodies support this notion. In

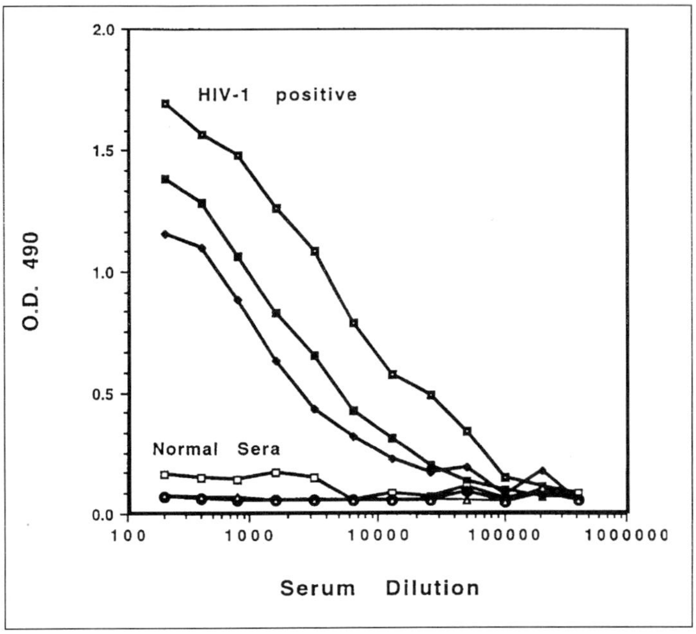

Fig. 13.4. ELISA using directly photo-biotinylated HIV-1 positive sera. Plates were coated with recombinant p17 core protein. HIV positive and negative sera were affinity-biotinylated and added to plates. After washing avidin-horse radish peroxidase was added and ELISA was developed.

addition the site can be used to insert reporter or effector molecules into antibodies without endangering the integrity of the antibody. This property can also be used for chemical antibody engineering.

References

1. Nisonoff A, Hopper JE, Spring SB. The antibody molecule. Academic Press NY, 1975.
2. Haas IG. BiP-A heat shock protein involved in immunoglobulin chain assembly. Curr Topics Microbiol Immunol 1991;167:71-82.
3. Haley BE. Nucleotide photoaffinity labeling of protein kinase subunits. Methods Enzymol 1991; 20:477-487.
4. Maloney DG, Kaminski MS, Burowski D. Monoclonal anti-idiotype antibodies against murine B cell lymphoma 38C13: Characterization and use as probes for the biology of the tumor in vivo and in vitro. Hybridoma 1985; 4:191-209.
5. George JT, Stevenson FK. Prospects for the treatment of B cell tumor using idiotype vaccination. Intern Rev Immunol 1989, 4:271-310.
6. Cheseboro B, Metzger H. Affinity labeling of a phosphorylcholine binding mouse myeloma protein. Biochemistry 1972; 11:766-771.
7. Potter RL, Haley B. Photoaffinity labeling of nucleotide binding sites with 8-azidopurine analogs: techniques and applications. Methods Enzymol 1983; 91: 613-633.
8. Pokkuluri PR, Bouthiller F, Li Y et al. Preparation, characterization and crystallization of an antibody Fab fragment that recognizes RNA. Crystal structure of native and three Fab-mononucleotide complexes. J Mol Biol 1994; 243:283-297.
9. Rajagopalan K, Pavlinkova G, Levy S et al. Novel unconventional binding site in the variable region of immunglobulins. Proc Natl Acad Sci US 1996; in press.

CHAPTER 14

Superantigen-Induced Stimulation of Rheumatoid-Factor Producing B Cells

Jörg J. Goronzy, Xiaowen He and Cornelia M. Weyand

INTRODUCTION

The term "superantigen" was introduced for a number of antigens that are able to stimulate a large fraction of the total T cell repertoire. Most superantigens are of microbial origin and often function as bacterial toxins. The staphylococcal products, enterotoxin A through E, have been studied in detail for their superantigenic activity. In contrast to mitogens, stimulation of T cells by superantigens requires the presence of an MHC class II antigen presenting cell. Also, superantigens do not stimulate the total T cell repertoire but only a fraction of 5-30%. The molecular basis for these observations are well defined.[1] Superantigens function by building a bridge between the T cell receptor (TcR) on the T cell and a major histocompatibility (MHC) class II molecule on the antigen presenting cells. The binding is largely specific for the TcR Vβ element and only to a lesser degree influenced by TcR polymorphism within the α-chain or the junctional region of the β-chain. The binding site on the MHC class II molecule is located outside of the peptide binding cleft and is therefore not influenced by allelic polymorphisms.

By virtue of their ability to stimulate T cells and to build a bridge between T cells and cells expressing MHC class II molecules, superantigens have been shown to be a potent stimulator of T cell dependent polyclonal B cell activation.[2] Applying this model to an in vivo situation, superantigen stimulation may mimic a chronic graft-versus-host disease, which can lead to clinical manifestations of autoimmunity, including IgG autoantibody production.[3] It has been proposed that different superantigens differ in their ability to act as T cell dependent B cell stimulators.[4] We have, therefore, compared the ability of different superantigens

Human B Cell Superantigens, edited by Moncef Zouali.

to promote B cell help and to induce autoantibody production.[5] In these studies, we have found that the T cell superantigen staphylococcal enterotoxin D (SED) in the presence of T cells expressing the appropriate TcR Vβ element activates a subset of B cells which is characterized by a high frequency of immunoglobulins expressing rheumatoid factor (RF) specificity.

Several models can account for the finding that a T cell superantigen activates a particular subset of B cells. It is possible that the selective B cell stimulation by SE D reflects the repertoire of T cells which are activated by the superantigen and are competent to provide B cell help and that the superantigen itself is only a surrogate marker for this subset of functionally selected T cells. Alternatively, this superantigen may have a direct effect on the B cell population. Binding of the superantigen to the MHC class II molecules expressed on B cells mediates transmembrane signaling which may even be enhanced by the cross-linking of class II molecules occurring during superantigenic stimulation.[6] Evidence has been provided that B cell activation as well as B cell apoptosis may be influenced by MHC mediated signals.[7,8] B cell subsets may differ in their susceptibility to these signals, which could explain the preferential stimulation of RF producing B cells with SED. A third possibility implies that SED does not only selectively bind to certain TcR molecules, but also to selected immunoglobulins. In this context, it is of particular interest that human T cells express MHC class II molecules and that an additional bridging between cell bound immunoglobulins on B cells and MHC class II molecules on T cells is possible.

To address these questions, we have characterized the molecular diversity of the immunoglobulin heavy chains expressed by B cells which proliferate in response to SED stimulated T cell clones. Our results show that the V_H gene segment repertoire of SED stimulated B cells is unique compared to polyclonally stimulated B cells, suggesting that SED directly targets immunoglobulin molecules.[9] The V_H repertoire of SED stimulated B cells shares many features with the repertoire of B cells which spontaneously secrete antibodies with RF specificities in patients with rheumatoid arthritis (RA) and primary Sjögren's syndrome (pSS).[10] These results suggest that SED targets a B cell subset which is activated and produces autoantibodies in RA and pSS patients.

STIMULATION WITH THE BACTERIAL SUPERANTIGEN SED PREFERENTIALLY INDUCES RF PRODUCTION

Human T cell clones were established and characterized for their response pattern to a series of bacterial superantigens. 1×10^5 T cell clones were then cocultured with 10^4 B cells and the T cell clones were either activated by an appropriate superantigen or by immobilized anti-CD3. Supernatants were harvested after 11 days, and the concentrations of secreted IgM, IgG, and antibodies with RF specificity was determined. In the anti-CD3 driven cultures, antibodies with RF activity were only detectable in coculture systems utilizing B cells from patients with RA.[5] In contrast, stimulation with SED resulted in a preferential stimulation of B cells secreting RF. A representative experiment is shown in Figure 14.1 with B cells from a normal individual. Although anti-CD3 and SED driven cultures induced similar amounts of IgM and anti-CD3 driven cultures were generally superior in the induction of IgG, significant levels of RF were only found in the SED driven cultures. Compared to other bacterial enterotoxins which function as superantigens, this effect was most pronounced for SED. The T cell clone used in the experiment in Figure 14.1 equally proliferated to SEC3 and SED. Immunoglobulin secretion was reduced in the SEC3 driven cultures, however, RF production was completely absent.

To examine whether RF production was influenced by the T cell clone used, a panel of T cell clones were tested.[5] These experiments showed that the induction of

RF production correlated with the superantigen and not with the T cell clone used. SED was clearly superior to the other superantigens tested in its potency to induce RF production. In these experiments, the supernatants were adjusted for the total amount of IgM secreted and the RF activity was compared in the adjusted samples (data not shown).

Subsequently, we addressed the question whether the selective induction of RF depended on the SED binding to the T cell or the B cell. If T of B cells were separated by permeable membranes, RF production was not induced regardless of whether the SED was incubated with the T cell or the B cell.[5] We utilized a T cell clone which did not proliferate in response to SED. This T cell clone was activated with anti-CD3 and cocultured with B cells incubated with SED at the appropriate concentrations (Fig. .14.2). RF producing B cells were activated under these tissue culture conditions, suggesting that binding of the SED to the B cell is important in the preferential stimulation of RF producing B cells.

To further analyze the functional repertoire of B cells stimulated with SED, the frequency of RF producing B cells stimulated under the two culture conditions, coculture with anti-CD3 stimulated T cells and coculture with SED stimulated T cells were compared.[11] Replicate cultures of serial dilutions of B cells were incubated with 1 x 10^5 cloned T helper cells and the frequency of immunoglobulin producing cells and RF producing cells was determined after 15 to 16 days. Upon activation of the

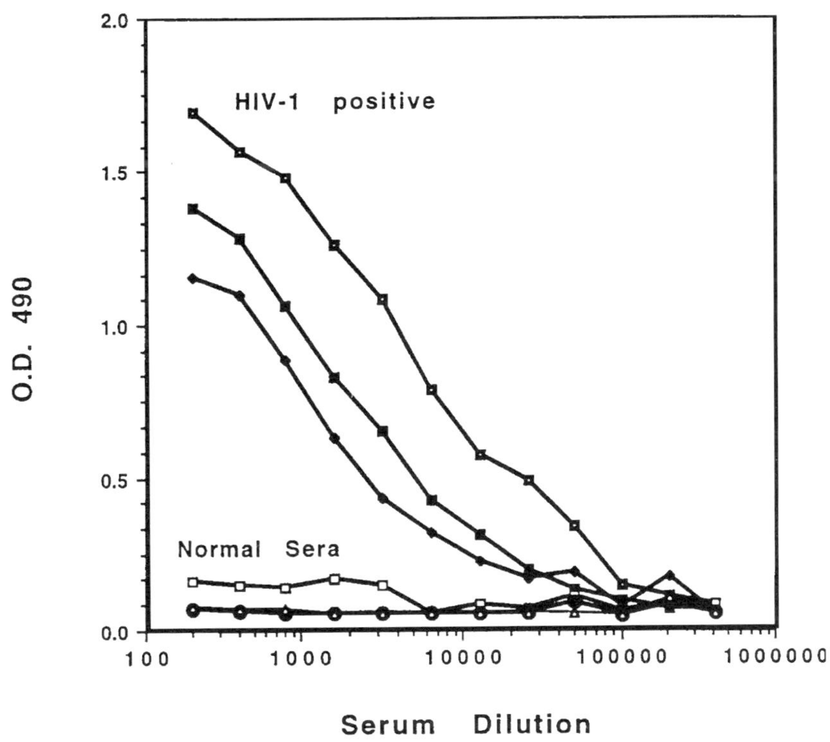

Fig. 14.1. Selective stimulation of RF producing B cells by the bacterial enterotoxin SE D. 10^4 B cells from a normal donor were cocultured with 1 x 10^5 activated cloned T cells. T cell activation was performed with immobilized anti-CD3 (left), 0.5 µg/ml SE C3 (middle) and SE D (right). The T cell clone proliferated equally to all three stimuli (data not shown). Culture supernatants were analyzed for IgM (open bars), IgG (shaded bars) and RF (solid bars) by ELISA. (Modified with permission from: He X et al. J Clin Invest 1992; 89: 673-80. ©1992 The American Society for Clinical Investigation, Inc.)

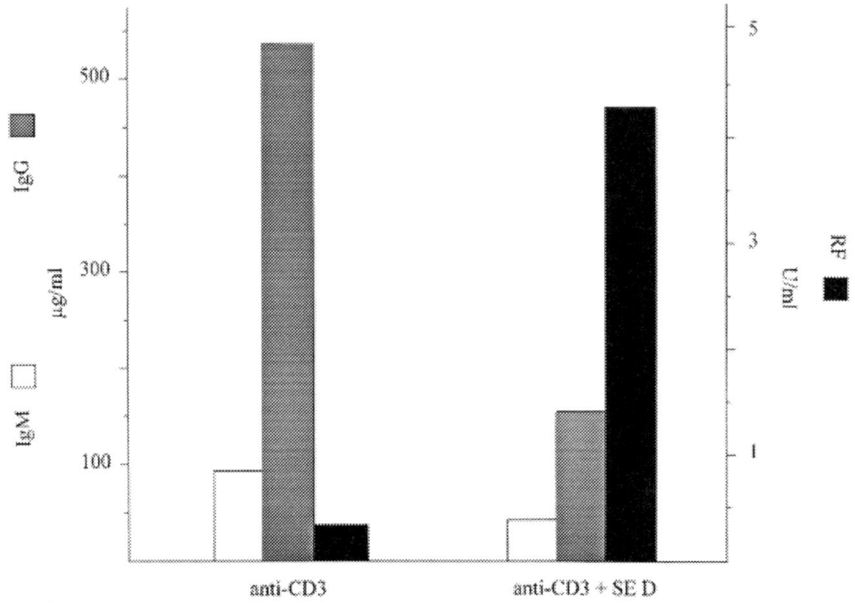

Fig. 14.2. Induction of RF is Independent of the Binding of SE D by the TCR. 10^4 B cells were cocultured with 1×10^5 cells of a T cell clone which did not proliferate to SE D. T cells were stimulated with immobilized anti-CD3 and the production of IgM (open bars), IgG (shaded bars) and RF (solid bars) was determined. The addition of SE D (right panel) suppressed total immunoglobulin production and selected for B cells secreting antibodies with RF specificities. (Reprinted with permission from: He X, Goronzy J, Weyand C. J Clin Invest 1992; 89: 673-80. ©1992 The American Society for Clinical Investigation, Inc.).

T cells with cross-linked anti-CD3, approximately 2-10% of B cells from normal donors' peripheral blood started to proliferate and to synthesize IgM and IgG. Only approximately 1 out of 500 of these B cells produced antibodies with RF specificity. In contrast, stimulation of the T/B cell cultures with SED induced the preferential outgrowth of RF^+ B cells, approximately 1 out of 3, to 1 out of 4 IgM producing B cells produced antibodies with RF specificity.[11] Patients with RA had higher frequencies of RF^+ B cells which could be activated in the anti-CD3 driven cultures. The repertoire of SED responsive B cells was, however, indistinguishable in normal controls and in patients with RA in that approximately 30% of IgM antibodies detected in the culture supernatant had RF activity. These data suggest that SED activates a subset of B cells which is characterized by a high frequency of RF producing B cells. This subset of B cells is present in similar frequencies in normal individuals and in RA patients. In normal individuals, these B cells do not respond to anti-CD3 activated T cells. However, it was unclear whether there is a relationship between B cells spontaneously synthesizing RF and SED responsive B cells in RA patients.

MOLECULAR CHARACTERIZATION OF IMMUNOGLOBULIN HEAVY CHAIN SEQUENCES OF SED STIMULATED B CELLS

To investigate whether SED targets RF producing B cells by immunoglobulin specific mechanisms, B cell clones were established from three different donors and characterized for their immunoglobulin heavy chains.[9] In these experiments, a T cell clone was cocultured with a limited number of B cells (1-3 cells/well). The T cells were either activated by immobilized anti-CD3 monoclonal antibody or by SE D. IgM producing and RF producing microcultures were identified and the B cells were analyzed for V_H gene segment usage by V_H specific RT-PCR. Under both culture conditions, V_H3 gene segments were most frequently used (43% in the anti-CD3 driven cultures versus 48% in the SE D stimulated cultures). Specifically, most of the RF producing B cells obtained after SE D stimulation expressed a V_H3 gene element.

Figure 14.3 shows a comparison between RF^- B cells after coculture with anti-CD3 stimulated T cells and RF^+ B cells derived from the three different donors after SE D stimulation. Eighty percent of the RF^+ versus 43% of the RF^- B cells utilized a V_H3 gene segment. The subsequent, more detailed analysis of the immunoglobulin genes were therefore restricted to the V_H3^+ B cell clones. The PCR amplified products were directly sequenced and the sequences were compared with published germline sequences for both sets of B cell clones. The majority of sequences had a high homology with the germline sequences. In those sequences for which sequence deviations were found, the replacement/silent ratio was low and there was no clustering of mutations in the complimentarity determining regions (CDR), suggesting that the B cell clones established under both culture conditions do not show extensive evidence of somatic mutation.

The distribution of V_H, D_H, and J_H gene segment usage in V_H3^+ B cell clones

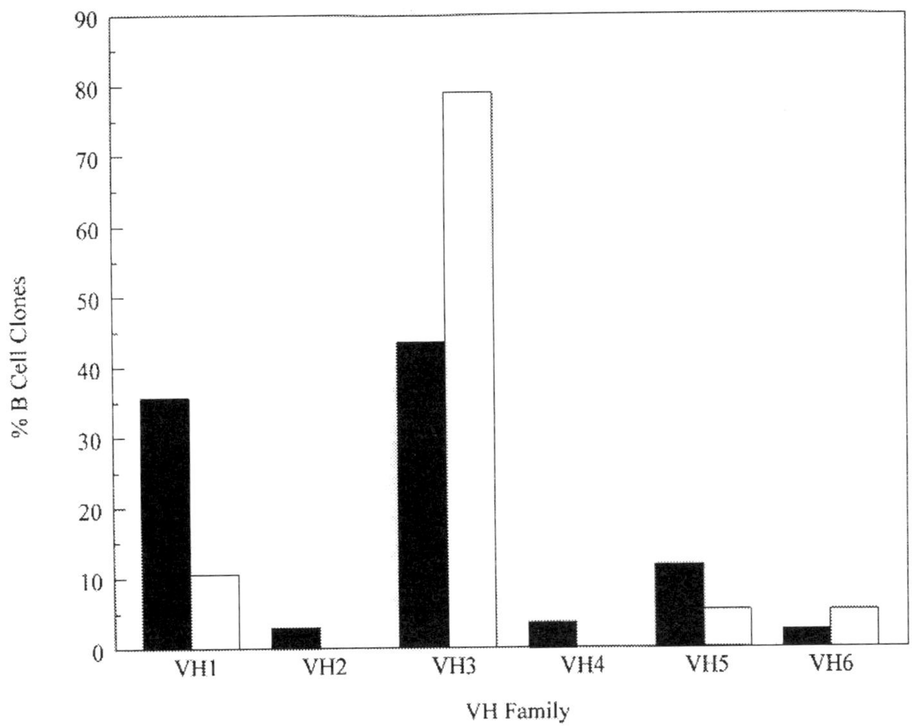

Fig. 14.3. V_H3 gene family usage of SE D responsive RF^+ R. B cell clones were established by coculture with anti-CD3 stimulated cloned T cells (solid bars) and by coculture with T cells and SE D (open bars). SE D responsive B cells were characterized for their ability to produce RF and only RF^+ microcultures were selected. VH gene family usage was determined by RT-PCR. Compared to the polyclonally activated B cells (solid bars), the RF^+ B cells from the SE D driven cultures preferentially used a VH3 gene element. (Modified with permission from: Xie C et al. International Immunol 1995; 7: 425-434. ©1995 Oxford University Press).

Table 14.1. Comparison of the distributions of V_H, D_H and J_H elements in VH3+ B cell clones

	% B cel clones				
	V3-23	**V3-21**	**V3-30**	**V3-48**	**Others**
anti-CD3	33	0	26	13	29
SE D	17	28	39	0	17

	JH1	JH2	JH3	JH4	JH5	JH6
Anti-CD3	0	4	4	67	13	13
SE D	0	0	6	50	17	28

	DXP	DA	DLR	DK	DN	DM	DHFL16	DHQ	DIR	Unassigned
anti-CD3	29	0	21	17	25	4	4	0	4	4
SE D	17	11	28	22	6	11	6	6	0	17

Distribution of V_H elements is idfferent at p = 0.01
(Modified with permission from Xie C et al. International Immunol 1995; 7:425-434. ©1995 Oxford University Press.)

are shown in Table 14.1. Under both culture conditions, anti-CD3 and SE D activated T cell clones, the J_H4 gene segment was most frequently used. Also, there was no difference in the distribution of D_H gene segment usage when the two culture conditions were compared. However, V_H gene segment usage could distinguish the two modalities of stimulation. The most striking difference was the usage of V3-21 which was not found at all in the anti-CD3 driven cultures but was present in 28% of the SED driven cultures encountered. In contrast, the V3-23 gene segment, which has been described to be frequent in the human B cell repertoire[12] and which was expressed by 33% of all B cell clones established with anti-CD3 activated T cells was less frequently utilized in the SED driven cultures. The distributions of V_H elements used by the B cell clones established under the two different culture conditions was significantly different at the p = 0.001 level.

These results suggest that SED may directly target immunoglobulin heavy chain sequences. Preferential usage of the V_H3 gene segment family would be consistent with the notion that it may act as a B cell superantigen. However, the skewing within the V_H3 family and the preferential usage of certain V_H3 elements, in particular V3-21, suggests that the interaction must be more complex than the binding of a superantigen to a framework determinant as the framework is conserved for all V_H3 elements. The major differences between V3-21 which was enriched in the SED driven cultures and V3-23 which was decreased resides within the CDR1 and CDR2. In particular, V3-21 is characterized by a stretch of five serines in the CDR2, raising the possibility that the binding of SED to the immunoglobulin heavy chain is not as straightforward as postulated for a superantigen and that CDR2 encoded determinants are important in SED binding.

COMPARISON OF RFS PRODUCED BY RA AND PSS PATIENTS AND SED INDUCED RFS FROM NORMAL CONTROLS

The repertoire of SED responsive B cells which produce immunoglobulins with RF specificities is not different when RA patients and normal individuals are compared. In contrast, only RA patients carry a highly frequent B cell subset which responds to anti-CD3 stimulated T helper cells with the production of RF. The SED responsive RF^+ B cells preferentially utilize certain members of the V_H3 gene family. To examine whether the RF producing B cells generated under the two different culture conditions (SED stimulation in normal versus coculture with anti-CD3 activated T cells in RA patients) are related, we have examined whether the RF^+ B cells derived from patients show the same preference for selected V_H3 elements. We have established clonal B cell populations from the peripheral blood of normal donors (127 B cell clones), RA patients (113 RF^- and 60 RF^+ B cell clones) and patients with pSS (82 RF^- and 47 RF^+ B cell clones) by coculturing with anti-CD3 stimulated T helper cell clones.[10] The cross-reactivity pattern of the RF antibodies secreted by the B cell clones was determined by ELISA on a panel of antigens (Ig Fc, actin, keratin, denatured DNA, thyroglobulin, and tetanus toxoid). Only 8 of the 68 antibodies were truly polyreactive and had a broad cross-reactivity pattern. Forty-five antibodies were monospecific for Fc fragments and within the panel of antigens tested, no cross-reactivity was detected.

The molecular structure of the IgM heavy chain was again characterized by V_H family specific RT-PCR and sequencing of the amplified product. The V_H gene segment usage of the IgM heavy chains from RF^+ and RF^- B cells are shown in Table 14.2. RF specificity was associated with a preferential usage of V_H3. Members of the V_H3 gene family were used in 42% of RF^- B cells from normals compared to 77% in RF^+ B cells from RA patients. This difference was significant at the $p = 0.001$ level. The preferential usage of V_H3 is very similar to the results obtained for RF^+ B cells from SED driven cultures in normal individuals (Fig. 14.3). In these experiments, 80% of SED stimulated RF^+ B cells utilized V_H3 compared to 42% of B cell clones which were derived from normal individuals by coculture with anti-CD3 stimulated B cells and which did not secrete immunoglobulins with RF specificity.

IgM heavy chains which expressed a member of the V_H3 family were again sequenced and the V_H3 subtypes were determined. The results are summarized in Table 14.3. The two germline gene segments, V3-23 and V3-30, accounted for approximately two-thirds of all the V_H3^+ B cell clones analyzed. The usage of V3-23 was decreased in both, patients with RA and patients with pSS. In both patient subsets, the usage of V3-21 was increased. This gene segment was not found at all in RF^- B cells from normal controls but was used by B cells derived from pSS and RA patients. The usage of V3-21 correlated with RF specificity in both patient sub-

Table 14.2. V_H genesegment usage in IgM heavy chains from RF^+ and RF^- B cells

Donors	Specificity	No. of clones	Frequency % V_H1	V_H2	V_H3	V_H4	V_H5	V_H6	p patients vs normal controls
Normal controls	RF^-	127	30.7	3.9	42.5	8.7	12.6	1.6	N/A
RA patients	RF^-	113	23.0	3.5	50.4	16.8	4.4	1.8	n.s.
	RF^+	60	13.3	1.7	76.7	3.3	3.3	1.7	0.001
pSS patients	RF^-	82	24.4	2.4	43.9	12.2	11.0	6.1	n.s.
	RF^+	47	21.3	2.1	61.7	6.4	4.3	4.3	n.s.

Table 14.3. Usage of V_H3 gene segment in IgM heavy chains from RF^+ and RF^- B cells

Donors	Specificity	No. of clones	Frequency % V3-23	V3-30	V3-21	V3-15	Others	p patients vs normal controls
Normal controls	RF^-	33	39.4	27.3	0	3.0	30.3	N/A
RA patients	RF^-	34	17.6	20.6	5.9	8.8	47.1	n.s.
	RF^+	31	16.1	13.0	19.4	16.1	35.5	0.007
pSS patients	RF^-	27	18.5	25.9	7.7	3.7	44.4	n.s.
	RF^+	27	11.1	37.0	14.8	0	37.0	0.03

(Reprinted with pemission from He X et al. Molecular Med 1995; 1:768-780. ©1995 Molecular Medicine.)

sets. The distribution of the different V_H3 family members in the RF^+ B cells derived from RA and pSS patients were significantly different from the distribution in normal individuals. As it was also the case for the SED stimulated B cells, no differences in J_H and D_H gene segment usage were observed when RF^+ B cell clones from RA patients and from pSS patients were compared with RF^- B cells from normal individuals.

The molecular analysis of RF^+ B cells obtained from normal individuals after SED stimulation and of RF^+ B cells obtained from RA and pSS patients showed striking similarities. For both subsets of B cells, a preferential transcription of members of the V_H3 families is characteristic. For both subsets, the V_H3 gene segment V3-23, which is abundantly used in a random B cell population, is diminished while the gene segment V3-21 is found in increased frequencies. These results suggest that there is a structural relationship between the SED responsive B cells in normal individuals and the RF^+ B cells which are preactivated in the peripheral blood of patients with RA. V3-21$^+$ B cells are present in the repertoire of normal individuals and can be stimulated with SED. However, they remain nonresponsive to anti-CD3 stimulated T cell clones. To directly address this issue, we have compared the proliferation of V3-21$^+$ and V3-23$^+$ B cells under the two culture conditions (Fig. 14.4). B cells from normal individuals were cocultured with anti-CD3 activated T cells or with T cells and SED. Microcultures were harvested after 20 days and V_H3 frequencies were amplified by V_H3 family specific PCR. The usage of V3-23 and V3-21 was semiquantified in the amplified product by hybridization with oligonucleotides specific for the sequence polymorphism within the CDR2. Both, stimulation in the presence of anti-CD3 activated T cells and stimulation with SED, resulted in the proliferation of V3-23 B cells as concluded from the high concentration of V3-23 transcripts. A different picture emerged for V3-21$^+$ B cells. In the anti-CD3 driven cultures, the V3-21 sequences virtually disappeared while they were present in high frequencies after SED stimulation. These data suggest that the B cells, which are targeted by SED via a V_H specific mechanism, are anergic in normal controls but responsive in patients with RA and pSS.

DISCUSSION

Immunity against pathogenic microbes is one of the fundamental functions of the immune system. The success of host defense is not only determined by the mobilization of natural and acquired immune responses but also by strategies developed by the microorganism. Pathogenicity of microbes may relate to their ability to invade and colonize the host, the production of toxins and the induction of tissue injury. Equally important for the survival of the pathogen is their capability to resist and evade host defense mechanisms. The common pathogen, the gram-positive bacterium *Staphylococcus aureus* produces exotoxins which have been classified based upon their distinct serology and include SEA, SEB, SEC, SED and SEE. These proteins derived from bacteria have recently attracted the interest of immunologists, not because of their immunogenicity, but because of their ability to stimulate T lymphocytes. Their superantigenic potential resulting in the activation of a substantial fraction of the T cell compartment might actually represent a pathogenic factor. The functional consequences of T cell stimulation includes the release of high concentrations of cytokines which could be responsible for manifestations like fever, cardiovascular leakage and shock. Also, functional implications of broad T cell activation might actually involve the induction of T cell nonresponsiveness. One of the fascinating aspects of superantigens derived from bacteria is the potential to link infection and autoimmunity.[1] Self tolerance is maintained by clonal deletion of potentially autoreactive lymphocytes and also by the induction of anergy. If superantigens can reactivate silenced T or B cells and thus break tolerance, they would represent a unique mechanism through which an infectious organism could eventually cause autoimmunity. Guided by these consider-

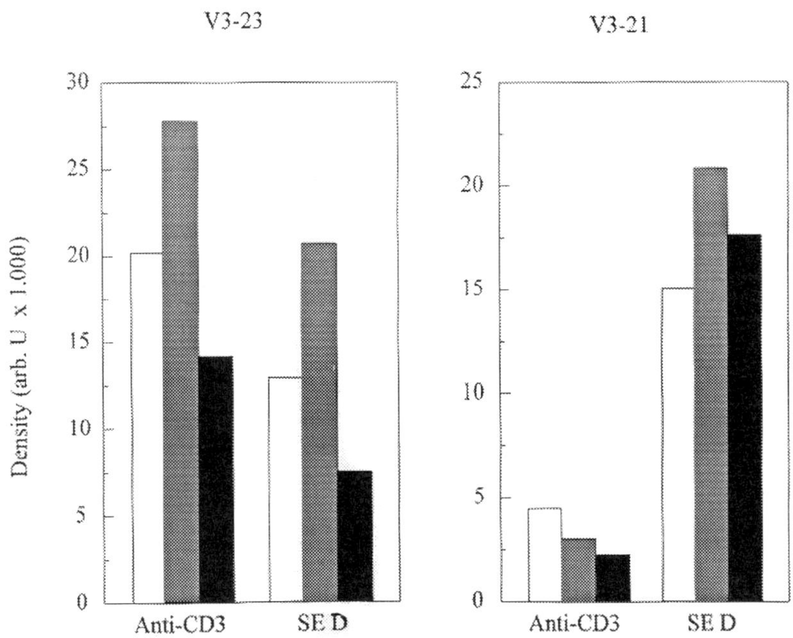

Fig. 14.4. V3-21 B Cells are nonresponsive to Anti-CD3 activated T cells but can be activated by coculture with SE D and T cells. B cells from three normal donors (open, shaded and solid bars) were cultured with anti-CD3 and SE D stimulated T cells as described in Fig. 14.1. Total RNA was obtained, amplified by RT-PCR with VH3 and IgM specific primers. V3-21 and V3-23 sequences were semiquantified by oligonucleotide hybridization. At the onset of culture, V3-21 sequences were present in high frequencies (data not shown). Only SE D and not anti-CD3 stimulated T cells were able to activate the V3-21⁺ B cells. (Reprinted with permission from: He X et al. Molecular Med 1995; 1: 768-780. ©1995 Molecular Medicine).

ations, we have focused on analyzing the functional consequences of superantigenic activity for T/B cell interaction. These studies have led to the observation that the staphylococcal product SED can selectively induce the synthesis and release of antibodies with RF specificity. Molecular analysis of SED induced RFs provides evidence that they are similar to RF spontaneously secreted in patients with RA and pSS. Our data are best compatible with a direct action of SED on a responsive B cell subset mediated through sequence polymorphisms encoded by the CDR1 and CDR2. In essence, these data support the model that exposure to the bacterial product SED could induce pathological events typically seen in some autoimmune syndromes.

Stimulation of B cells from normal individuals in the presence of the T cell superantigen, the bacterial enterotoxin SED and activated T cells resulted in the preferential proliferation of B cells which secrete antibodies with RF specificity. The finding that B cells with the potential to release RF are frequent in the repertoire of normal individuals is not surprising. It has long been known that chronic exposure to bacteria can induce RF positivity which is reversible with successful treatment of the infection. Thus, RF production is typical for patients with certain autoimmune syndromes such as RA and pSS but not pathognomic. Over the last decade, evidence has accumulated that RF^+ B cells are actually a critical component of normal immune responses. Kipps and Duffy[13] have shown that B cells which express immunoglobulins with RF specificity on their surface are characterized by a unique localization in the mantle zone of the lymph node, suggesting that they might be involved in antigen presenting events. Studies utilizing RF^+ lymphoblastoid lines have documented that RF^+ B cells are excellent antigen presenting cells.[14] Their capability to bind IgG containing immune complexes equips them with the ability to capture and enrich antigens contained in these immunocomplexes. Carson et al[15] have suggested that pathology of RF^+ B cells is linked to secretion of RF molecules but not their surface expression. Support for this model has come from experiments in RF transgenic mice.[16] B cells from these mice can function as potent antigen presenters but serum concentrations of RF were low. Inbreeding with MLR-lpr mice resulted in the abundant secretion of RF molecules, suggesting that RF expressing and RF secreting B cells are functionally distinct and underlie different regulatory mechanisms. Data presented here indicate that SED stimulation was capable of causing the secretion of immunoglobulins with IgG binding specificity.

The high frequency of SED-responsive B cells as determined by limiting dilution experiments suggests that the SED induced response does not represent a conventional antigen specific response. The SED induced shift in the antibody repertoire correlates with a distinct pattern of V_H gene segment usage in SED activated B cell clones compared with B cells grown in the presence of anti-CD3 activated T cells. SED is primarily a T cell superantigen,[17,18] however, these observations raise the possibility that it may also function as a B cell superantigen. B cell superantigenic activity has been exemplified for protein A which has been shown to bind to framework 3 determinants shared by all members of the V_H3 family and thus selectively activates V_H3 expressing specificities.[19] SED responsive RF^+ B cells also preferentially utilized a V_H3 gene segment.[9] Sequence analysis of V_H3^+ IgMs showed that most of these molecules were in germline configuration and that there was no biased usage of J_H and D_H gene elements. These observations are consistent with SED functioning as a B cell superantigen. In contrast to protein A, SED responsive B cells have a preferential usage of certain members of the V_H3 family. V3-23, which is enriched in SED responsive B cells, and V3-21, which is diminished, share a conserved framework sequence but are distinct in CDR1 and CDR2. These data would suggest that the CDR1 and/or CDR2 loops are involved in the interaction between SED and the Ig molecule, similar to responses to conventional antigens. A V_H restriction is not completely unusual for antibody responses to antigens and has been described for the response to the capsular polysaccharides of *Hemophilus influenza* type b.[20] The lack of restriction in the CDR3 could be compatible with an antigen specific response for which the sequence polymorphism in the CDR1 and CDR2 are most important. In contrast to the B cell response to conventional antigens, which is usually only detected after in vivo vaccination and even then in a low frequency, the number of SED responsive B cells which start to proliferate and to produce RF is high, at least in the order of several percent of the total B cell repertoire.[11] These data would suggest that while the interaction between SED and immunoglobulins involves the CDRs, it is broader and less selective than usually seen for responses to conventional antigens.

SED preferentially stimulates B cells which display RF specificity. The correlation between V_H gene segment usage and fine specificity would suggest that determinants encoded by the V_H gene elements are crucial for this antigenic profile. A correlation between V_H gene segment and, in particular, $V\kappa$ gene segment usage, has been described for RFs which are preferentially found in lymphoproliferative diseases.[21] We have not studied the molecular diversity of the Ig light chains after SED stimulation, however, the repertoire of V_H gene segment usage in the RFs derived from lymphoproliferative diseases such as chronic lymphocytic leukemia, Waldenström's macroglobulinemia, and mixed cryoglobulinemia and after SED stimulation are clearly distinct.

The RFs seen in patients with RA and pSS have a different molecular structure and are polyclonal.[22,23] It was therefore surprising to find that the SED induced RFs had structural similarities to the RFs seen in patients with RA and pSS. Peripheral blood mononuclear cells from RA patients and from pSS patients have a high frequency of B cells secreting RF which can be expanded in cultures stimulated with anti-CD3 activated T cells.[11,24] Under the same culture conditions, such B cells cannot be stimulated in normal individuals. Although most of the immunoglobulins with RF specificity established from the peripheral blood of RA and pSS patients are of the IgM isotype and are in germline configuration, the majority of these antibodies are rather selective for IgG Fc and do not cross-react in multiple antigens. The molecular analysis of the Ig heavy chain of these antibodies showed a very similar molecular structure compared to the SED responsive B cells. These antibodies preferentially utilize a V_H3 gene segment and within the V_H3 family the V3-21 gene segment is overrepresented and the V3-23 segment is underrepresented. In contrast to the V_H gene segment usage, the usage of J_H and D_H gene segments was not different from a randomly selected B cell population. These results raise the provocative possibility that the mechanisms underlying the induction of RFs in RA and pSS patients may share features with the selective activation of a B cell subset by SED under in vitro culture conditions. In this model, B cells which frequently use the V3-21 gene segment and which express RF specificity are frequent in the peripheral blood of healthy individuals, but they are anergic to conventional T cell dependent stimuli. This state of nonresponsiveness in normal individuals can be broken by superantigenic stimulation. A similar mechanism may function in RA and pSS patients. At this stage, the immunoglobulins are in germline configuration. Only subsequently somatic mutation occurs as a consequence of a T cell dependent antigen driven process.[22,23,25,26]

Acknowledgments

The authors appreciate the secretarial support of Toni L.Higgins. This work is supported in part by grants from the National Institutes of Health (RO1 AR71974 and RO1 AR42527), a Clinical Science grant (NAF #14) and a Biomedical Science grant (NÅÏ #16) from the Arthritis Foundation and by the Mayo Foundation.

References

1. Kotzin BL, Leung DYM, Kappler J et al. Superantigens and their potential role in human disease. Adv Immunol 1993; 54:99-166.
2. Mourad W, Mehindate K, Schall TJ et al. Engagement of major histocompatibility complex class II molecules by superantigen induces inflammatory cytokine gene expression in human rheumatoid fibroblast-like synoviocytes. J Exp Med 1992; 175:613-16.
3. Portanova JP, Kotzin BL. Lupus-like autoimmunity in murine graft-versus-host disease. Concepts. Immunopathol 1988; 6:119-40.
4. Tumang JR, Posnett DN, Cole BC et al. Helper T cell-dependent human B cell differentiation mediated by a mycoplasmal superantigen bridge. J Exp Med 1990; 171:2153-58.
5. He X, Goronzy J, Weyand C. Selective induction of rheumatoid factors by superantigens and human helper T cells. J Clin Invest 1992; 89:673-80.
6. Fuleihan R, Mourad W, Geha RS. Engagement of MHC-class II molecules by staphylococcal exotoxins delivers a comitogenic signal to human B cells. J Immunol 1991; 146:1661-66.
7. Nabavi N, Freeman GJ, Gault D et al. Signaling through the MHC class II cytoplasmic domain is required for antigen presentation and induces B7 expression. Nature 1992; 360:266-68.
8. He X, Zhong W, Goronzy JJ et al. Induction of B cell apoptosis by TH0, but not TH2, CD4+ T cells. J Clin Invest 1995; 95:564-70.
9. Xie C, Brühl H, He X et al. Selective activation of L3A10+ rheumatoid factor producing B cells by the staphylococcal enterotoxin D. Internatl Immunol 1995; 7:425-34.
10. He X, Goronzy JJ, Zhong W et al. VH3-21 B cells escape from a state of tolerance in rheumatoid arthritis and secrete rheumatoid factor. Molecular Med 1995; 1:768-80.
11. He X, Goronzy JJ, Weyand CM. The repertoire of rheumatoid factor producing B cells responsive to bacterial superantigen and bystander help in normals and patients with rheumatoid arthritis. Arthritis Rheum 1993; 36:1061-69.
12. Huang C, Stewart AK, Schwartz RS et al. Immunoglobulin heavy chain gene expression in peripheral blood B lymphocytes. J Clin Invest 1992; 89:1331-43.
13. Kipps TJ, Duffy SF. Relationship of the CD5 B cell to human tonsillar lymphocytes that express autoantibody-associated cross-reactive idiotypes. J Clin Invest 1991; 87:2087-96.
14. Lanzavecchia A. Receptor-mediated antigen uptake and its effect on antigen presentation to class II-restricted T lymphocytes. Annu Rev Immunol 1990; 8:773-93.
15. Carson DA, Chen PP, Kipps TJ. New roles for rheumatoid factor. J Clin Invest 1991; 87:379-83.
16. Tighe H, Chen PP, Tucker R et al. Function of B cells expressing a human immunoglobulin M rheumatoid factor autoantibody in transgenic mice. J Exp Med 1993; 177:109-18.
17. Choi Y, Kotzin B, Herron L et al. Interaction of *Staphylococcus aureus* toxin "superantigens" with human T cells. Proc Natl Acad Sci U.S.A. 1989; 86:8941-45.
18. Goronzy JJ, Oppitz U, Weyand CM. Clonal heterogeneity of superantigen reactivity in human V(6+ T cell clones. Limited contributions of V(sequence polymorphisms. J Immunol 1992; 148:604-11.
19. Hillson JL, Karr NS, Oppliger IR et al. The structural basis of germline-encoded V_H3 immunoglobulin binding to staphylococcal protein A. J Exp Med 1993; 178:331-6.
20. Silverman GJ. Human antibody responses to bacterial antigens: studies of a model conventional antigen and a proposed model B cell superantigen. Int Rev Immunol 1992; 9:57-78.
21. Carson DA, Chen PP, Fox RI et al. Rheumatoid factors and immune networks. Annu Rev Immunol 1987; 5:109-26.
22. Sasso EH. Immunoglobulin V genes in rheumatoid arthritis. Rheum Dis Clin N Am

1992; 18:809-36.

23. Randen I, Thompson KM, Pascual V et al. Rheumatoid factor V genes from patients with rheumatoid arthritis are diverse and show evidence of an antigen-driven response. Immunol Rev 1992; 128:49-71.

24. He X, Zhong W, McCarthy TG et al. Increased frequencies of rheumatoid factor producing B cells in seronegative rheumatoid arthritis. Arthritis Rheum In press.

25. Olee T, Lu EW, Huang D-F et al. Genetic analysis of self-associating immunoglobulin G rheumatoid factors from two rheumatoid synovia implicates an antigen-driven response. J Exp Med 1992; 175:831-42.

26. Randen I, Brown D, Thompson KM et al. Clonally related IgM rheumatoid factors undergo affinity maturation in the rheumatoid synovial tissue. J Immunol 1992; 148:3296-301.

CHAPTER 15

Superantigen-Dependent Helper T Cell/B Cell Interaction: A Model for Helper T Cell-Mediated B Cell Activation and Apoptosis

Elaine J. Schattner, Dae-Hyun Yoo, Mary K. Crow and Steven M. Friedman

INTRODUCTION

The superantigens (SAgs) are a fascinating group of microbial products that impact the immune system by virtue of their affinity for T cell and B cell antigen receptor variable (V) region gene products.[1,2] The first SAg to be recognized selectively trigger T cell mitogenesis, and include gene products of the 3' long terminal repeat open reading frame of mouse mammary tumor virus (previously known as minor lymphocyte-stimulating (Mls) antigen),[3-7] the *Staphylococcus aureus* enterotoxins,[8] the *Streptococcus* M protein,[9] and a gene product of *Mycoplasma arthritidis*, termed MAM.[10] These T cell SAgs share a number of features that distinguish them from conventional peptide antigens. In particular, SAgs bind avidly to major histocompatibility complex class II (MHC-II) molecules at a site distinct from the conventional antigen-binding cleft, in the absence of antigen processing. In contrast to regular antigens, which bind selectively to antigen-specific T cell receptor (TcR) complementarity determining regions (CDRs), SAgs have affinity for the products of one or more TcR Vβ gene families. As many as 5-30% of an individual's T cell pool is activated in this manner, such that SAgs are potent Vβ selective T cell mitogens.

Human B Cell Superantigens, edited by Moncef Zouali. © 1996 R.G. Landes Company.

Careful examination of specific B cell mitogens has provided convincing evidence that some of these agents represent B cell SAgs. While it has been generally recognized that Staphylococcal protein A (SpA) can bind to IgG at the Fc region, it is now understood that SpA can also bind via a second, immunoglobulin (Ig)-interactive domain.[11-13] By specifically engaging Ig heavy chain variable V_H3 gene products, SpA serves as a selective B cell mitogen. Similar findings have been observed for other microbial gene products that bind to Ig V gene products. For example, the human immunodeficiency virus (HIV) gp120 molecule also appears to target V_H3 positive B cells.[14] Similarly, Protein L of *Peptococcus magnus* binds specifically to selected kappa light chain V gene families.[15] Finally, as discussed in other chapters in this volume,[16] there is experimental evidence to suggest that the Staphylococcal enterotoxins, which have a clear role as T cell SAgs, may also function as B cell SAgs.

Our laboratory has developed a model system which uses microbial SAgs to examine the effects of cognate helper T cell (Th)-B lymphocyte interactions on B cell activation and function.[17] Direct (cognate) interaction between antigen-specific B of $CD4^+$ T cells is essential for initiation of humoral immune responses. In conventional cell culture systems, analysis of the consequences for the B cell of cognate interaction is hampered by the fact that Th cells and B cells specific for any particular antigen are present at very low frequency. The approach we have applied takes advantage of the dual affinity of microbial SAgs for MHC-II molecules expressed on the B cell surface and particular TcR β chain V gene products. According to this model, any B cell, regardless of its specificity for antigen, may bind SAg to surface MHC class II antigens and be rendered a target for cognate T cell help by SAg-reactive Th cells. The SAg "bridge" facilitates a nonphysiologic form of cognate T/B cell interaction between SAg-bearing B cells and SAg-reactive $CD4^+$ T cells, such that the B cell response can be analyzed at the population level.

Initially, we explored the potential for SAg-induced Th/B cell interactions to effect positive B cell responses, proliferation and Ig secretion.[18-20] More recently we have shown that SAg-mediated Th/B cell interaction can promote T cell-dependent apoptotic deletion of B cells.[21] Experimental data pertaining to these two areas of investigation are outlined below.

SAGS MEDIATE PRODUCTIVE TH/B CELL INTERACTION

Gleichmann and co-workers have proposed that abnormal interactions of Th and B cells provide the cellular basis for graft versus host disease (GVHD).[22-23] This disease is characterized by acute and chronic immunologic abnormalities, due to donor Th cells specific for recipient MHC class II alleles which interact with recipient B cells in a cognate manner. This process drives both polyclonal and antigen-specific antibody production, particularly in response to multivalent foreign and autoantigens. We have suggested that the dual affinity of SAgs for MHC class II molecules and selected TcR Vβ gene products promotes an abnormal form of cognate Th/B cell interaction which mimics that seen during GVHD. This hypothesis is supported by a number of in vitro experiments that demonstrate a clear, T cell dependent immunostimulatory effect of some microbial SAgs on the humoral arm of the immune response.

Some of the background for this work comes from experiments in our laboratory in which a panel of microbial SAgs were used to activate peripheral blood mononuclear cells, and diverse T and B cell responses were observed.[18,20] In our experience, the *S. aureus* enterotoxins elicit vigorous T cell mitogenic responses but do not usually stimulate Ig production. In contrast, the *Mycoplasma arthritidis* SAg, MAM, is a less potent mitogen for peripheral human T cells, and yet triggers a strong, T cell-dependent polyclonal IgM and IgG response. Further analyses of specific *S. aureus* toxins (SEB and SEE) and toxic shock syndrome toxin (TSST-1) indicate that these SAgs can, in fact, trigger Th cell-dependent B cell activation of autologous B cells, if the T cells have been x-irradiated or if their proportion is extremely small in relation to the target B cells. These observations suggest that the strong T cell response induced by SAgs to which a high proportion of Vβs react may actually dampen the humoral response.

Based on the analogy between SAg-mediated Th/B cell collaboration and aberrant Th/B association in GVHD, we sought to assess the effects of SAg and compare them with GVHD sequelae in vivo, by extending our investigations concerning Th-mediated, SAg-induced B cell activation to the murine system. First, we demonstrated that murine B cells can be activated by syngeneic SAgs-reactive Th cells and SAg in vitro, resulting in polyclonal IgG and IgM production. Here, the presence of specific antigens in culture, such as heterologous erythrocytes, promoted the production of antigen-specific antibodies. We also found that splenic B cells, isolated from BALB/c nude mice which had been treated in vivo with the SAg TSST-1, efficiently and selectively induce the in vitro proliferation of TSST-1 specific, syngeneic Th cells and, in turn, are driven to proliferate and differentiate into antibody producing cells. These results suggest that B cells that bind bacterial SAg in vivo are rendered effective stimulators of and targets for SAg-reactive Th cells.

To extend the analysis of SAg's capacity to promote productive Th/B cell collaboration in vivo, we performed adoptive transfer experiments in which 20 x 10^6 purified BALB/c splenic B cells were transferred into SCID recipients. After a four week interval, which allowed for B cell engraftment and the production of low levels of serum IgG, the mice also received 10 x 10^6 TSST-1-reactive BALB/c Th cells and 50 μg of TSST-1 intravenously. As shown in Figure 15.1, the transfer of Th cells and TSST-1 resulted in a rapid and striking increase in serum IgG concentrations in both recipients. The SCID mice were then rechallenged with TSST-1 on three separate occasions over a nine month period. In each case, there was a prompt increase in serum IgG levels.

The role of TSST-1 and TSST-1-reactive Th cells in stimulating IgG production was further delineated by experiments using TSST-1 in four groups of SCID mice that were reconstituted with BALB/c B cells, as described above. In the first group, the SCID mice were injected with 50 μg of active TSST-1 four weeks after they were given B cells. As shown in Figure 15.2, these B cell-reconstituted SCID mice failed to show an increase in serum IgG levels in response to the administration of TSST-1 alone. These three mice received 50 μg of active TSST-1 at four distinct time points (Fig. 15.2A), and although the serum IgG concentrations rose somewhat over the course of the experiment, this change was not temporally associated with administration of SAg. In contrast, B cell reconstituted mice that also received 10 x 10^6 TSST-1 reactive syngeneic Th cells, responded to each subsequent TSST-1 challenge with a prompt increase in serum IgG levels (Fig. 15.2B). Panels C and D show the results of similar experiments using an inactive form of TSST-1. As shown, heat-inactivated TSST-1 did not affect serum IgG levels, even in the presence of TSST-1 reactive Th cells. Taken together, these results suggest that both SAg reactive Th cells and biologically active SAgs are required to effect SAg-dependent B cell activation in vivo.

Given the putative role of SAg-induced B cell activation in autoimmune disease,[23] we examined the sera from the mice shown in Figures 15.1 and 15.2 for the presence of autoreactive antibodies that are characteristic of autoimmune diseases such as systemic lupus erythematosus (SLE). Antinuclear antibodies (ANA's) were negative during the first three months in all mice tested. However, 4-8 months after B cell engraftment, there was weak staining (1^+) of the nuclear membrane using sera obtained from mice that received the active form of TSST-1 and TSST-1 reactive Th cells, but not in any of the other test groups. IgG anti-DNA antibodies were not detected in the sera of any test group. It should be noted that TSST-1-reactive Th cells were readily detected in the spleen of these mice at the time of sacrifice (data not shown).

Taken together, our studies demonstrate that repetitive exposure to certain microbial SAg can promote Th cell-dependent B cell activation in vivo. This strengthens the analogy between SAg-mediated Th/B cell interactions and allo-specific Th/B cell interactions which are responsible for autoimmune sequelae of GVHD. Following exposure to microbial SAg that do not induce anergy in the CD4+ subset, SAg-reactive Th cells may provide an abnormal form of cognate help for B cells. In particular, B cells that react with multivalent self-antigens, which comprise the targets of autoantibodies in SLE, may become fully activated and differentiated such that they efficiently generate and secrete antibody. In this regard, we note that the SCID recipients reconstituted with normal BALB/c B cells, TSST-1 reactive Th cells, and TSST-1 produced low levels of anti-nuclear autoantibodies, but not anti-DNA antibodies. One explanation may be the absence of pathogenic autoreactive B cells in the splenic B cell pool of normal BALB/c donors. Alternatively, under

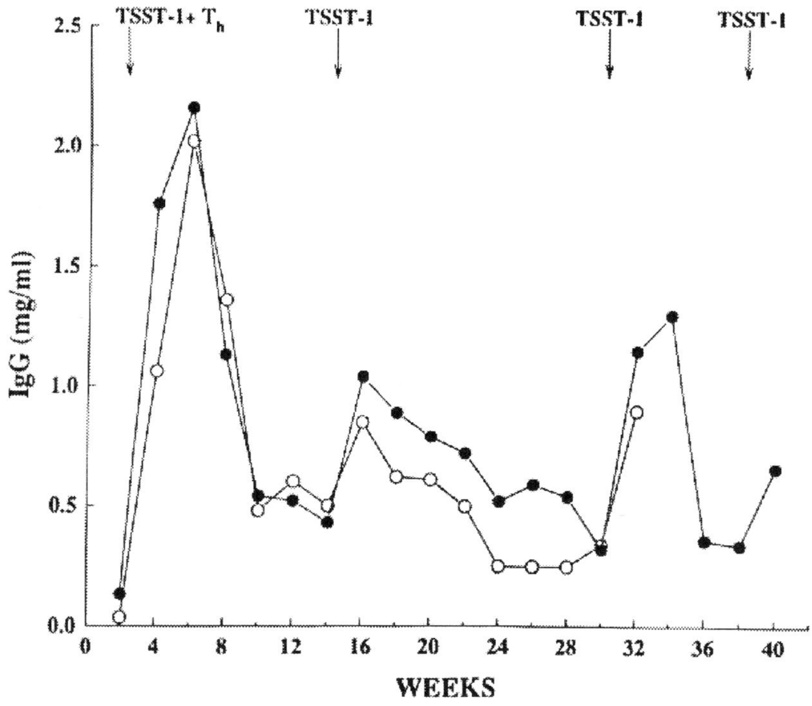

Fig. 15.1. Microbial SAg activate B cells in vivo. 20 x 10^6 purified BALB/c splenic B cells were adoptively transferred into two, six week-old syngeneic SCID recipients. After four weeks, which allowed B cell engraftment, the mice received 10 x 10^6 TSST-1-reactive BALB/c Th cells and 50 µg TSST-1 by intravenous injection. The mice were rechallenged with TSST-1 alone at subsequent points (arrows) and serum IgG levels assayed by ELISA at the time points indicated. (Note that one mouse died at week 32, two weeks following TSST-1 administration). Each curve (open or closed circles) represents the results for an individual mouse.

these experimental conditions, there may be an inherent resistance of BALB/c B cells to breaking tolerance.

SAg-DEPENDENT TH/B CELL INTERACTION CAN RESULT IN B CELL APOPTOSIS

The negative effects of some bacterial products on the immune system and, in particular, on B cell growth, have been appreciated for some time, but the specific mechanisms have been elucidated only recently. In one of the first reports on the effects of SAg in vivo, Marrack and Kappler's group observed that SEB injection into mice resulted in a toxic condition characterized by weight loss and immune suppression that is mediated by T cells with Vβ-reactivity to SEB.[8] The capacity of some SAg to specifically reduce growth of a tumor cell population was suggested by Newell and co-workers, who reported that SEB injection suppressed growth of a xenografted skin tumor, in an effect that was mediated by activated, SEB-reactive T cells.[24] This observation was extended to lymphocytic tumors by Ochi et al, who used SEB conjugated to anti-idiotype antibody against an IgM-expressing, MHC-II negative murine B cell lym-

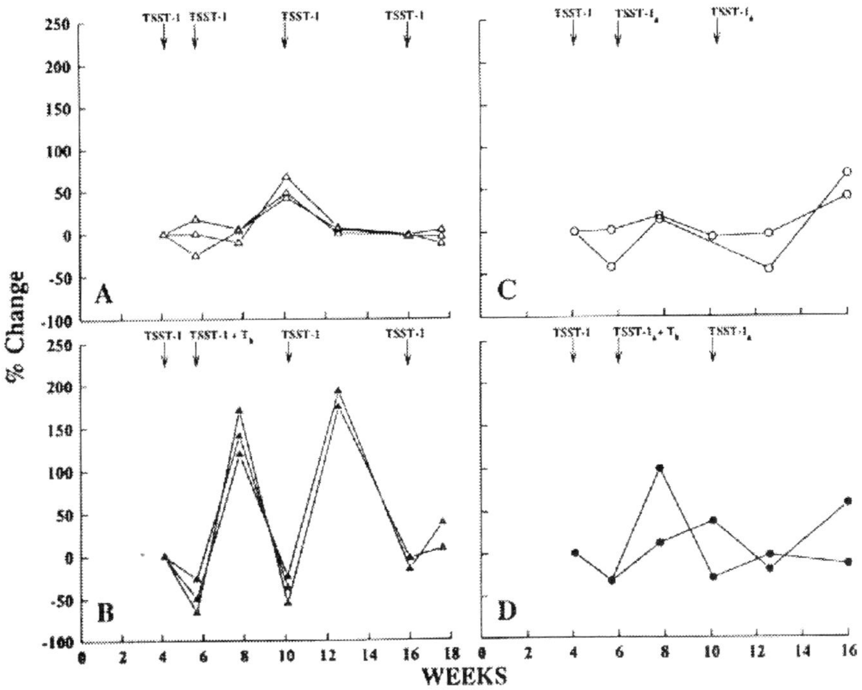

Fig. 15.2. TSST-1-dependent B cell activation in vivo requires SAg-reactive Th cells and biologically active TSST-1. SCID mice were engrafted with 20 x 10^6 purified BALB/c B cells as described for Fig. 15.1. Four weeks later, all mice were challenged with 50 μg of active TSST-1. Two weeks later, two groups (B, D) received 10 x 10^6 TSST-1-reactive BALB/c Th cells while the remaining groups (A, C) were injected with medium alone. At the time points indicated (arrows), mice received active TSST-1 (A, B) or heat inactivated (Δ) TSST-1 (C, D). As shown, the plots reflect the percent change in serum IgG concentrations as compared to the preceding IgG level. (Note that one mouse treated with active TSST-1 and TSST-1-reactive Th cells died at week ten, following TSST-1 administration (B)). Closed symbols, mice receiving Th cells; open symbols, mice receiving media alone; triangles, mice receiving biologically active TSST-1; circles, mice receiving heat-inactivated TSST-1.

phoma line, and found that this combination offered significantly more anti-tumor effect than either SEB or anti-idiotype antibody alone.[25]

Although T cell-mediated cytotoxicity and anti-tumor effects are often attributed to $CD8^+$ cytotoxic T cells (CTL's),[26,27] several lines of evidence have clarified the cytolytic capacity of $CD4^+$ T cells. In 1986, Schmid and co-workers reported that certain Th clones induce apoptotic destruction of target cells by secretion of a soluble factor.[28] Romagnani's group established that *Toxicara canis*-reactive Th1 cells have cytolytic capacity and actually reduced Ig production by autologous Epstein-Barr virus (EBV)-transformed B cells pulsed with that antigen.[29] Subsequent investigations have demonstrated that the majority of $CD4^+$ T cell-mediated apoptosis is mediated by Fas ligand. These results contrast with those observed for $CD8^+$ T cells, which exercise cytotoxicity of target cells by processes that are predominantly calcium-dependent, and perforin-mediated.[30] Fas (CD95, APO-1) is a 48-kDa cell surface antigen of the tumor necrosis factor/nerve growth factor (TNF/NGF)-receptor superfamily[31] that can mediate apoptosis of lymphocytes and certain other cell types, including cells of lymphocyte cell lines and some solid tumor cell lines.[32,33] Fas ligand is expressed or secreted by activated Th1 type $CD4^+$ T cells, and when bound to the Fas receptor on the lymphocyte induces their apoptotic destruction.[34-37] We and others have reported that $CD4^+$ T cells are important in immune regulation of some B cell malignancies by means of the Fas-Fas ligand cytotoxicity pathway.[21,38]

In our laboratory, the link between $CD4^+$ T cells, Fas ligand, and B cell cytotoxicity was established in the course of investigations concerning SAg-induced cognate interaction between $CD4^+$ T cells and target B cells. Using MAM and MAM-reactive $CD4^+$ T cells, we observed the induction of B cell apoptosis as a consequence of SAg-induced Th cell-B cell interaction. We initially obtained this result using human tonsillar B cells in coculture with SAg-reactive T cells and SAg. These B cells were observed to express augmented levels of the Fas antigen, and underwent accelerated apoptosis in vitro. Because nontransformed, in particular germinal center B cells, undergo spontaneous apoptosis in vitro, the human Burkitt's lymphoma (BL) Ramos cell line cells were used as B cell targets for most of the subsequent studies. The Ramos B cell line was chosen for these experiments because the BL cells represent the malignant outgrowth of resting germinal center B cells.[39,40] The Ramos cells are the oncologic equivalent of early B cells that express CD10, CD40, and CD54 (ICAM). They express low levels of the Fas antigen.[41] As shown in Table 15.1, when

Table 15.1. SAg-induced cognate T-B signaling upregulates Fas expression and apoptosis of Ramos Burkitt's lymphoma B cells

Description of culture	Mean fluorescence channel (MFC) Fas staining	Cell viability after 72 hours (x 10^6/ml)
Ramos + media	31	2
Ramos + MAM (1:80,000)	31	1.6
Ramos + T_{MAMxr}	82	1.1
Ramos + MAM (1:80,000) + T_{MAMxr}	420	0.4

Ramos B cells were cultured for 72 hours with media, MAM, irradiated, $CD4^+$, MAM-reactive T cells (T_{MAMxr}), or MAM + T_{MAMxr}. After staining with a biotin-conjugated antibody to Fas, followed by FITC-avidin, or with a biotin-conjugated control antibody, followed by FITC-avidin, the cells were analyzed by flow cytometry. The mean channel fluorescence for each Fas stain is indicated. Note that at the time of analysis, >99% of the gated cells were B1 positive, and <1% CD4 positive. Viabilities were determined by hemocytometry after diluting each cell suspension in trypan blue.

Ramos B lymphocytes are cultured in the presence of polyclonal, CD4$^+$ SAg-reactive T cells and the relevant SAg (in this case MAM), they are induced to express high levels of the Fas antigen and undergo apoptosis. This does not occur when B cells are exposed to SAg without SAg-reactive T cells, in which case, there is no increase in B cell Fas expression and, for most SAg, there is no effect on B cell viability. When the B cells are exposed to SAg-reactive T cells in the absence of SAg, or in the presence of an extraneous SAg, there is a slight to moderate upregulation of the Fas antigen on the target B cells, but B cell death does not occur. In contrast, when SAg-reactive T cells and the relevant SAg are both present with the B cells, B cell Fas expression is markedly enhanced and the cells undergo apoptosis. To demonstrate the functionality of increased Ramos B cell Fas expression, we used an IgM anti-Fas preparation that induces apoptosis via Fas receptor crosslinking, and found that apoptosis of the SAg and SAg-reactive T cell-stimulated B cells was specifically augmented by the anti-Fas monoclonal antibody. In addition, there was partial inhibition of apoptosis using a blocking, nonsignaling $F(ab')_2$ anti-Fas antibody preparation.[21] Importantly, these results do not rule out the activity of other cytotoxic pathways that may be induced by the SAg bridge in the setting of a polyclonal SAg-reactive CD4$^+$ T cell population, such as apoptosis induced by perforins or TNFα.

Investigations in our laboratory and others have demonstrated that Fas expression alone is not sufficient for B cell death. Rather, in B cells that are sensitive to Fas-mediated death signals and express the Fas receptor at their surface, Fas must be triggered by either antibody to Fas, or by the physiologic ligand for Fas, Fas ligand, for apoptosis to occur. In our system (and in vivo), an important determinant of the B cell's fate may be the relative abundance of Th1 and Th2 cells in coculture. Th1 cells secrete cytokines central to the cellular immune response, such as IL-2 and IFN-γ, and selectively express Fas ligand following activation. In contrast, Th2 cells secrete cytokines such as IL-4 and IL-10, which support the humoral immune response.[42]

Based on the fact that Fas ligand mediates Th1 CD4$^+$ T cell-induced cytotoxicity, we predicted that although any SAg-reactive CD4$^+$ T cells might upregulate Fas on target B cells when SAg is present, only the Th1 cells would induce apoptosis of the activated B lymphocytes. To test this hypothesis, we employed MAM-reactive Th1 and Th2 CD4$^+$ T cell clones derived from one normal donor, and compared the efficacy of these clones in their capacity to upregulate Fas on Ramos B cell targets and to induce apoptosis. As shown in Figure 15.3, when either MAM-reactive Th1 or Th2 cells are present with Ramos B cells, but without MAM, there is no significant upregulation of Fas on the B cells. When MAM is added to the culture system, Fas is upregulated in each case, as expected, due to the effects of cognate signaling induced by T cells in the presence of SAg. However, B cell death occurs only in the presence of Th1 type CD4$^+$ T cells. This specific activity of the Th1 cells in inducing apoptosis of activated, Fas-expressing B cells supports the role of these cells and Fas ligand in SAg-mediated B cell death.

Once antigen-specific T cells have bound to B cells that express antigen in the context of MHC-II, or have bound due to a SAg "bridge" effect between the TcR and MHC-II on the B cell, cognate signals are transmitted between the T of B cells by at least two pairs of costimulatory molecules. These include CD40 ligand (CD40L), which is transiently expressed on CD4$^+$ T cells following T cell activation, and the CD40 molecule, which is constitutively expressed at the B cell surface.[43] The other well-described costimulatory pair is CD28 on the T cell and B7 (BB1) on the B cell.[44] Until recently, the interaction of CD40L and CD40 were understood to have positive effects on the B cell. Ligation of CD40 on resting germinal center B cells has been shown to cause B cell activation characterized by tyrosine kinase activity, increased DNA synthesis, and expression of activation antigens including CD23.[45,46] Unstimulated germinal center B cells, usually die within a few days in culture, but can be rescued from apoptosis by exposure to anti-CD40 antibody, or to CD40L.[47] SAg-induced T cell activation promotes B cell growth by cytokine production and also by upregulating CD40L.

Based on the capacity of SAg to link T of B cells in a cognate interaction, we examined whether the CD40-CD40L component of cognate signaling was responsible for Fas upregulation in the B cell. Using CD40L⁺ Jurkat T cell line mutants which constitutively express this molecule (D1.1), and CD40L⁻ mutants which cannot express CD40L (B2.7),[48] we observed that the CD40L⁺ cells selectively induce Fas upregulation on Ramos B cells. Subsequent studies, using monoclonal antibody to CD40, demonstrated that CD40 cross-linking at the B cell surface results in Fas upregulation and renders the cells susceptible to Fas-mediated death. This result was reported by our laboratory using the Ramos human BL cell line, by Marshak-Rothstein's group using murine splenic B cells, and by Banchereau's group using human tonsillar B cells.

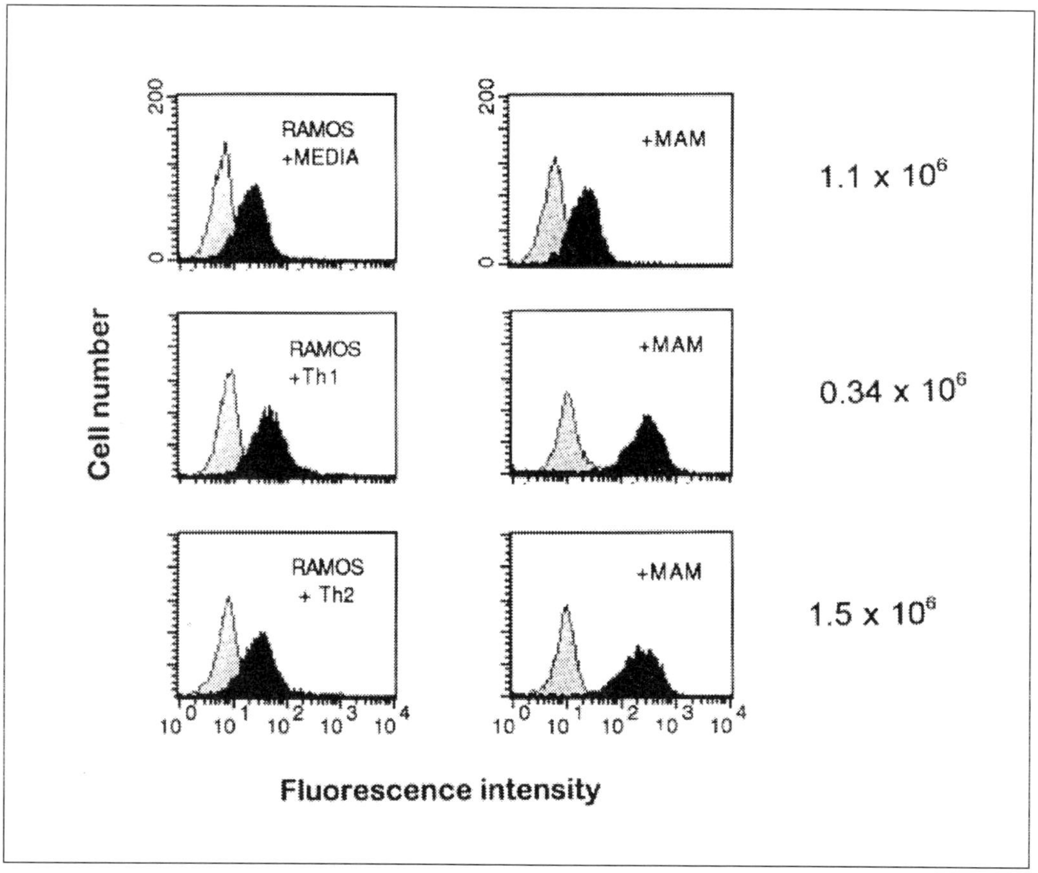

Fig. 15.3. Both Th1 and Th2 MAM-reactive CD4⁺ T cells induce Fas expression on target B cells in the presence of MAM, but only the Th1 cells induce apoptosis. Ramos B cells were cultured in the presence of media (upper panel), with a CD4⁺, MAM-reactive Th1 clone (M19, middle panel) or Th2 clone (M26, lower panel) derived from peripheral blood T cells of a healthy donor. The cells were grown in culture without (left) or with (right) MAM, and analyzed by flow cytometry and fluorescence staining. Shown are stains with a negative control (CD4, pale histograms), and Fas (dark histograms). Histograms depict cell number versus intensity of fluorescence staining. The number to the right of each MAM histogram pair represents the viability of cells, in millions of cells per ml, after three days of culture with MAM, as indicated.

Under some circumstances, B cells induced to upregulate Fas are rendered resistant to death signals, particularly when they are stimulated by concomitant crosslinking of the surface antigen receptor. In our experimental system using MAM and MAM-reactive CD4+ T cells in the presence of target Ramos B cells, there is a striking protective effect of surface immunoglobulin (sIg) crosslinking (Fig. 15.4). As we have demonstrated before, when the B cells are exposed to MAM and MAM-reactive CD4+ T cells, there is dramatic cell death. In the presence of anti-human IgM, however, apoptosis is reduced, in a process that is inversely dose-dependent. The rescue effect of sIg crosslinking occurs when anti-IgM is added as late as 48 hours into the coculture experiment (panel B), but not after 72 hours (data not shown).

Taken together, these results indicate that SAg-induced cytotoxicity of human B cells by CD4+ T cells is reduced in the presence of antigen-receptor crosslinking. The findings are consistent with a multistep model for antigen-specific B cell activation. In the presence of either antigen receptor crosslinking or T cell stimulatory signals alone, the B cells are deleted. However, when both antigen and antigen-specific Th cell signals are provided, the B cells are protected from Fas-mediated apoptotic deletion. At the same time, Fas expression on the B cells is upregulated by CD40 ligation, which allows for subsequent, Fas-mediated elimination once antigen is no longer present. In addition, by upregulating Fas and facilitating elimination of those B cells that have not seen antigen, the multistep process offers protection in the germinal center from bystander B cells that may become inappropriately activated by CD4+ T cells.

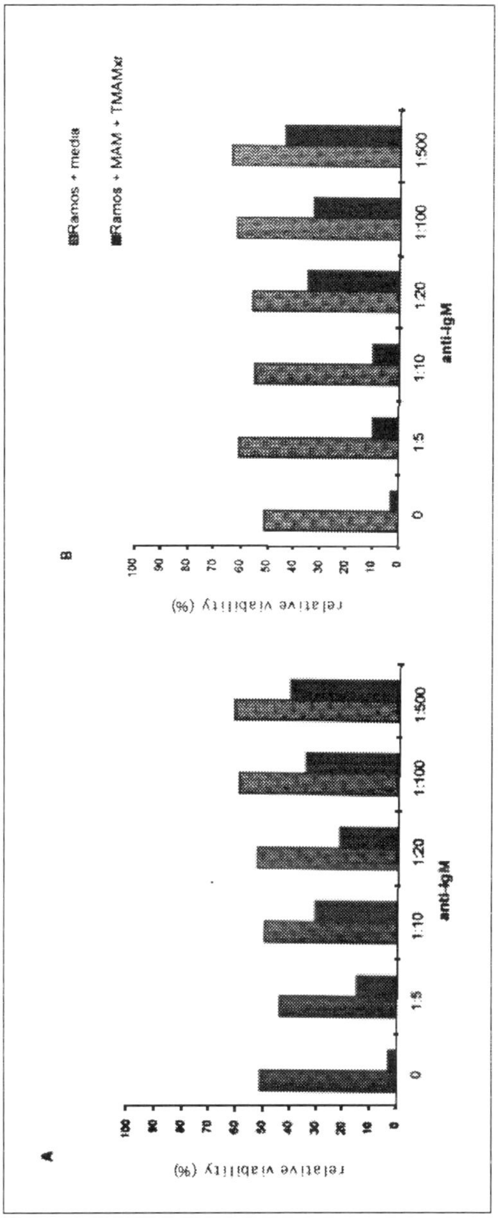

Fig. 15.4. Crosslinking of the surface antigen receptor by anti-IgM reduces SAg-induced, T cell mediated apoptosis of target B lymphocytes. Ramos B cells were cultured with media alone, or with MAM and MAM-reactive CD4+ T cells (T_{MAMxt}), in the absence or presence of varying dilutions of culture supernatant containing the murine anti-human IgM monoclonal antibody, HB57. As shown, there is only a minor effect of sIg crosslinking on Ramos B cells with media. In contrast, when the SpA bridge system is used to induce B cell apoptosis (MAM + T_{MAMxt}), B cell viability is improved in the presence of anti-IgM added at either t_0 (panel A) or t_{48}h (panel B). The reduction of SpA-induced B cell apoptosis relates inversely to the dose of crosslinking anti-IgM.

POTENTIAL ROLE FOR SAG IN AUTOIMMUNE DISEASE PATHOGENESIS

The association of particular TcR Vβ gene family usage among pathogenic T cells in a variety of autoimmune diseases is suggestive that SAg may be important in the pathophysiology of those diseases. Moreover, there is some direct evidence for SAg-activity in Kawasaki's disease and also in juvenile diabetes.[49,50] The potent but selective T and B cell-stimulatory effects of SAg suggest several distinct mechanisms by which SAg may be pathogenic in inflammatory and autoimmune diseases. First, SAg may trigger damage to the host by massive cytokine release, such as that which occurs in the toxic shock syndrome induced by the Staphylococcus SAg, TSST-1. Another possibility is that SAg may activate autoreactive T cells that are normally quiescent. Presumably, such clones that have escaped thymic deletion have too low an affinity for self-antigen to be activated by self-antigen that is present in the periphery. However, following an encounter with SAg, self-reactive T cells that have been activated and express high levels of adhesion molecules would interact readily with tissues expressing the relevant self-antigen, and would accordingly drive an organ specific autoimmune response. Finally as discussed above, SAg can promote an aberrant form of Th/B cell interaction analogous to that which occurs in GVHD, and in this manner may play a role in systemic autoimmune disease such as systemic lupus erythematosus (SLE).

In this context, it is pertinent that the Fas/FasL system is implicated in SLE. This is based on observations of several strains of mice that develop SLE-like features and bear defects in expression or function of Fas (*lpr*) or FasL (*gld*). These mice accumulate double-negative ($CD4^-$, $CD8^-$) T cells in the peripheral lymphoid organs, produce autoantibodies, and develop systemic immune-complex disease.[51-53] Since it was known that these murine models of SLE arise due to defects in the Fas-FasL system, we sought to examine Fas-Fas ligand function in humans with SLE by utilizing our assay for SAg-dependent $CD4^+$ T cell-induced Fas-mediated apoptosis of B cells. For these experiments, short-term cultures of $CD4^+$ T cells reactive with MAM were generated from the peripheral blood lymphocytes of SLE patients, and from normal donors.

Ramos B cells, which we know to be sensitive to Fas upregulation and apoptosis in the SAg system, were cocultured with irradiated MAM-reactive $CD4^+$ T cells in the presence or absence of MAM. In each case, Fas antigen expression and viability of Ramos cells were assessed after 48 hours. We found that MAM-reactive $CD4^+$ T cells derived from the peripheral blood of 12 SLE patients functioned quite similarly to the MAM-reactive $CD4^+$ T cells derived from healthy human controls. For example, Figure 15.5 demonstrates the results using SAg-reactive T cells from one patient. As shown, the interaction of MAM-reactive $CD4^+$ T cells, MAM, and Ramos B cells, resulted in marked upregulation of Fas expression on the B cells, which suggests that CD40L is expressed in the SLE patient's T cells and can transmit cognate signals. Moreover, it is clear from these observations that the SLE $CD4^+$ T cells, like those derived from healthy controls, can induce efficient, Fas-mediated death of the Ramos-B cell targets. We would point out that, in collaboration with Dr. Keith Elkon's group, we have observed that peripheral B cells from SLE patients express normal levels of the Fas antigen. It remains to be formally established, however, whether SLE B cells that express Fas undergo apoptosis as usual. The SAg bridge system provides an opportunity for examining $CD4^+$ T cell-induced cytotoxicity of a variety of B cell targets, and could in principal be applied to the SLE B cells.

SAg AND SAg-T $CD4^+$ T CELLS INDUCE FAS-MEDIATED APOPTOSIS OF MALIGNANT HUMAN B CELLS

The SAg bridge system provides a window for observing $CD4^+$ T cell-mediated regulation of B cell tumors. Using T cell lines (TCLs) of known SAg-reactivity, cognate stimulatory capacity, and Fas ligand function, we can use this model to evaluate malignant B cell resistance to $CD4^+$ T cell-mediated Fas upregulation and apoptosis. In the SAg bridge system, failure of B cell apoptosis can occur due to

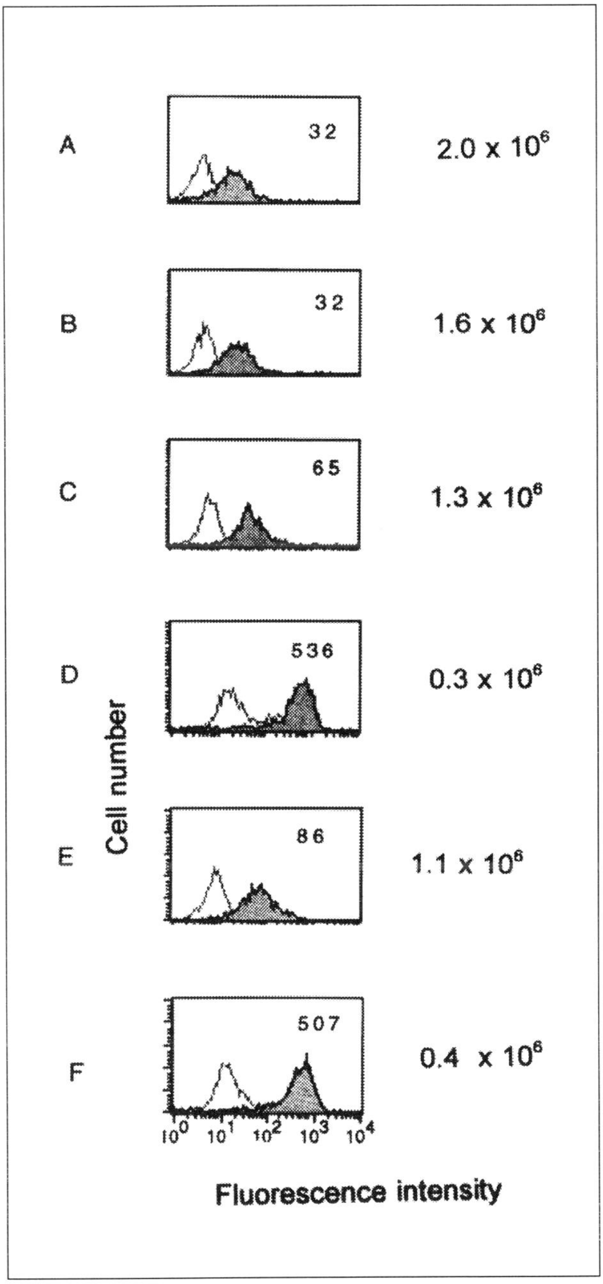

Fig. 15.5. SAg reactive T cells from an SLE patient upregulate Fas on target B cells and effect Fas-mediated cytotoxicity. MAM-reactive TCLs from a patient with SLE were generated and used in the SAg bridge system. Fas expression on target Ramos B cells (A) is not affected by MAM alone (B), or by MAM-reactive SLE-derived CD4⁺ TCLs (C). When the target B cells are exposed to SLE-derived MAM-reactive CD4⁺ TCLs in the presence of MAM, there is dramatic upregulation of the Fas antigen and apoptosis (D). These results are similar to those obtained with MAM-reactive CD4⁺ TCLs derived from a healthy donor without (E) and with MAM (F). Each histogram shows the background fluorescence staining with an isotype-matched control antibody, the staining for Fas expression (overlay), and the mean channel fluorescence staining with anti-Fas (upper right corner). Histograms depict cell number versus intensity of fluorescence staining. To the right of each histogram is the viable cell number, as determined by trypan blue exclusion and hemocytometry, for each culture circumstance after 72 hours.

signaling defects at several points. First, there may be deficient Fas upregulation after CD40 ligation. This might occur due to defects in the CD40 receptor itself, or to changes affecting elements of the CD40 signaling pathway. Alternatively, Fas may be upregulated, but apoptosis might not occur, due to defects intrinsic to the Fas receptor, due to defects in the immediate, death domain-associated signaling pathway molecules such as FADD,[54] or to problems with the more distal signaling elements, such as the ICE-like protease. Clearly, the identification of specific molecular defects that result in failed cell death signals is an important goal in understanding mechanisms of tumor development and resistance.

We have begun to apply the SAg bridge model to check T cell induced Fas upregulation and death in specific B cell malignancies. One example of such a study was performed using the malignant cells from a patient with a refractory, EBV negative Burkitt's lymphoma that progressed to a leukemic phase. For these experiments, leukemic cells were isolated from the peripheral blood and then exposed in culture to media alone, to MAM, to irradiated MAM-reactive T cells (MAMTxr), or to the combination of MAM and MAMTxr. The results were similar to those we have reported with the Ramos BL cell line. In this case, Fas was upregulated on the tumor B cells consequent to SAg-induced cognate interaction with SAg-reactive T lymphocytes, and the cells were induced to undergo apoptosis (Table 15.2). In contrast, malignant B cells from a second case appear to be resistant to Fas-mediated cytotoxicity despite good Fas upregulation consequent to CD40 ligation, which suggests that those tumor B cells may have defective Fas-associated signaling.

One can also use this system to study $CD4^+$ T cell function in patients with B cell malignancies by generating SAg-reactive TCLs from the peripheral blood mononuclear cells. As described above for TCLs from SLE patients, induction of activation antigens such as Fas on well-characterized, target B cells such as the Ramos cell line, can be assessed by flow cytometry after coculture with SAg-reactive TCLs, and presumably would reflect the capacity of the patient's T cells to instigate cognate signals via CD40L. A second parameter to measure is B cell apoptosis consequent to cognate interaction with SAg-reactive T cells. If Fas-upregulated and Fas-mediated death were to occur in well-characterized target B lymphocytes that are induced to express the Fas antigen, this would imply that Fas ligand expression and function is intact in the TCLs.

DISCUSSION

The effects of T cell SAg on B cell activation and apoptosis are pronounced and specific. Using the SAg bridge as a model for cognate interaction between antigen-specific T cells and B cells, we are able to analyze the effects of antigen, and the T cell response to antigen, on the B cell. By separating T of B cells purified from

Table 15.2. SAg signaling induces apoptosis of fresh Burkitt's lymphoma cells in vitro

Culture condition	Viable cell number after 3 Days (x 10^6/ml)	% Viable cells
Easter + media	0.99	92%
Easter + MAM	1.05	84%
Easter + T_{MAMxr}	1.4	77%
Easter + MAM + T_{MAMxr}	0.44	35%

Malignant B cells from the patient (termed "Easter") were isolated and demonstrated to be of Burkitt's (small, noncleaved cell) type by flow cytometry (CD10, CD19, CD40, IgM positive) and cytogenetic analysis (+t8;14). Cells from passage 0 were grown in culture with media, MAM, irradiated, $CD4^+$, MAM-reactive T cells (T_{MAMxr}), or MAM + T_{MAMxr}, and viabilities determined at 72 hours by hemocytometry after diluting each cell suspension in trypan blue.

the peripheral blood of patients with autoimmune disease and with lymphocytic malignancies, we are able to monitor B cell activation, Fas expression, and apoptosis as is induced by a particular patient's SAg-reactive CD4$^+$ T cells. Along similar lines, we can evaluate how the B cells from a particular patient can be manipulated to express Fas and undergo apoptosis in our SAg-dependent system.

The model can be applied to malignant B cells from a variety of B cell tumors, each of which represents the malignant outgrowth of B cells at a particular stage of B cell ontogeny. In this way, we can use the system not just to evaluate the susceptibility to Fas-mediated cytolysis among different B cell malignancies, but also to gain insights in our understanding of the stages of B cell differentiation when the Fas-Fas ligand system is important in regulating B cell apoptosis. Careful analysis of failed B cell apoptosis in the system will be a useful tool for dissecting out specific mechanisms of resistance to Fas-mediated cytotoxicity, and may provide critical information regarding the etiology of some B cell malignancies.

It is intriguing to speculate whether the anti-tumor effects reported by some groups that have used SEB and other SAg are in fact due to CD4$^+$ T cell mediated Fas upregulation on the tumor cells, with subsequent B cell apoptosis due to Fas ligand expression by activated, SAg-reactive T cells. In vivo studies are needed, similar to those we have performed, to evaluate the positive effects of T cell SAg on B cell isotype switching and antibody production and to assess the effects of SAg and SAg-reactive T cells on apoptosis of xenografted B cell tumors.

Acknowledgment

This work was supported with funds from The William H. Kearns Foundation and The Dorothy Rodbell Cohen Foundation for Sarcoma Research (E.S), The Westvaco Foundation (S.F.), and NIH AI32634 and P50 AR42588-02 (Specialized center of research in systemic lupus erythematosus).

References

1. Dellabona P, Peccoud J, Kappler J et al. Superantigens interact with MHC class II molecules outside of the antigen groove. Cell 1990; 62:1115-1121.
2. Herman A, Kappler JW, Marrack P et al. Superantigens: mechanism of T cell stimulation and role in immune responses. Ann Rev Immunol 1991; 9:745-72.
3. Marrack P, Kushnir E, Kappler J. A maternally inherited superantigen encoded by a mammary tumor virus. Nature 1991; 349:524-26.
4. Frankel WN, Rudy C, Coffin JM et al. Linkage of Mls to endogenous mammary tumor viruses of inbred mice. Nature 1991; 349:526-28.
5. Woodland DL, Hap MP, Gollob KJ et al. An endogenous retrovirus mediating deletion of α/β T cells? Nature 1991; 349: 529-30.
6. Dyson PJ, Knight AM, Fairchild S et al. Genes encoding ligands for deletion of Vβ11 T cells cosegrate with mammary tumor virus genomes. Nature 1991; 349:531-32.
7. Pullen A, Wade T, Marrack P, Kappler J. Identification of T cell receptor β chain that interacts with the self superantigen Mls-1a. Cell 1990; 61:1365-74.
8. Marrack P, Blackman M, Kushir E et al. The toxicity of staphylococcal enterotoxin B in mice is mediated by T cells. J Exp Med 1990; 171:455-64.
9. Watanabe-Ohnishi R, Aelion J, LeGros L et al. Characterization of unique human TCR V beta specificities for a family of streptococcal superantigens represented by rheumatogenic serotypes of M protein. J Immunol 1994; 152:2066-73.
10. Atkin CL, Wei S, Cole BC. The *Mycoplasma arthritidis* superantigen MAM: Purification and identification of an active peptide. Infect Immun 1994; 62:5367-15.
11. Inganas M. Comparison of mechanism of interaction between protein A from *Staphylococcus aureus* and human monoclonal IgG, IgA, and IgM in relation to the classical Fc and alternative F(ab')2 protein A interactions. Scand J Immunol 1981; 13:343-52.
12. Vidal MA, Conde FP. Alternative mechanism reactivity of protein A-immunoglobulin reaction: the VH-associated reactivity

of a monoclonal human IgM. J Immunol 1985; 135:1232-38.
13. Hilson J, Karr NS, Oplinger II et al. The structural basis of germline-encoded VH3 immunoglobulin binding to staphylococcal protein A. J Exp Med 1993; 178:331-36.
14. Berberian L, Goodlick L, Kipps TJ et al. Immunoglobulin VH3 gene products: Natural ligands for HIV gp120. Science 1993: 261:1588-91.
15. Nilson BHK, Solomon A, Bjorck L. Protein L from peptostreptococcus magnus binds to the light chain. J Biol Chem 1993:267:2234-39.
16. Domiati-Saad R, Lipsky PE. Staphylococcal protein A and staphylococcal enterotoxins: Two-model B cell superantigens. In: Zouali M, B cell superantigens, Austin: RG Landes Co., 1996.
17. Tumang JR, Posnett DN, Cole BC et al. Helper T cell-dependent human B cell differentiation mediated by a mycoplasmal superantigen bridge. J Exp Med 1990; 171:2153-58.
18. Crow MK, Zagon G, Chu Z et al. Human B cell differentiation induced by microbial superantigens: Unselected peripheral blood lymphocytes secrete polyclonal immunoglobulin in response to *Mycoplasma arthritidis* mitogen. Autoimmunity 1992; 14:23-32.
19. Friedman SM, Crow MK, Tumang JR et al. Characterization of human T cells reactive with the Mycoplasma arthritidis-derived superantigen (MAM): Generation of monoclonal antibody against Vβ17, the T cell receptor gene product expressed by a large fraction of MAM-reactive human T cells. J Exp Med 1991; 174:891-900.
20. Friedman SM, Posnett DN, Tumang JR et al. A potential role for microbial superantigens in the pathogenesis of systemic autoimmune disease. Arthritis Rheum 20.1991; 34:468-80.
21. Schattner E, Elkon KB, Yoo D-H et al. CD40 ligation induces Apo-1/Fas expression on human B lymphocytes and facilitates apoptosis through the Apo-1/Fas pathway. J Exp Med 1995; 182:1557-65.
22. Gleichmann E, Gleichmann H, Wilke W. Autoimmunization and lymphomagenesis in parent → F1 combinations differing in the major histocompatibility complex. Transp Rev 1976; 31:156-224.
23. Gleichmann E, van Elven EH, van der Veen JP. A systemic lupus erythematosus (SLE)-like disease in mice induced by abnormal T-B cell cooperation. Preferential formation of autoantibodies characteristic of SLE. Eur J Immunol 1982; 12:152-159.
24. Newell KA, Ellenhorn JDI, Bruce DS et al. In vivo T cell activation by staphylococcal enterotoxin B prevents outgrowth of a malignant tumor. Proc Natl Acad Sci USA 1991; 88:1074-78.
25. Ochi A, Migita K, Xu J et al. In vivo tumor immunotherapy by a bacterial superantigen. J Immunol 1993; 151:3180-86.
26. Fearon ER, Pardoll DM, Itaya T et al. Interleukin-2 production by tumor cells bypasses T helper function in the generation of an anti-tumor response. Cell 1990; 60:397-403.
27. Kuge S, Miura Y, Nakamura Y et al. Superantigen-induced human $CD4^+$ helper/killer T cell phenomenon. J Immunol 1995; 154:1777-85.
28. Schmid DS, Tite JP, Ruddle NH. DNA fragmentation: Manifestation of target cell destruction mediated by cytotoxic T cell lines, lymphotoxin-secreting helper T cell clones and cell-free lymphotoxin containing supernatant. Proc Natl Acad Sci USA 1986; 83:1881-86.
29. Del Prete GF, De Carli M, Ricci M et al. Helper activity for immunoglobulin synthesis of T helper type II (Th1) and Th2 human T cell clones: the help of Th1 clones is limited by their cytolytic capacity. J Exp Med 1991; 174:809-13.
30. Kagi D, Vignaux F, Ledermann B et al. Fas and perforin pathways as major mechanisms of T cell-mediated cytotoxicity. Science 1995; 265:528-530.
31. Oehm A, Behrmann I, Falk M et al. Purification and molecular cloning of the Apo-1 cell surface antigen, a member of the tumor necrosis factor/nerve growth factor receptor superfamily. J Biol Chem 1992; 267: 10709-15.
32. Owen-Schaub LB, Yonehara S, Crump WL III et al. DNA fragmentation and cell death are selectively triggered by activated

human lymphocytes by Fas antigen engagement. Clin Immunol 1992; 140:197-205.

33. Owen-Schaub L, Radinsky R, Kruzel E. Anti-Fas on non-hematopoietic tumors: levels of Fas/Apo-1 and bcl-2 are not predictive of biological responsiveness. Cancer Res 1994; 54:1580-86.
34. Ju S-T, Cui H, Panka DJ et al. Participation of target Fas protein in apoptosis pathway induced by CD4+ Th1 and CD8+ cytotoxic T cells. Proc Natl Acad Sci USA 1994; 91:4185-89.
35. Dhein J, Walczak H, Baumler C. Autocrine T cell suicide mediated by Apo-1/(Fas/CD95). Nature 1995; 373:438-40.
36. Brunner T, Mogil RJ, LaFace D. Cell autonomous Fas (CD95)/Fas ligand interaction mediates activation-induced apoptosis in T cell hybridomas. Nature 1995; 373:441-44.
37. Ju S-T, Panka DJ, Cui H et al. Fas (CD95)/FasL interactions required for programmed cell death after T cell activation. Nature 1995; 373:444-48.
38. Trauth BC, Klas C, Peters AMJ et al. Monoclonal antibody-mediated tumor regression by induction of apoptosis. Science 1989; 245:301-5.
39. Gregory CD, Tursz T, Edwards CF et al. Identification of a subset of normal B cells with a Burkitt's lymphoma (BL)-like phenotype. J Immunol 1987; 139:313-18.
40. Klein G. Epstein-Barr virus strategy in normal and neoplastic B cells. Cell 1994; 77:791- 93.
41. Schattner E, Mascarenhas J, Bishop J et al. CD4+ T cell induction of Fas-mediated apoptosis in Burkitt's lymphoma B cells. Blood, in press, 1996.
42. Cherwinski HM, Schumacher JH, Brown KD et al. Two types of mouse helper T cell clone. III. Further differences in lymphokine synthesis between Th1 and Th2 clones revealed by RNA hybridization, functionally nonspecific bioassays and monoclonal antibodies. J Exp Med 1987; 166:1229-44.
43. Lederman S, Yellin MJ, Krichevsky A. Identification of a novel surface protein on activated CD4+ T cells that induces contact-dependent B cell differentiation (help). J Exp Med 1992; 175:1091-1101.
44. Sharpe AH. Analysis of lymphocyte activation in vivo, using transgenic and knockout mice. Curr Op in Immunol 1995; 7:389-95.
45. Rousset F, Garcia E, Banchereau J. Cytokine-induced proliferation and immunoglobulin production of human B lymphocytes triggered through their CD40 antigen. Ann Rev Immunol 1994; 12:881-920.
46. Faris M, Gaskin F, Parsons JT, Fu SM. CD40 signaling pathway: Anti-CD40 monoclonal antibody induces rapid dephosphorylation and phosphorylation of tyrosine-phosphorylated proteins including protein tyrosine kinase lyn, fun, and syk and the appearance of a 28 kDa tyrosine phosphorylated protein. J Exp Med 1994; 179: 1923-31.
47. Liu Y-J, Joshua DE, Williams GT et al. Mechanism of antigen-driven selection in germinal centers. Nature 1989; 342:929-31.
48. Yellin MJ, Lee JJ, Chess L et al. A human CD4- T cell leukemia subclone with contact-dependent helper function. J Immunol 1991:147:3389-95.
49. Abe J, Kotzin BL, Meissner C. Characterization of T cell repertoire changes in acute Kawasaki disease. J Exp Med 1993; 177:791-96.
50. Conrad B, Weidmann E, Trusso G et al. Evidence for superantigen involvement in insulin-dependent diabetes mellitus etiology. Nature 1994; 371:351-355.
51. Watanabe-Fukunaga R, Brannan CI, Copeland NG et al. Lymphoproliferation disorder in mice explained by defects in Fas antigen that mediates apoptosis. Nature 1993; 356:314-17.
52. Drappa J, Brot N, Elkon KB. The Fas protein is expressed at high levels on double-positive thymocytes and activated mature T cells in normal but not MRL/lpr mice. Proc Natl Acad Sci USA 1993; 90: 10340-44.
53. Takahashi TM, Tanaka CI, Brannan NA et al. Generalized disease in mice caused by a point mutation in the Fas ligand. Cell 1994; 76:969-76.
54. Chinnaiyan AM, O'Rourke, Tewari M. FADD, a novel death domain-containing protein, interacts with the death domain of Fas and initiates apoptosis. Cell 1995; 81:505-12.

CHAPTER 16

Variable Region Genes of Human Antibodies to Red Blood Cells: Potential Targets for Superantigen Interaction

Kathleen N. Potter, J. Donald Capra and Virginia Pascual

INTRODUCTION

Induction of antibodies to red blood cells can be the result of either intentional or unintentional miss-match blood inoculations. The so-called "natural" autoantibodies to red blood cells (RBC) which are found in the sera of healthy people are thought to be produced either in response to similar structures which are on the surface of foreign infectious agents, and/or result from the random rearrangement of immunoglobulin germline genes. The production and analysis of human monoclonal antibodies to RBC antigens, and the production of transgenic mice expressing an anti-mouse RBC autoantibody,[1] have also aided the characterization of the human autoimmune and alloimmune response to these antigens. It is often difficult to establish the relationship between autoantibodies with positive physiological function and those which are pathogenic. Anti-RBC autoantibodies potentially function to maintain homeostasis in the form of eliminating autoantigens or scenescent cells.[2,3] There are many examples, however, where anti-RBC antibodies cause disease.

It was first proposed by Pascual and Capra[4] that there could be B cell superantigens which would interact with soluble and membrane-bound immunoglobulins outside of the conventional binding-sites, equivalent to the interaction of superantigens with specific T cell receptor Vβ chains. The existence of B cell superantigens is now well accepted. They include staphylococcal protein A (SpA) interacting with V_H3 encoded antibodies,[5] HIV gp120 interacting with V_H3 encoded antibodies,[6] CD4,[7]

Human B Cell Superantigens, edited by Moncef Zouali. © 1996 R.G. Landes Company.

protein L from *Peptococcus magnus*,[8] and human liver protein Fv.[9] The criteria for being classified as a B cell superantigen include (i) the simultaneous stimulation of a large percentage of B cells compared with conventional antigens, (ii) restricted use of V_H or V_L gene segments resulting in polyclonal responses, and (iii) binding as intact proteins outside of the conventional antigen binding site. In this chapter we will examine the heavy and light chain variable region gene segments used by human antibodies in response to red blood cell antigens. The possible role of superantigens interacting with these variable regions will be discussed.

RED BLOOD CELL ANTIGENS

Over 254 different antigens have been reported on the surface of the human RBC, with the majority of these being distributed within 22 blood group systems (reviewed in refs. 10-11). The antigens in three of the systems, ABH, P and Lewis, are carbohydrate in nature, while those in the remaining 19 systems are proteins. While some of these antigens are exclusively found on red blood cells, the ABH and related antigens Le^a, Le^b, Le^x, Le^y, I, i, P^k, P and P1 are also found in other tissues and secretions.

The ABH antigens are the most clinically important blood group antigens followed by the Rh antigens. The A, B, and H antigens are determined by allelic genes on chromosome 9. The H antigen in blood group O consists of a fucose residue joined by an α1-2 linkage to galactose, [Fuca1-2]Gal, one form of the blood group A antigen is a branched trisaccharide with a GalNac residue attached α1-3 to the H structure forming GalNAcα1-3 [Fucα1-2]Gal, and one form of the blood group B antigen is a trisaccharide with a Gal residue attached α1-3 to the H structure forming Galα1-3[Fucα1-2]Gal trisaccharide. The only difference between these two forms of A and B antigens is the N-acetyl group. The A and B antigens are also found in pancreatic and gastrointestinal mucosal tissue and on the surface of some microorganisms.[12]

The antigens of the Rh blood group system (D, C/c and E/e) are the products of a single gene complex located on chromosome 1. They are nonglycosylated polypeptides of approximately 30 kDa and are found only on red blood cells in association with a membrane glycoprotein which has similar membrane topology. The carbohydrate component of this glycoprotein is an N-linked glycan with ABH/Ii activity. The E/e polymorphism results from a mutation of proline 226 in Rh E to alanine in Rh e. The C/c polymorphism results from a serine 103 mutation in Rh C to a proline in Rh c on a polypeptide which is the same or very similar to that which expresses the E/e antigens. The D antigen is the most immunogenic of the common blood group antigens after A and B. Of the Rh antigens, anti-D antibodies are the most often cause of hemolytic transfusion reactions and hemolytic disease of the newborn. The use of human Rh D monoclonal antibodies caused accelerated clearance of Rh-D^+ red blood cells and suppressed Rh D immunization in Rh D^- volunteers indicating that blood group monoclonal antibodies have therapeutic utility.[13]

The Lewis-y (Le^y) Fuc(α1-2)Gal(β1-4) [Fuc(α1-3)]GlcNAc antigen is expressed on the surface of RBC, and detected in greater than 70% of epithelial cancers such as breast, ovary, colon, and lung. The Knops/McCoy (Kn/McC) human erythrocyte blood group antigens generate antibodies in high titer, but which have low avidity. The Kn/McC antigens were detected on the complement receptor C3b/C4b (CR1),[14] which is found on the surface of erythrocytes, monocytes, granulocytes, B cells, some T cells, macrophages, splenic follicular dendritic cells and glomerular podocytes. CR1 mediates the binding and processing of immune complexes, endocytosis and immune adherence as well as a complement regulatory function.[15]

ANTI-I/i ANTIBODIES

Cold agglutinins (CA) are autoantibodies with specificity for several carbohydrate determinants. Historically CA were identified as anti-red blood cell antibodies causing hemagglutination and lysis of red blood cells below 37°C (reviewed in refs. 16-17). The CA activity of these antibodies is directly responsible for the pathogenic effects seen in the cold agglutination syndrome. However, since several of the carbohydrate determinants involved in cold agglutination are not specific to red blood cells, but are found on several cell types, the agglutination of RBC, while perhaps clinically the most significant, is probably only one of several biological activities of these antibodies.

The most common carbohydrate specificities of CA are the I/i antigens, which are repeating N-acetyllactosamine subunits attached to either ceramide or protein. The i antigen is a linear oligosaccharide chain, while the I antigen is a branched oligosaccharide formed when a β1-6 branch attaches to a galactose residue of the i chain by a branching transferase. Fetal and newborn red blood cells express mostly i antigen, whereas after the first year of life, red blood cells express mostly I antigen. I/i antigens are also expressed on the oligosaccharides which form the backbones for the ABH blood group antigens. The surface of red blood cells of many species display the I/i antigens.[18] In addition to red blood cells, the I/i antigens are also found on the surface of human granulocytes, macrophages, platelets and lymphocytes.[19] Bacteria such as *Listeria monocytogenes* [20] and *Streptococcus pneumoniae* Type XIV[21] display I related antigens on their surfaces. The I/i antigens are not sensitive to proteases such as papain or ficin and are resistant to sialidase treatment.

The precise antigenic determinants recognized by many CA have not been determined. With respect to the I/i antigens, inhibition assays with chains longer than tetramer oligosaccharides suggest that anti-I/i antibodies bind oligosaccharides larger than trisaccharides.[22] Inhibition studies also indicate that several epitopes are recognized by multiple monoclonal antibodies within the I/i carbohydrate structure.[23]

The H chains of cold agglutinins specific for the I/i carbohydrate antigens and produced under chronic lymphoproliferative conditions, are almost always encoded by the V_H4-34 (V_H4-21) gene segment (Table 16.1).[24,25,26,27,28,] This nearly universal use of a single gene segment in antibodies directed against an antigen is very striking and suggests that the V_H4-34 gene segment is required to encode the anti-I/i specificities of CA.[24]

The rat monoclonal antibody 9G4, produced in response to a human IgM monoclonal protein obtained from a lymphoma patient, exclusively reacts with V_H4-34 encoded antibodies[29,30] The 9G4 idiotope (Id) is a cross-reactive idiotypic (CRI) marker for V_H4-34 encoded antibodies. Antibodies derived from gene segments from the other six V_H families, as well as the other members of the V_H4 family, are unreactive.[31,32] The phenomenon of CRI was first described in 1968 [33] when it was demonstrated that many human CA reacted with absorbed rabbit polyclonal antisera. The antisera did not react with other macroglobulins lacking the ability to agglutinate red blood cells at low temperature. This result suggested the presence of V region antigenic structures shared by CA and was the first demonstration of shared Id among nonidentical antibodies derived from unrelated individuals. The binding of 9G4 blocks the interaction of V_H4-34 antibodies to the I/i, A,D, C, c, E, of e Rh antigens.[30,31] These data suggest that the CRI and the antigen binding site are in close proximity. The localization of the 9G4 CRI to FR1 implicates FR1 in antigen binding more than previously thought.

The V_H4-34 gene segment is only one out of the approximately 100 V_H gene segments in the human heavy chain locus.[34,35] While the 9G4 Id is formed by the H chain alone, the determinant is detected only when a V_H4-34 H chain is paired with a L chain. The 9G4 Id, i.e., V_H4-34 encoded antibodies, is expressed by approximately 6% of B cells in normal human fetal spleen at 20 weeks of gestation, and is found in various normal adult lymphoid

Table 16.1. V region genes used in responses to red blood cell antigens

Clone	Specificity	V_H family	GL donor	D_H	J_H family	V_L donor	GL	J_L	9G4	Ref
Anti–ABH										
ABO.B1	B	V_H3	V_H3–23			κ1	hk102			65
ABO.HI1	HI	V_H3	V_H3–23			λ3	IGLV3S1			65
A–1	A	mu				λ			–	31,64
A–2	A	mu				λ			-	31,64
Anti–I/i										
FS–1	I	V_H4	V_H4–34	DXP'1	J_H3	κ2	GM607	Jκ2	+	24,26
FS–2	I	V_H4	V_H4–34	DXP'1	J_H4	κ3b	305	Jκ5	+	24,26
FS–4	I	V_H4	V_H4–34	DLR2	J_H4	κ3b	KAP	Jκ2	+	24
FS–6	I	V_H4	V_H4–34	D5–64/CO5	J_H4	κ3b	305	Jκ1	+	24
FS–7	I	V_H4	V_H4–34	DN1	J_H4	κ1	HK102	Jκ1	+	24
FS–9	I	V_H4	V_H4–34		J_H4	κ3b			+	55
FS–10	I	V_H4	V_H4–34		J_H4	κ			+	55
FS–11	I	V_H4	V_H4–34		J_H4	κ			+	55
KAU	I	V_H4	V_H4–34	DXP'1	J_H4	κ3b	325	Jκ4		27
VOG(20A)	I	V_H4	V_H4–34	?	J_H4	κ3a	328	Jκ4	+	25,51
P3	I	V_H4	V_H4–59			κ1			-	51
P4	I	V_H4	V_H4–59			κ3			-	51
P16	I	V_H4	V_H4–59			κ3			-	51
P7	I	V_H4	V_H4–39			κ4			-	51
Sp1	I	V_H3	V_H3–15	DXP1	J_H4	κ1	L11		-	50
4G	I	V_H3	V_H3–48		J_H4	κ3a	Vg		-	50
A14	i	V_H4	V_H4–34			κ1			-	51
A37	i	V_H4	V_H4–34			κ				51
A71	i	V_H4	V_H4–34			λ				51
A141	i	V_H4	V_H4–34			κ				51
A150	i	V_H4	V_H4–34			λ				51
A185	i	V_H4	V_H4–34			λ				51
A483	i	V_H4	V_H4–34		J_H4	λ			∠	51
CAP(15A)	i	V_H4	V_H4–34	?	J_H4	κ1	JK1		+	25,51
DP2C	i	V_H4	V_H4–34	?	J_H4	λ2a	DPL11	Jλ2/3	+	46
F14	i	V_H4	V_H4–34	DXP1	J_H3					105
FS–3	i	V_H4	V_H4–34	DN–1	J_H4	λ1	VIS2		+	24
FS–5	i	V_H4	V_H4–34	D21–9	J_H4	κ1	16K		+	24
H19	i	V_H4	V_H4–34	DN1	J_H3					105
HY18	i	V_H4	V_H4–34	DK1	J_H4	λ			+	28
LWA10	i	V_H4	V_H4–34	DK1	J_H6	κ		ND		28
MG2B	i	V_H4	V_H4–34	DXP'1/D2	J_H4	κ4	kIV	Jκ2	+	47
MH4	i	V_H4	V_H4–34	?	J_H4	κ3	325	Jκ2	+	47
MH7	i	V_H4	V_H4–34	DXP'1/D2	J_H4	λ1b	DPL2	Jλ2/3	+	47
N6	i	V_H4	V_H4–34		J_H4	κ3b				51
N26	i	V_H4	V_H4–34		J_H6	κ3				51
N115	i	V_H4	V_H4–34		J_H4	κ				51
N127	i	V_H4	V_H4–34		J_H4	κ1				51
N184	i/I	V_H4	V_H4–34		J_H4	λ				51
O15	i	V_H4	V_H4–34		J_H3	λ			+	51
O26	i	V_H4	V_H4–34		J_H6	κ3			+	51
P5	i	V_H4	V_H4–34		J_H4	κ1			+	51
RT2B	i	V_H4	V_H4–34	D4	J_H1	λ11a	DPL11	Jλ2/3	+	47
RT5A	i	V_H4	V_H4–34	D4	J_H6	κ3	KV3g	Jκ4	+	47
Sp2	i	V_H4	V_H4–34	DXP4	J_H6	λ2.1			+	50

Table 16.1. (Continued) V region genes used in responses to red blood cell antigens

Clone	Specificity	V_H family	GL donor	D_H	J_H family	V_L donor	GL	J_L	9G4	Ref
Anti–Rh										
MS-4	C	$\gamma1$				κ			-	31
MS-23	C	$\gamma1$				κ			-	31
MS-24	C	mu				κ			-	31
MS-25	c	V_H1				κ			-	31
MS-28	c	$\gamma3$				κ			-	31
MS-30	c	V_H4*	V_H4-34*			λ			+	31
MS-31	c	V_H4*	V_H4-34*			l			+	31
MS-32	c	V_H4*	V_H4-34*			l			+	31
MS-33	c	V_H4*	V_H4-34*			l			+	31
MS-34	c	V_H4*	V_H4-34*			l			+	31
MS-35	c	V_H4*	V_H4-34*			l			+	31
MS-36	c	V_H4*	V_H4-34*			l			+	31
MS-37	c	$\gamma3$				κ			-	31
MS-40	c	$\gamma1$				κ			-	31
MS-41	c	V_H4*	V_H4-34*			l			+	31
MS-42	c	V_H4*	V_H4-34*			l			+	31
MS-43	c	V_H4*	V_H4-34*			λ			+	31
MS-44	c	V_H4*	V_H4-34*			λ			+	31
MS-45	c	V_H4*	V_H4-34*			λ			+	31
MS-46	c	V_H4*	V_H4-34*			λ			+	31
MS-47	c	V_H4*	V_H4-34*			λ			+	31
MS-48	c	$\gamma3$				κ			-	31
MS-49	c	V_H4*	V_H4-34*			l			+	31
MS-50	c	V_H4*	V_H4-34*			l			+	31
MS-51	c	V_H4*	V_H4-34*			λ			+	31
MS-52	c	$\gamma1$				κ			-	31
MS-54	c	V_H4*	V_H4-34*			l			+	31
AD6	D	V_H4	V_H4-34			λ				60
AD8	D	V_H4	V_H4-34	DA1/4	J_H6					60
AD9	D	V_H4	V_H4-34		J_H6	λ				60
AD14	D	V_H4	V_H4-34	DXP1'	J_H6	λ				60
AD17	D	V_H4	V_H4-34	D2inv	J_H4	$\lambda3$	DPL-16			60
AD21	D	V_H4	V_H4-34	DXP1'	nd	λ				60
BAG-1	D	$\gamma1$				κ			-	31
BRAD 3	D	V_H3	V_H3-30			$\kappa3$	325			59
FOG 3	D	V_H3	V_H3-30	DK1		κ	02		-	31
FOG 1	D	V_H4	V_H4-34	DA1/4		κ	L11		-	31
FOG A	D	$\gamma3$				κ			-	31
FOG B	D	V_H4	V_H4-39			λ			-	31
FOM 1	D	V_H4	V_H4-34	DLR5inv		$\lambda3.1$	IGLV3S1		+	31
FOM A	D	V_H4	V_H4-34			$\lambda3.1$	IGLV3S1		+	31
GAD 2	D	V_H3	V_H3-30			$\lambda3.1$	IGLV3S1		-	31
GED-1	D	$\gamma1$				κ			-	31
HAM 1	D	V_H3				κ			-	31
HAM2	D	mu				λ			-	31
HAMA	D	V_H4*	V_H4-34*			κ			+	31
HAM B	D	V_H3	V_H3-30			λ			-	31
KEG-1	D	$\gamma1$				κ			-	31
MAD 2	D	V_H4	V_H4-34	DIRinv		$\lambda3.1$	IGLV3S1		+	31
MS-2	D	$\gamma3$				κ			-	31
MS-3	D	$\gamma1$				κ			-	31
MS-26	D	$\gamma1$				κ			-	31

Table 16.1 continues on next page

Table 16.1. (Continued) V region genes used in responses to red blood cell antigens

Clone	Specificity	V_H family	GL donor	D_H	J_H family	V_L donor	GL	J_L	9G4	Ref
NELP1	D	mu				λ			-	31
NELP2	D	V_H4*	V_H4-34*			λ			+	31
NELP3	D	V_H4*	V_H4-34*			λ			+	31
NELP4	D	V_H4*	V_H4-34*			λ			+	31
NELP5	D	V_H4*	V_H4-34*			λ			+	31
NELP6	D	V_H4*	V_H4-34*			λ			+	31
Og-31	D	V_H4	V_H4-34	DN1		λ3.1	IGLV3S1		+	58
PAG 1	D	V_H4	V_H4-59			λ			-	31
REG-A	D	V_H3	V_H3-30			κ3	325		-	31
Rh.D1	D	V_H5	V_H5-51			λ3	IGLV3S1			65
Rh.E1	E	V_H3	3005f3			λ2	DPL11			65
MS-5	E	mu				κ			-	31
MS-6	E	mu				κ			-	31
MS-10	E	mu				κ			-	31
MS-11	E	mu				κ			-	31
MS-12	E	V_H4*	V_H4-34*			λ			+	31
MS-14	E	mu				κ			-	31
MS-27	E	mu				κ			-	31
MS-16	e	V_H4*	V_H4-34*			λ			+	31
MS-17	e	V_H4*	V_H4-34*			κ			+	31
MS-19	e	V_H3							-	31
MS-21	e	V_H1				κ			-	31
MS-22	e	γ1				κ			-	31
MS-1	G	γ3				λ			-	31
Anti-Kidd										
MS-15	Jka	VH4*	VH4-34*			κ			+	31
MS-7	Jkb	VH4*	VH4-34*			κ			+	31
MS-8	Jkb	VH4*	VH4-34*			λ			+	31
MS-9	Jkb	VH4*	VH4-34*			κ			+	31
Anti-Pr2										
Spleen	Pr2	V_H1	V_H1-18							76
Node 3	Pr2	V_H1	V_H1-18							76
Node 4	Pr2	V_H1	V_H1-18							76
LS1	Pr2	V_H1	1-1		J_H4	κ3	KVL			72
LS2	Pr2	V_H1	1-1		J_H4	κ3	KVL			72
LS4	Pr2	V_H1	1-1		J_H4	κ3	KVL			72
LS5	Pr2	V_H1	1-1		J_H4	κ3	KVL			72
LS6	Pr2	V_H1	1-1		J_H4	κ3	KVL			72
LS7	Pr2	V_H1	1-1		J_H4	κ3	KVL			72
LS8	Pr2	V_H1	1-1		J_H4	κ3	KVL			72
Anti-Gd										
IgMGAS	Gd	V_H5	V_H5-51			κ	15AVK1			85
Anti-Kell										
K.Kpb1	Kp	V_H3	V_H3-13			λ2				65

*; V_H4-34 gene segment usage determined from 9G4 reactivity. Heavy chain gene segment nomenclature is from Matsuda et al[34] and Cook et al[35] when known.

tissues such as 10.8% of bone marrow B cells, 6.9% in peripheral blood B cells, 2.9% of total tonsil B cells, 5.0% of spleen cells, 3.2% of lymph node B cells and curiously, less than 1% of circulating IgM and IgG proteins.[30,36] At both the DNA and protein levels, the V_H4-34 gene is overrepresented in the peripheral B cell repertoire of normal adults and accounts for 7.8% and 10.3% of IgM clones in two cDNA libraries.[36] The V_H4-34 gene segment is also overrepresented in the autoimmune repertoire,[37] but expressed only at an incidence of 3.7% by tumor cells from patients with chronic lymphocytic leukemia (CLL), indicating that there is no preferential usage of the gene segment in this neoplasm compared with 14.5% in other B cell lymphomas.[38]

Anti-i antibodies bind over 50% of all B cells, whereas anti-I antibodies react with less than 10% of either tonsillar or blood B cells. V_H4-34 anti-i antibodies (HY18 and LWA10) selectively bind to a subset of human tonsil B lymphocytes within the mantle zone of secondary follicles,[28] suggesting that V_H4-34 encoded antibodies potentially play a role in B cell maturation. While B cells demonstrate strong expression of i antigens, normal T cells express I/i antigens on sialoglycoproteins at low levels.[39] The B cell CD45 (B220) leukocyte common antigen has both the linear and branched O-glycosidically linked poly-N-acetyllactosamine residues that form the i and I determinants respectively.[40,41] CD45 is a glycoprotein tyrosine phosphatase thought to be involved in regulating B of T lymphocyte activation and proliferation.[42] Antibodies to CD45 on B or T cells can either inhibit or augment lymphocyte activity in vitro depending on what other membrane receptors are in proximity.[43] Anti-CD45 antibodies are reported to influence T-dependent B cell isotype switching.[44] It is possible, therefore, that some B cells are simultaneously producing the i antigen on their surface and the corresponding V_H4-34 encoded anti-i antibody. Autoanti-I/i antibodies, therefore, have a potential regulatory role in lymphocyte function, and the I/i antigen may be involved in intercellular interactions, especially between B cells.

Pathogenic CA are generally of the IgM isotype and derived from monoclonal B cell expansions, as found in cold agglutinin disease, Waldenstrom's macroglobulinaemia and some B cell lymphomas.[45] They are both mutated and unmutated, although in general anti-i antibodies are less mutated than their anti-I counterparts.[24,25,26,27,28] Naturally occurring CAs with anti-I/i activities are found in low titers in cord blood[46] and normal adult sera,[30,36] but levels rise transiently following infections with agents such as Epstein-Barr virus in infectious mononucleosis (anti-i specificity),[47] cytomegalovirus (anti-I specificity), rubella virus (anti-PR specificity)[16] and *Mycoplasma pneumoniae.*[48] Since it is rare to find anti-i activity and 9G4 reactive antibodies in the sera of normal individuals, it has been postulated that B cells with membrane bound autoantibody receptors are anergic B cells which do not secrete autoantibodies into the blood.[49] Transiently occurring CA are found to be monoclonal or oligoclonal IgM. The data suggest that these microorganisms can either directly or indirectly stimulate B cells with V_H4-34 encoded surface antibodies to begin to produce the antibodies in soluble form.

While patients with cold agglutinin disease produce CA which are uniformly V_H4-34 encoded, naturally occurring, nonpathogenic anti-I/i CA from normal sera have been shown to be encoded by the V_H3 gene segments V_H3-15 and V_H3-48 (WHG26),[50] and in addition to V_H4-34, anti-I antibodies can use other V_H4 family gene segments including V_H4-59 (71-4) and V_H4-39 (2-1).[51] The V_H4-59 (71-4) and V_H4-39 (2-1) encoded antibodies, however, are reported to react with the I antigen on normal adult red blood cells with lower avidity compared with V_H4-34 encoded antibodies. The anti-i antibodies from the normal B cell repertoire were V_H4-34 encoded, similar in molecular composition to the pathogenic antibodies.[50]

ANTI-RH D, C, c, E, e ANTIBODIES

The specificity of V_H4-34 encoded antibodies is not limited to the I/i antigens. V_H4-34 encoded antibodies have been isolated with specificities for IgG (rheumatoid factors; RF),[52,53] DNA,[54-56] lipid A,[57] the Smith (Sm) antigen (I. Sanz, personal communication), striated muscle,[58] several of the structurally distinct protein antigens on the surface of red blood cells,[59,60] as well as polyspecific antibodies of IgG and IgA isotypes.[61,62] Some of these V_H4-34 encoded antibodies do not exhibit any measurable CA activity. Only one anti-D antibody out of a panel of 30 IgM V_H4-34 encoded anti-D antibodies had demonstrable CA activity,[60] indicating that the V_H4-34 encoded protion of an antibody does not guarantee I/i binding.

A panel of 72 human monoclonal alloantibodies specific for human blood group antigens including the A, Rh C, c, D, E, e, G and the Kidd antigens Jka and Jkb was established [63] and tested for 9G4 reactivity.[31] The results are shown in Table 16.1. The 9G4 CRI was expressed by 64% (28/44) of the IgM and 21%(6/28) of the IgG anti-blood group antibodies compared with 7.7% (3/39) of control IgM antibodies. The two anti-A antibodies were 9G4 negative. The 9G4 Id was detected on 9/13 anti-D IgM antibodies and 0/13 anti-D IgG antibodies. Of this group, only FOG-1 (γ1κ) is known to be V_H4-34 encoded but is 9G4 negative due to a mutation in FR1. Twelve out of 13 anti-c and 0/1 anti-C IgM antibodies were 9G4 reactive, while 6/11 anti-c and 0/2 anti-C IgG antibodies were Id positive. One out of seven anti-E and 2/4 anti-e IgM antibodies were Id positive, and the one anti-e IgG antibody was Id negative. The single IgG anti-G antibody was 9G4 negative, while the one anti-Jka IgM antibody was Id positive, as were the three anti-Jkb antibodies. These data indicate that the human alloimmune response to blood group Rh and Kidd antigens is biased for usage of the V_H4-21 gene segment. Many of the IgM antibodies were polyreactive, as were some of the IgG antibodies, but to a lesser degree.[64]

Fourteen (4 IgM and 10 IgG) of the anti-D antibodies heavy and light chain V regions were sequenced to determine gene segment usage and extent of hypermutation.[59] Three out of the four IgM antibodies used the V_H4-34 gene segment, and one the V_H3-30 (1.9III) gene segment. Two out of the 10 IgG antibodies used the V_H4-34 gene segment, four were encoded by V_H3-30 (1.9III), and the remaining four each used one of either the V_H3-30 (1.9III), DP-58, V_H3-30 (GL-SJ2), V_H4-59 or V_H4-39 gene segments. The IgM light chains were Vλ3.1 encoded, with five different light chains being used in the IgG antibodies. The sequences confirm that minimally mutated V genes can encode anti-Rh D specific antibodies. An analysis of the patterns of hypermutation in allo- and autoanti-RBC antibodies indicated that anti-I autoantibodies are significantly more mutated than anti-D antibodies.[60]

Human antibody fragments specific for human antigens in the ABH blood group system, and the C, c, D, E and e antigens of the Rh system, were isolated from a phage display library.[65] The amino acid sequences of 6 anti-RBC single-chain (sc)Fv with specificities for the antigens HI, D and Kp^b were deduced from nucleotide sequences. The H chain gene segments used were from the V_H3 and V_H5 families and the L chain gene segments were from the κ1, λ2 and λ3 families. A summary of the results indicating the closest germline genes is shown in Table 16.1. These antibodies are considered autoantibodies as the red cells of the donors expressed the three antigens. It is interesting to note that the anti-E scFv cross-reacted with Rh E negative RBC. A Fab library was also generated by Siegel and Silberstein[66] who developed a method for library screening with intact RhD-positive RBC.

Human-mouse hybridomas were established using peripheral blood lymphocytes from healthy individuals immunized against Rh alloantigens.[67] Of 55 monoclonal alloantibodies, 11 reacted with intracellular self-antigens. Ten of these eleven antibodies were of the IgM isotype. Therefore, during an immune response against a foreign antigen, B cells often produce polyreactive antibodies, indicating that the polyreactive autoantibodies present in the sera of healthy individuals may be the result of induction by foreign antigens.

ANTI-PR_2 ANTIBODIES

Another category of CA have specificity for the PR antigens. PR antigens are O-linked oligosaccharides located on the α and δ sialoglycoproteins (reviewed in refs. 68,69). The PR antigen sub-group is determined by linkage of the terminal sialic acid residue to the oligosaccharide chain and is expressed in high levels on both fetal and adult red blood cells. They are widely distributed on different cell types, including human lymphocytes, granulocytes, and monocytes, kidney, liver, stomach, pancreas, lung and brain tissue,[70,71] and are equally expressed on adult and newborn red blood cells. PR antigens are sensitive to neuraminidase and proteases (hence the name PR) such as papain or ficin.[72,73] The sialic acid contributes to the epitope recognized by anti-PR antibodies. The anti-PR_2 autoantibody recognizes glycoprotein determinants found on a subset of both T of B lymphocytes.

The V_H and V_L region gene segments of seven Epstein Barr virus (EBV) transformed B cell lines with anti-PR reactivity (LS1, LS2, LS4, LS5, LS6, LS7, LS8) from a single patient were cloned and sequenced.[73] The V_H sequences were V_H1 encoded with 88% homology to the germline V_H1 gene segment GL1-1. The light chain sequences were 97% homologous to the Vκ3 germline gene GL-KVL. The seven clones shared the same gene segments and junctional elements confirming their clonal origin. It was determined through the establishment of Id-negative mutant clones, that a single V_H CDR3 mutation (Cys to Tyr) altered both the idiotype and anti-PR_2 specificity of the antibody LS2.[74]

When two anti-PR_2 CA were sequenced from a PR_2 specific lymphoma, the V_H was 92% homologous to a V_H1 germline gene, while the V_L was 97% homologous to a Vκ3 germline gene.[75] Three anti-PR_2 antibodies were sequenced from a B cell lymphoma; one from the spleen and two from lymph node relapses.[76] The antibodies were V_H1 encoded with the closest germline gene being V_H1-18 (VH1GRR). The D region was DLR2 encoded in all three antibodies. There was no information on the V_L gene segment usage. It would appear from the limited number of sequenced anti-PR_2 antibodies that the human V_H response to PR_2 is predominantly V_H1 and Vκ3 family mediated, although the sample size is too small to establish whether there is a restricted usage of particular gene segments.

ANTI-MN ANTIBODIES

The MN human blood group antigens are determined by the amino-terminal octaglycopeptide of glycophorin A, the most abundant sialoglycoprotein on the human RBC membrane. MN antigens are inactivated by neuraminidase treatment. The M (Ser-Ser-Thr-Thr-Gly-) and N (Leu-Ser-Thr-Thr-Glu-) antigens differ in the first and fifth positions and both are O-glycosylated at positions 2 through 4.[77,78] To analyze the fine specificity of antibodies recognizing these antigens, recombinant glycophorin A molecules were expressed in Chinese hamster ovary cells.[79] Three polyclonal human anti-M sera were partially sialic acid dependent, recognized Ser_1 as the immunodominant amino acid, and did not require Gly_5. Two monoclonal mouse anti-N antibodies required Leu_1 but Glu_5 was not essential. Some anti-MN antibodies are specific for the peptide backbone, however, most MN specific antibodies recognize complex epitopes involving both protein and carbohydrate structures.[79,80,81]

The antibodies to the Miltenberger antigens Mi.I and Mi.II are named anti-Vw and anti-Hut respectively.[82] The Mi antigens are peptide blood group antigens on glycophorin A. They are present in less than 0.1% of the population but can cause hemolytic disease of the newborn.[83]

ANTI-SA, LUD, FL, VO, LI, AND GD ANTIBODIES

Some IgM antibodies to the Sa, Lud, Fl, Vo, Li and Gd (glyco[lipid]-dependent) gangliosides are cold reacting. Fl, Vo, Sa and Gd antigens are sialo-dependent groups. The Gd antigen[84] is found on glycolipids and expressed on both newborn and adult RBC. The Fl antigen is found on glycoproteins and glycolipids and is expressed on adult RBC. Vo antigens are also found on glycoproteins and glycolipids and are expressed on neonatal RBC. A monoclonal CA with anti-Gd activity was V_H5-51 encoded and used the J_H4 gene segment.[85] The D_H gene segment was not homologous with any reported D_H gene segment. The L chain was 15AVK1 and Jκ2 encoded.

The above is a general summary of the antibodies specific for red blood cell antigens. The research in our laboratory, together with our collaborators, has concentrated on the study of V_H4-34 encoded cold agglutinins with I/i specificity. The results described below summarize our findings

Expression of the 9G4 idiotope among EBV-transformed B cell clones and heterohybridomas from patients with cold agglutinin disease

Eight patients with clinically diagnosed CA disease were studied.[24,26] Seven patients had a detectable monoclonal IgM in the serum, and all had elevated CA titers. 9G4 Id positive cells were raised above normal levels in all patients, including one with no detectable serum paraprotein. B cells were immortalized with EBV (FS-1 to FS-8) and FS-3 to FS-8 were fused to mouse myeloma cells to generate hybridoma cell lines. IgM secreted by the selected clones were more than 95% 9G4 Id positive and agglutinated red cells in the cold with high efficiency. Six of the selected clones displayed preferential agglutination of adult (anti-I) rather than cord (anti-i) red blood cells. The two remaining clones (FS-3 and FS-5) showed a slight preference for cord red blood cells.

Mutational analysis using antibodies produced in the baculovirus expression system was used to localize the 9G4 Id.[86] Localization of this Id potentially identifies a structural requirement for I/i binding and explains the unusual restricted use of V_H4-34 for I/i binding. We exchanged H chain regions by PCR-SOEing between an Id positive cold agglutinin and an Id negative antibody. PCR-SOEing involves two sequential PCR reactions. In the first set of reactions, the DNA products to be fused are individually generated by PCR using oligomers with overlapping ends. In the second set of PCR reactions the two fragments are fused as a result of the overlapping ends annealing to each. The 3' overlap of each strand serves as a primer for the extension of the complementary strand. Once the two fragments are fused, the combined product is amplified during the second PCR. Figure 16.1 illustrates the H chain constructs with FR1, CDR1 and CDR2 regions exchanged between the germline V_H4-34 encoded CA FS-7 and the closely related gene segment V_H4-61 (V71-2), which is a member of the V_H4 family, but not associated with 9G4 binding. The close similarity of the two sequences shown in

Figure 16.2 indicates differences in amino acid sequence are localized to FR1, CDR1 and CDR2. The swap of FR1 in mutant A3 led to the loss of 9G4 binding. Exchanges of CDR1 and CDR2 in mutants A4, A5 and A6, had no effect on 9G4 binding. This result localized the 9G4 Id to FR1 of V_H4-34 encoded antibodies. 9G4 was still able to bind to antibodies which were composed of the FS-7 μ chain paired with seven different light chains from different L chain families. The 9G4 reactivity of the combinatorial antibodies is shown in Table 16.2. The sequences of the L chains are shown in Figure 16.3.[87,88,89] Direct and inhibition ELISA indicated that disruption of FR1 at either positions 6-12 or 23-25 drastically reduced 9G4 binding (Fig. 16.1; A7 and A8). The sequences at these two positions in V_H4-34 encoded

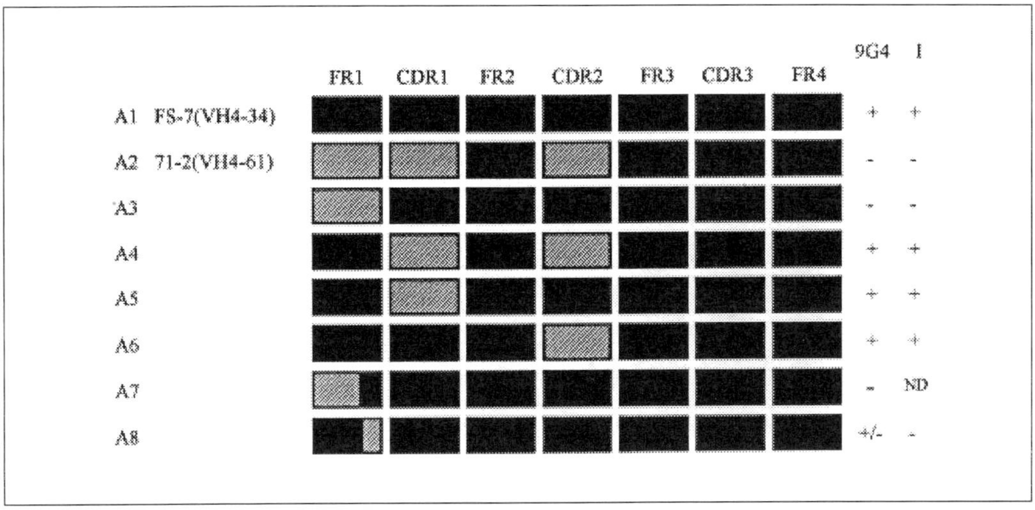

Fig. 16.1. 9G4 reactivity and I binding activity of V_H4-34 mutant antibodies. FS-7 H chain mutants were constructed by PCR-SOEing mutagenesis. All H chains were paired with the FS-7κ chain. V_H4-34 (black areas), V_H4-61 (hatched areas). (Reprinted with permission from Potter KN et al. The Journal of Experimental Medicine, 1993;178:1419-1428. ©1993 The Rockefeller University Press and Li Y-C et al. J Mol Biol 1996; 256(3):577-589. ©1996 Academic Press.)

Table 16.2. Reactivity of CA FS-7 and combinatorial antibodies with 9G4

Light Chain	V_L Family	Heavy Chain	$-V_H$ Family	9G4 Reactivity
–	–	FS-7μ	4	-
FS-7κ	κ1	FS-7μ	4	+
RF-TS2κ	κ3a	FS-7μ	4	+
RF-TMC1κ	κ3	FS-7μ	4	+
37-2κ	κ3b	FS-7μ	4	+
91A3κ	κ10	FS-7μ	4	+
HBVκ	κ5	FS-7μ	4	+
FS-3λ	λ1	FS-7μ	4	+
FS-3λ	λ1	FS-6μ	4	+
FS-7κ	κ1	FS-6μ	4	+
FS-7κ	κ1	FR1(4-34)μ	4	+
FS-3λ	λ1	FR1(4-34)μ	4	+
RF-TS2κ	κ3a	FR1(4-34)μ	4	+
FS-7κ	κ1	Ab25μ	3	-
37-2κ	κ3b	Ab25μ	3	-
RF-TSκ	κ3a	RF-TS2μ	3	-
HBVκ	κ5	HBVμ	3	-

Combinatorial antibodies were produced by coinfecting Sf9 cells with the H chain and L chain producing viruses indicated. Purified antibodies were tested for reactivity with 9G4 by ELISA. RF-TS2κ is a rheumatoid factor L chain (87), 37-2 is an anti-acetylcholine receptor L chain (88), HBVκ (119) is an anti-hepatitis B virus surface antigen antibody and 91A3κ is a mouse anti-arsonate antibody L chain (89). Ab25μ is an anti-thyroglobulin antibody H chain (61). FS-6 is a mutated CA H chain (24). FR1(4-34)μ is a V_H4-61 H chain with has the FR1 sequence of V_H4-34.
+ = OD_{405} 0.8-1.0; - = OD_{405} < 0.2.

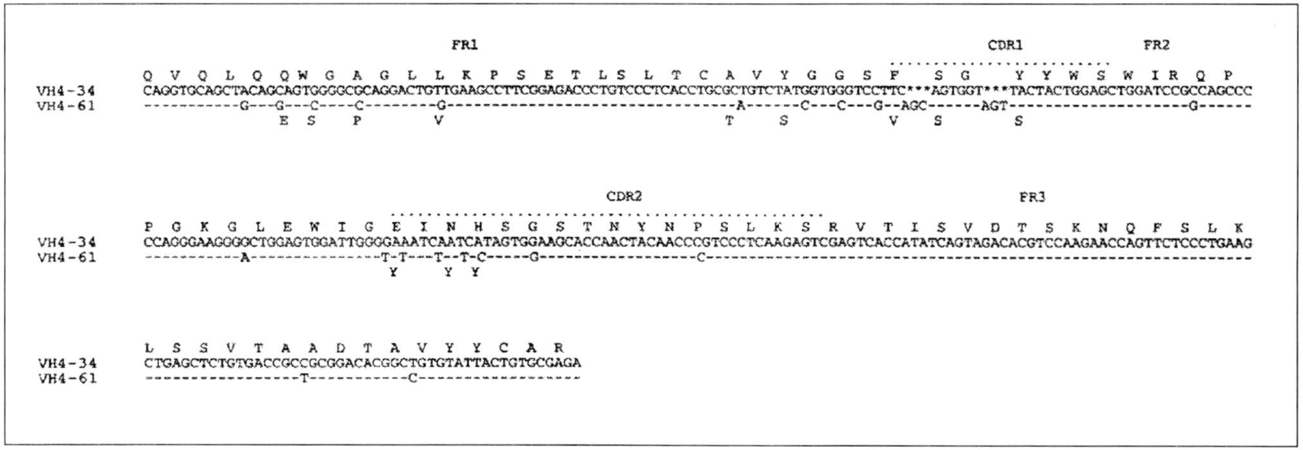

Fig. 16.2. Comparison of the nucleotide and amino acid sequences of germline V_H4-34 and V_H4-61 (71-2) gene segments. Dashes indicated identical amino acids and dots indicate the CDR1 and CDR2. Sequence differences are indicated. Stars correspond to extra base pairs in the V_H4-61 sequence. (Reprinted with permission from Potter KN et al. The Journal of Experimental Medicine, 1993; 178:1419-1428. ©1993 The Rockefeller University Press).

	FR1	CDR1	FR2	CDR2
FS-7κ	DIQMTQSPSTLSASVGDRVTITC	RASQSIS.SWLA	WYQQKPGKAPKLLIY	KASSLES
FS-6κ	E-VL----G---L-P-E-A-LS-	-----V-S-H--	-------Q--R----	AT--RAT
RF-TS1κ	E-VL----G---L-P-E-A-LS-	-----V-S-Y--	-------Q--R----	G---RAT
37-2κ	E-VL----G---L-P-E-A-LS-	-----V-S-Y--	-------Q--R----	G---RAT
RF-SJ3κ	E-VL----G---L-P-E-A-LS-	-----V-S-Y--	----R--Q--R----	G---RAT
RF-TS2κ	E-V-----A---V-P-E-A-LS-	-----V-.TN--	-------Q--R----	G--TRAT
RF-TMC1κ	E-VL----A---LFP-EKA-LS-	-----V-.RH--	-------Q--R----	D--KRAT
91A3κ	------T--S----L------S-	----D-N.NY-N	--R---DGTV-----	YT-R-H-
FS-3λ	QSVV--P--VSG-PGQRVA--S-	TG-S-NIGAGYDVH	----L--T-------	GN-NRP-
HBV1λ	QS-L--P--VSV-PGQTAR.---	GGDNIG-K-VN	-F-----Q--V-VV-	DDNERP-

	FR3	CDR3	FR4	Ref.
FS-7κ	GVPSRFSGSGSGTEFTLTISSLQPDDFATYYC	QQYNSYSR..T	FGQGTKVEIKR	24
FS-6κ	-I-D---------D------R-E-E---V---	---GRSP-..-	-----------	24
RF-TS1κ	-I-D---------D------R-E-E---V---	---G-SPG..-	--H--------	87
37-2κ	-I-D---------D------R-E-E---V---	---G-SPM.Y-	--H--------	88
RF-SJ3κ	-I-D---------D------R-E-E---V---	---G-SLGGY-	------L----	87
RF-TS2κ	-I-A--------------------SE---V-F-	----NWPP.I-	--H--------	87
RF-TMC1κ	-I-A---------D-S-IV---E-E---V---	-HR-NWPPSI-	--H--------	87
91A3κ	-------------DYS----N-EQE-IS--F-	--G-ALP-..-	--G---L----	89
FS-3λ	---D-----K---SAS-A-TG--AE-E-D---	-S-D-SLSGYV	--T----TVLG	24
HBV1λ	-ISE-----N--NTA-----RVEAG-E-D---	-VWD-SSDHVV	--G---LTVL	119

Fig. 16.3. Light chain sequences. The sequences of the light chains expressed in the baculovirus system and used in combinatorial antibodies are shown. (Reprinted with permission from: Li Y-C et al. J Mol Biol 1994; 256(3):577-589. ©1996 Academic Press.)

antibodies are QWGAGLL and AVY respectively. In all other members of the V_H4 family, these sequences are ESGPGLV and TVS. These two regions of FR1 are highlighted in the three dimensional structure of an immunoglobulin shown in Figure 16.4. Residues 6-12 form a loop structure which is also capable of interacting with CH1 of the constant region,[90] which may influence antibody specificity or binding avidity. Several V_H4-34 encoded antibodies which do not react with 9G4 have been sequenced. Table 16.3 lists the FR1 sequences of antibodies with mutations in the FR1 and the corresponding 9G4 reactivity. Antibodies FOG1 and HBL-2[91] lost 9G4 reactivity. The mutations at positions 3, 5 and 9 are also present in 9G4 reactive antibodies. The mutations at positions 24 in FOG1 and 23 in HBL-2 are likely responsible for rendering these antibodies 9G4 unreactive.

Antibodies were tested for I binding in an ELISA using a phenol/saline I extract from adult red blood cells kindly provided by Dr. D. Roelcke (University of Hamburg, Germany).[92] Since IgM antibodies are produced only as four chain monomers and not pentamers in insect cells, hemagglutination of red blood cells in the cold could not be performed. We attempted to cross-link the monomeric IgM antibodies with IgG antibodies, but this proved unreliable. The H chain mutants described in Figure 16.1 were used in the I binding assay. As demonstrated by mutants A4, A5 and A6, CDR_H1 and CDR_H2 are not involved in I binding. Only when FR1 was V_H4-34 encoded was there I binding. In mutant A3 where only the FR1 is V_H4-61 in sequence, the antibody did not bind I. A V_H4-34 encoded V region has a potential N-linked glycosylation site at position N52. Since this site is mutated in mutants A4 and A6, which retain the ability to bind the I antigen, the indication is that this V_H region glycosylation is not a strict requirement for producing a protein structure required for I binding.

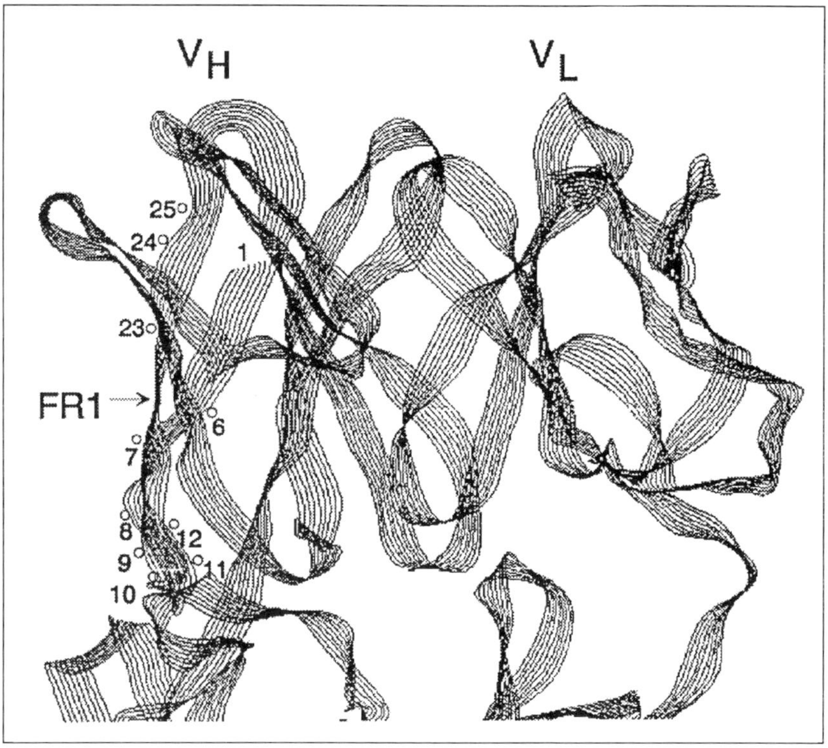

Fig. 16.4. A ribbon drawing of the crystal structure of the Fab portion of the V_H2 encoded antibody New[90] from the Brookhaven database using the HyperChem computer software (Waterloo, Canada). The FR1 regions 6-12 and 23-25 are indicated.

Table 16.3. Mutated V_H4-34 FR1 sequences and their 9G4 reactivity

Antibody	FR1 sequence	9G4 reactivity	Ref.
V_H4-34 (GL)	QVQLQQWGAGLLKPSETLSLTCAVYGGS	+	
Ab17	............V-------A-------	+	61
Ab28	----------V-S-------------A-	+	61
FOG1	--H-----T---------------H---	–	31,59
FS-2	--H-----T-------------------	+	24,26
FS-4	-------------------P--------	+	24
FS-6	----H-----------------------	+	24
HBL-3	--D--------QT----T----------	+	91
HBL-2	----E---E--------------I----	–	91
LES	--H-----------------N-------	+	25
MAD2	-G---es---------------------	+	31,59
O15	----------------------T-----	+	51
O26	----E-----------------------	+	51
SA4A	---H------------------------	+	58
VOG(20A)	--------------------N-------	+	25

Comparison of the FR1 amino acid sequences of V_H4-34 encoded antibodies and the corresponding 9G4 reactivity. Dashes indicate homologous residues and dots indicate unsequenced positions. Lower case indicates residues from sequencing oligomer. GL:Germline

Table 16.4. FR1 sequences used in FR1 exchanges

Family	Antibody	Gene Segment	FR1 Sequence	Ref.
V_H4	FS-6	V_H4-34	QVQLHQWGAGLLDPSETLSLTCAVYGGSFS	24
V_H1	RF-TS1	V_H1-69	L---V-S--EVKK-GSSVKVS-KAS-DT--	52
V_H2	HiH10	V_H2-26	--T-KEP-PV-VK-T---T---T-S-FA--	120
V_H3	RF-SJ3	V_H3-30	---MVES-G-VVQ-GRS-R-S--AS-FT--	52
V_H4	71-2	V_H4-61	----QES-P--VK---------T-S---V-	24
V_H4	SG	V_H4-39	-L--QES-P--VK---------T-S---I-	93
V_H5	B5	V_H5-51	E---V-S--EVKK-G-S-KIS-KGS-Y--T	116
V_H6	HBp2	V_H6-1	----Q-S-P--VK--Q-------IS-D-V-	120

Dashes indicate identical amino acids.

The role of FR1 in I binding was studied by replacing the FR1 of FS-6, a V_H4-34 encoded CA with I specificity, with the FR1 sequences from the other 6 V_H families, as well as two non-V_H4-34 members of the V_H4 family. The FR1 sequences are listed in Table 16.4.[93] All of the mutant H chains were paired with the FS-6κ L chain. As shown in Figure 16.5, only antibody B1 with the V_H4-34 encoded FR1 was able to bind I. All of the other antibodies, B2 through B7, did not bind I even though the CDR_H3 sequence was that of FS-6, a demonstrated I binder. Therefore, even when an appropriate CDR_H3 sequence is present, an inappropriate FR1 sequence is able to abrogate I binding.

Molecular analyses of the Ig variable region genes expressed by the heterohybridomas derived from each of the patients with CA disease discloses restriction in the usage of the V_H and J_H gene segments and high diversity in the heavy chain CDR_H3

Nucleotide sequence analysis of CA variable region genes to the I/i antigens revealed the universal usage of the V_H4-34 gene segment in association with different D_H, J_H and J_L gene segments with the result that each CDR_H3 and CDR_L3 has a unique sequence with no evident sequence motifs. When compared to the reported germline V_H4-34 gene segment, half of the

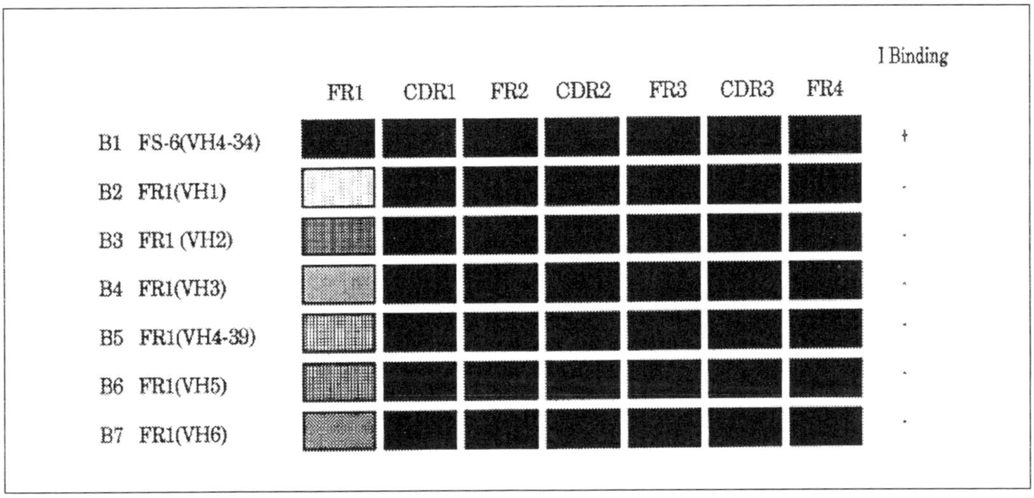

Fig. 16.5. I binding by FR1 exchange mutants. The FR1 of FS-6 (V_H4-34) H chains were exchanged with the FR1 sequence from the other V_H families by PCR-SOEing. The I binding activity as determined by ELISA is indicated. (Reprinted with permission from: Li Y-C et al. J Mol Biol 1994; 256(3):577-589. ©1996 Academic Press.)

clones showed 100% identity, while the other half display a variable degree of somatic diversification ranging from 94.4%-96% homology. There is a preponderant usage of J_H4 (6/8 clones), although other J_H segments are also used.[24] A list of several CA CDR_H3 sequences is shown in Table 16.5. The total of amino acid residues in the CDR_H3 and CDR_L3 of several CA is shown in Table 16.6. It is seen that the H and L chains CDR3s in this selection of CA have a combined length ranging from 16 to 26 amino acids.

We studied the role of the CDR_H3 in I binding by producing several mutant mu chains in the baculovirus system. As shown inFigure 16.6, we produced the CA FS-3 H chain, with its natural CDR_H3 sequence, and in a second mutant, replaced the CDR_H3 of FS-7 with that of the monoreactive rheumatoid factor RF-SJ4. In addition, two mutants were generated in which the first seven (Ala1) and the last six (Ala2) residues of the FS-6 CDR_H3 were replaced by alanine residues. All four antibodies were 9G4 reactive, however, only antibody Ala1 bound I antigen. This result indicates that the CDR_H3 sequence, while it can be quite diverse, cannot be of any sequence or uninvolved in I binding. The CA FS-3 is an i binder, and does not bind I in our assay. It would appear from mutants Ala1 and Ala2 that the last six residues of the FS-6 CDR_H3 are more involved in contacting the I antigen than are the first seven.

Within a population of CA, no single light (L) chain is utilized, but rather a number of L chains derived from a variety of V_L families of both⊇κ and⊇λ isotypes as indicated in Table 16.1. Using a panel of mouse anti-Id antibodies to the CA VOG 20A (V_H4-34/Vκ3a), a heterogeneity of L chain idiotype expression by cold agglutinins was observed and attributed to the use of at least three different Vκ3 · gene segments, kv328, kv325 and Vg, and/or somatic mutation of the variable region genes.[94] In I binding CA, L chains are predominantly derived from the Vκ3 family, although κ chains from the Vκ1 and Vκ2 families are also used.[95] While the CDR_L3 of most CA is uniformly 9 amino acids long (Table 16.7), they are all unique, with the QQY sequence being the closest to a common motif, although it is not present in all CDR_L3. While there are a number of different light chains associated with CAs, the evidence which we discuss below indicates that light chain utilization is not random, but the result of a selection process which pairs a specific L chain with an

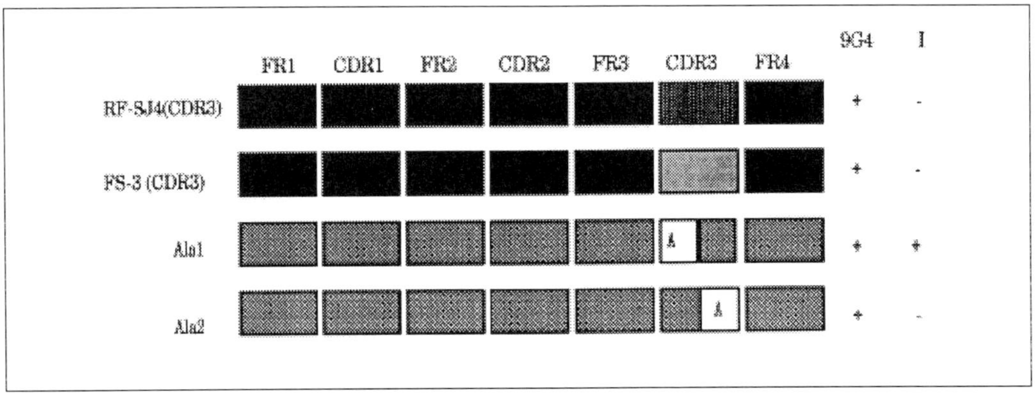

Fig. 16.6. The effect of CDR_H3 on I binding. In mutant RF-SJ4(CDR3) the CDR_H3 sequences of RF-SJ4 (V_H4-61) replaced the CDR_H3 of the FS-7 H chain. FS-3(CDR3) is the natural sequence of the FS-3 (V_H4-34) H chain from the CA FS-3λ which has anti-i specificity. The FS-7 and FS-3 H chains differ by one amino acid in CDR2 at position 53 (His in FS-7 to Y in FS-3) and have unrelated CDR3 sequences. Ala1 and Ala2 are FS-6 H chains with mutated CDR_H3 sequences having alanines replacing either the amino (Ala1) or carboxyl (Ala2) amino acids of the CDR_H3 of the FS-6 H chain. (Reprinted with permission from: Li Y-C et al. J Mol Biol 1994; 256(3):577-589. ©1996 Academic Press.)

Table 16.5. Comparison of CDR$_H$3 sequences between V$_H$4-34 encoded antibodies and antibodies encoded by other V$_H$ families

Antibody	Speci-ficity	V$_H$ family	CDR$_H$3 Sequence	CDR$_H$3 family	Ref.
FS-1	I	4-34	GQRGSGSDYRQGA--------------FDI	16	26
FS-2	I	4-34	EWGSGAYYPYY----------------FDY	14	26
FS-4	I	4-34	RLGSGSYPN------------------FDY	12	24
FS-6	I	4-34	ALGDGSTEGLP-----------------DY	13	24
FS-7	I	4-34	GREQWLVRGG----------------YFDY	14	24
20A	I	4-34	GFDLGPTNITSRP---------------DY	15	25
KAU	I	4-34	PPHDTSGHYWN------------------Y	12	27
Sp1	I	3-15	IRRSGYFGE-------------------DY	11	50
4G	I	3-48	DQRGLPR---------------------DY	9	50
FS-9	I	4-34	GPALMITG	8	55
FS-10	I	4-34	EDAFSRII		8
55					
FS-11	I	4-34	GDTVVVPSRP	10	55
A483	i	4-34	LRVRSGY-------------------YFDY	11	51
DP2C	i	4-34	QLVGG----------------------FDY	8	46
FS-3	i	4-34	GTRSWYPSD------------------FDY	12	24
FS-5	i	4-34	GPYYIDDSSGYYPG	14	24
F14	i	4-34	GKTDYYDILTGTLGGAFDI	19	105
H19	i	4-34	VGKQPQGVAFDI	12	105
MG2B	i	4-34	GSPKRYCSGGSCSD	14	47
MH4	i	4-34	SLKGHI---------------------FDY	9	47
MH7	i	4-34	VVTMVRGVITGRD-------------YFDY	17	47
N6	i	4-34	ELRSGSAG-------------------YFD	11	51
N26	i	4-34	GQRSSGYYS--------------YYYYMDV	16	51
N115	i	4-34	AFDQYYSY------------------YMDY	12	51
N127	i	4-34	ETGQWAG-------------------YSDY	11	51
N184	i	4-34	VRSNIVPAYYSGH----------------Y	14	51
N187	i	4-34	MTAPSSGSA-----------------YFDV	13	51
O15	i	4-34	APLDQYYDSSGYYHDA-----------FDI	19	51
O26	i	4-34	HCPIVYCSGGSCYSYYYYMDV	22	51
P5	i	4-34	GVVPAAKGH------------------FDY	12	51
RT2B	i	4-34	GRRQYQLTQ-----------------YFQH	13	47
RT5A	i	4-34	GGKVPAA--------------YYYYYYMDV	16	47
15A	i	4-34	ALMTAY--------------------YFDY	10	25,51
216	i/l A/B	4-34	GRMVRGAKYN	10	57
A6H4C5	i/l A/B	4-34	KAPRRLGL--------------YYYYGRDD	16	57
PAG-1	D	4-34	VLVSRTISQYS--------------YYMDV	16	31
FOM-A	D	4-34	ALDYISLDYG-----------------MDV	13	31
FOM-1	D	4-34	GLERPIRNQLLNRLGYY----------MDV	20	31
MAD-2	D	4-34	LWLDGHGYK------------------FDY	12	31
FOG-1	D	4-34	GRSRYSGYGFYSG--------------MDV	16	31
Og-31	D	4-34	SVAWYSSSWYKNYYYYSMDV	20	31
LES	RF	4-34	GPCEAYCTDDAPQAPQAG	15	25
PR-TS2	PR	4-34	GRRGAARLHYYY---------------MDV	15	52
410.7.f91	PR	4-34	GRYYHGSGRQPFQY	14	62
NE-1/NE13	DNA	4-34	RHVRPRVTR------------------MDV	12	56
T14	DNA	4-34	GWPYYYGAGSYYKRG-----------YFDY	19	54
RT-79	DNA/A	4-34	VRRSGRVVVPGARNRD	16	55
RT79/2	DNA/A	4-34	GRRITGTKRH	10	55
CAL-4G	DNA	4-34	RIMYCSGGSCYSAGWR	16	55
Hy18	i/B	4-34	GGFAATIVES-----------------FDY	13	28
LWA10	i/B	4-34	GVGSSGWYYYYGMDV	15	28
Ab17	PR	4-34	CAVITLLGLFANGDCDPGFEY	21	61
Ab63	PR	4-34	GGSVLRFLEWLLYPA------FDY	18	56

The CDR$_H$3 is arranged for maximal alignment of amino acid residues.

appropriate heavy (H) chain to generate I/i specificity.

We studied the role of the light chain in I binding by producing combinatorial antibodies composed of either the FS-6 or FS-7 H chain and ten different L chains. All of the combinatorial antibodies containing either the FS-6 or FS-7 H chain expressed the 9G4 Id. As a general conclusion, nonparental L chains paired with the H chains, had reduced I binding (Table 16.8). Modest binding occurs when the L chain is from the κIIIb family, irrespective of the original specificity of the donor L chain antibody. Therefore, even though the H chain FR1 and CDR_H3 are the major mediators of I binding, the L chain can also have a major effect on antigen binding activity. These results support the view that for every V_H gene segment and CDR_H3 in an expressed antibody, there is a L chain that has been coselected by antigen.

Table 16.6. Total number of amino acids in V_H and V_L CDR3s of some V_H4-34 encoded antibodies

Antibody	Specificity	CDR_H3 length	CDR_L3 length	Combined length	Ref.
FS-1	I	16	9	25	26
FS-2	I	14	9	23	26
FS-4	I	12	9	21	24
FS-6	I	13	9	22	24
FS-7	I	14	9	23	24
KAU	I	12	9	21	27
FS-3	i	12	11	23	24
FS-5	i	13	9	22	24
MG2B	i	14	9	23	47
DP2C	i	8	9	17	47
RT2B	i	13	9	22	47
RT5A	i	16	9	25	47
MH4	i	9	7	16	47
MH7	i	17	9	26	47

Table 16.7. Comparison of CDR_L3 sequences and lengths between some V_H4-34 encoded anti-I/i cold agglutinin light chains

Antibody	Specificity	CDR_L3 Sequence	CDR_L3 length	Ref
FS-1	I	MQALQSPYT	9	26
FS-2	I	QQYGTSPRP	9	26
FS-4	I	QQYDTSPYT	9	24
FS-6	I	QQYGRSPRT	9	24
FS-7	I	QQYNSYSRT	9	24
KAU	I	QQYGSSPLT	9	27
FS-3	i	QSYDSSLSGYV	11	24
FS-5	i	QQSYSTPWT	9	24
MH4	i	QQYGSSP	7	47
MH7	i	AAAWDDSLDG	9	47
RT5A	i	QQRSNWPPPM	9	47
MG2B	i	QQYSTOQS	9	47
RT2B	i	SSYTSSSTL	9	47
DP2C	i	SSYTSSSSV	9	47

Table 16.8. Effect of light chain exchanges on i binding

L Chain	Family			Heavy Chain (μ)		
		FS-6	**FS-7**	**FS-3**	**FR1(FS-7)**	**RF-SJ3**
FS-6κ	κ3b	++++	+/-	+/-	ND	ND
FS-7κ	κ1	+++	+	-	+	ND
FS-3λ	λ1	+/-	-	+/-	ND	ND
RF-SJ3κ	κ3b	++(+)	ND	ND	-	
RF-TS1κ	κ3b	+	-	ND	ND	ND
TMC-1κ	κ3	-	-	ND	ND	ND
37-2κ	κ3b	+	-	ND	ND	ND
RF-TS2κ	κ3a	-	-	ND	ND	ND
HBV1λ	λ5	-	-	ND	ND	ND
91A3κ	κ10	-	-	ND	ND	ND

ND; not done

DISCUSSION

Autoimmune hemolytic anemia (AHA) was one of the first recognized autoimmune diseases in humans. The molecular mechanisms underlying AHA, however, are still not completely elucidated, making it difficult to prevent or treat this disease. Also, due to the presence of some of the RBC antigens on cancerous tissue, there is considerable interest in the use of several of these mAb for imaging and therapy. In our laboratory we have analyzed a panel of human antibodies directed against a large array of self-antigens and found several instances where identical copies of germline V_H and J_H gene segments are rearranged to unique D segments to generate not only different, but also unique specificities highly restricted to patients. We were surprised to find a single human V_H gene segment, V_H4-34, encoding the H chain of eight antibodies with CA activity that were derived from different patients with hemolytic anemia. Interestingly, this restriction explained the former observation that antibodies with CA bear cross-reactive idiotypes, and suggested a relevant role for the product of the V_H gene segment in the interaction with the I/i antigens.

It is well established that the product of the V_H4-34 gene segment is necessary to generate anti-I/i specificities. Mutagenesis analyses in our laboratory have helped elucidate the role played by the V_H4-34 gene segment; it is now clear that FR1 residues uniquely encoded within this gene segment participate in the interaction with the red blood cell carbohydrates, and that CDR_H3 residues further define the fine specificity of V_H4-34 encoded antibodies. What remains to be addressed is the reason behind the overrepresentation of the V_H4-34 gene segment in the anti-Rh and anti-Kidd responses.

It would appear that the structures of the I/i antigens are such that they are bound predominantly by V_H4-34 encoded antibodies, to the near exclusion of all antibodies encoded by other V_H gene segments. It is this exclusive matching between antigen and antibody structures which is most unusual in the immune system. It is understandable that V_H4-34 encoded antibodies have additional specificities, this property being determined by the CDR_H3 sequences with involvement of the L chains. While anti-Rh antibodies are not exclusively V_H4-34 encoded, there is high utilization of this gene segment against these antigens as well as the I/i antigens.

The localization of the 9G4 Id to V_H4-34 FR1 provided information to help explain the near exclusive gene segment usage for the I/i antigens. The FR1 sequence of V_H4-34 encoded antibodies is unique from all the FR1 sequences in the other V_H families, including other members of the V_H4 family. Replacement of the V_H4-34 FR1 with FR1 sequences from gene segments representing the other V_H families resulted in loss of I binding. This result indicates that FR1 plays an important role in determining antigen specificity. An X-ray crystal structure of V_H4-34 encoded antibodies would shed more light on the structure of the antigen-combining site and its relationship with FR1. Antibodies interacting with carbohydrates are expected to encompass smaller interaction surfaces than those with globular protein antigens and are described as either pockets or grooves.[96] The results of some studies indicate that monoclonal anti-carbohydrate antibodies tend to have broad reactivity patterns, binding to both closely and distantly related structures.[97,98] It has been suggested that broad reactivity is possibly a general property of anti-carbohydrate antibodies. Human anti-GlcNAc monoclonal antibodies were shown to react with keratin from human skin and cytokeratin 14.[99] The cytokeratin peptide SFGSGFGGGY induced antibodies which expressed anti-GlcNAc activity, demonstrating that peptides can mimic carbohydrate antigens.

The role of FR1 in binding the I antigen, however, may not be limited to this interaction, but rather represents a prototypical interaction common to many antigen/antibody interactions. The involvement of FR in erythrocyte antigen binding has been shown for antibodies with other specificities,[100,101,102] and it has been suggested that when the antigen is a large molecule, both the CDR and FR residues are involved in the binding.[103]

An anti-digoxin antibody which had the first two amino acids of FR1 deleted, demonstrated enhanced antigen binding.[104] It is evident that certain exogenous and self proteins bind to conserved framework regions of the antibody molecule that are encoded within germline V_H gene segments and lie outside the conventional antigen binding sites. Therefore, several, or even the majority of expressed members of a given V_H family may share the ability to sustain such interactions due to their framework sequence similarity. Crystallographic and mutagenesis analyses of conventional antigen-antibody interactions reveal, however, that essential contact residues are usually the product of somatic diversification, and map to most or all five of the gene segments that encode the antibody variable region, with special emphasis on the CDRs within the V_H, D_H and V_L gene segments. Consequently, very few conventional antibody responses in the human are restricted in the usage of any of these five genetic elements.

Our experiments involving CDR_H3 swaps and mutations indicate that the CDR_H3 is also involved in determining the fine specificity of V_H4-34 encoded antibodies. After reviewing a large database of amino acid sequences of human and mouse immunoglobulin molecules, Kabat and Wu [104] evaluated the relative contribution of V_H and V_L regions to antibody specificity. These authors found several examples of antibodies with different specificities that shared identical V_H genes but displayed very distinct CDR_H3s. Additionally, a single CDR_H3 was expressed in the context of very different V_H and V_L gene segments in antibodies with identical specificity, supporting the relevance of the CDR_H3 in the interaction with antigen. When Parr et al[105] exchanged the CDR_H3 between a V_H4-34 encoded i binder and a V_H4-59 encoded non-i binder, the chimeric antibody composed of V_H4-34 attached to the CDR_H3 of the non-i binder, retained affinity for i antigen. This seemed to indicate that the CDR_H3 is not instrumental in determining antibody specificity. Our data, however, indicates that while a large number of unrelated CDR_H3 sequences permit I binding, there is a limit to the amino acid composition which allows I binding. It is the combination of the V_H4-34 encoded portion (especially FR1) and CDR_H3 structures which results in the specificity and affinity involved in I binding.

There are examples of antibodies that do not recognize the I/i antigens and yet express the product of this gene segment as a direct copy of the germline gene segment. Three-dimensional interactions within the different variable region elements as well as very likely between variable and constant region determinants may explain these observations. Antigens which are structurally similar to N-acetyl-lactosamine may interact with antibodies which are V_H4-34 encoded as well as antibodies encoded by gene segments from other V_H families. Lipid A, for example, which consists of β1-6 linked glucosamine disaccharide with fatty acid side chains attached to the amino groups, is structurally homologous to the i antigen, CD45 contains N-acetyl-lactosamine units, and DNA contains the carbohydrate deoxyribose and has a phosphate sugar backbone with an overall negative charge. The protein antigens potentially interact with V_H4-34 encoded antibodies by virtue of shape and not composition. The Rh antigens C, c, E and e are distinct, but structurally related to each other; as there are 36 amino acid substitutions that differentiate D from the CcEe proteins.[106] There appears to be a family of Rh-related glycoproteins carrying the ABO blood group and associated antigens which coimmunoprecipitate with Rh polypeptide using anti-Rh polypeptide antibodies.[107] It has been reported that this glycoprotein is a component of all Rh antigens immune complexes.[108] This carbohydrate perhaps provides the common denominator for the different Rh antigens and the I/i antigens, thus providing the structural requirement for using the V_H4-34 gene segment in the immune response. This antigenic shape, for which V_H4-34 encoded antibodies provides the best fit, could be referred to as unconventional, as most antigens can be bound by antibodies which are encoded by more than one gene segment. Therefore, antigens which are bound by V_H4-34 encoded antibodies can possibly form a structural group.

Since I binding involves the H chain FR1, CDR3 and the L chain, the binding largely represents a conventional antigen/antibody interaction. The presence of somatic mutations in the V genes encoding anti-I/i antibodies suggests an antigen-driven immune response. The involvement of the CDR_H3 in I binding indicates that the antigen cannot be classified as a superantigen which typically binds outside of the CDR_H3. If the antigens in this group are referred to as unconventional, then perhaps the V_H4-34 encoded antibodies which accommodates their structures, and which are overrepresented in the preimmune, immune and autoimmune repertoires, should also be referred to as unconventional or even superantibodies by virtue of their ability to bind antigens which no other antibodies can bind. Spellerberg et al[55] have referred to the V_H4-34 gene segment as a super-V_H gene.

It will be interesting to see whether this interaction between I/i antigens and V_H4-34 encoded antibodies remains an isolated example of exclusive human V_H usage or is the prototype of other exclusive antigen/antibody interactions. The anti-phosphorylcholine (PC) response in mice has some parallels with the human anti-I/i response. In mice, approximately 90% of the PC response express the T15 Id which is formed strictly from the association of the V1 gene of the S107 V_H gene family[109] with the DFL16.1 and J_H1 together with the Vκ22-Jκ5 encoded L chain.[110] The clonal nature of the response is similar to that of the monoclonal response in humans to I/i. This similarity continues in that B cells expressing the T15 Id are highly represented in a naive B cell repertoire.[111] It has been suggested that there is a limited number of ways to form an optimal PC binding site, hence explaining the restricted V gene segment usage.[108] Anti-PC antibodies protect mice and humans against lethal pneumococcal infections.[112] Anti-PC antibodies encoded by non-canonical V gene segments exhibited both anti-foreign and anti-self reactivities. In this example, it has been speculated that the idiotypically restricted response may serve to prevent the expression of antibodies that react with both foreign and self antigens and help maintain self-tolerance.[113] A second example of a restricted antibody response is the A/J mouse response to arsonate coupled to hemocyanin where the same V_H and $V\kappa$ variable germline genes are used.[114]

Out of over 254 red blood cell antigens, the V_H4-34 gene segment is overrepresented in response to nine of them (I, i, D, C, c, E, e, Jka and Jkb). V_H4-34 does not appear to be the predominant gene segment used against the ABH blood group antigens, nor against the other less clinically significant RBC antigens such as PR_2 (0/10), Gd (0/1) or Kell (0/1). While it is perhaps an overstatement to say at this time that the predominant response to RBC antigens in general is V_H4-34 mediated, the use of the V_H4-34 gene segment by anti- I (10/16) i (27/27), D (16/35), c (18/24), E (1/8), e (2/5) and anti-Kidd (4/4) antibodies is impressive. As a means of gaining a perspective on V_H4-34 gene segment utilization, 5/5 monoclonal antithyrotropin receptor antibodies from patients with Graves' Disease were all V_H3 encoded, and four clones with thyroid stimulating activity were derived from four V_H families; V_H2, 3, 4 (4-59) and 5.[115] When five human monoclonal antibodies with specificity for dihydrolipoamide acetlytransferase from patients with primary biliary cirrhosis were analyzed, the gene segments were from V_H families 2, 3, 4 and 5. None were V_H4-34 encoded.[116] One out of 20 (5%) IgM monoclonal anti-DNA antibodies was V_H4-34 encoded, and 2/13 (15%) IgG anti-DNA antibodies were V_H4-34 encoded.[117] None of 18 anti-HIV-1 human antibodies with specificities for gp41, gp120, or p24 utilized the V_H4-34 gene segment.[118] None of four human monoclonal antibodies to the hepatitis B virus were V_H4-34 encoded,[119] nor were seven antibodies to *Haemophilus influenzae* type b[120,121] or one antibody to *Bordetella pertussis*,[105] nor nine anti-insulin antibodies.[122,123]

It is significant, however, that a large proportion of B cells, as well as other cell types express V_H4-34 encoded H chains at any one time. This creates a situation whereby a potential superantigen, either on the surface of a microorganism or a self-antigen, could simultaneously interact with all the V_H4-34 expressing B cells resulting in polyclonal stimulation and apoptosis of a large portion of B cells. Auto-anti-idiotypic antibodies are self-molecules which bind antibodies in the variable region outside of the antigen combining site which could potentially function as superantigens. Polyclonal stimulation by a superantigen followed by antigen selection could lead to the development of monoclonal gammopathies such as cold agglutinin disease. Characterization of the structure, specificities and control of expression of V_H4-34 encoded antibodies is undoubtedly going to be of fundamental importance to understanding general mechanisms in the function of the human immune system.

Acknowledgments

We acknowledge the National Institutes of Health (AI-12127, GM-31689 and CA-44016) and the Robert Welch Foundation for financial support. JDC holds the Edwin L. Cox Distinguished Chair in Immunology and Genetics at the University of Texas Southwestern Medical Center at Dallas.

References

1. Okamoto M, Murakami M, Shimizu A et al. A transgenic model of autoimmune hemolytic anemia. J Exp Med 1992; 175:71-79.
2. Lutz HU, Bussolino F, Flepp R et al. Naturally occurring anti-band-3 antibodies and complement together mediate phagocytosis of oxidatively stressed human erythrocyts. Proc Natl Acad Sci USA 1987; 84: 7368-7372.
3. Garbar P. Autoantibodies and the physiological role of immunoglobulins. Immunol Today 1983; 4:101-122.
4. Pascual V, Capra JD. B cell superantigens? Current Biol 1991; 1:315-316.

5. Sasso EH, Silverman GJ, Mannik M. Human IgA and IgG F(ab')$_2$ that bind to staphylococcal protein A belong to the V_HIII subgroup. J Immunol 1991; 147: 1877-1883.
6. Berberian L, Goodglick L, Kipps TJ, Braun J. Immunoglonbulin V_H3 gene products: natural ligands for HIV gp120. Science (Wash DC) 1993; 261:1588-1591.
7. Lenert P, Kroon D, Spiegelberg H et al. Human CD4 binds immunoglobulins. Science (Wash DC) 1990; 248:1639-1643.
8. Nilson BHK, Solomon A, Bjorck L et al. Protein L from *Peptococcus magnus* binds to the κ light chain. J Biol Chem 1992; 267:2234-2239.
9. Bouvet JP, Pires R, Lunel-Fabiani F et al. Protein F. A novel F(ab)-binding factor, present in normal liver, and largely released in the digestive tract during hepatitis. J Immunol 1990; 145:1176-1180.
10. Anstee DJ, Mallinson G. The biochemistry of blood group antigens- some recent advances. Vox Sang 1994; 67(Suppl. 3):1-6.
11. Telen MJ. Erythrocyte blood group antigens: not so simple after all. Blood 1995; 85:299-306.
12. Springer GF, Horton RE. Blood group isoantibody stimulation in man by feeding blood group active bacteria. J Clin Invest 1969; 48:1280-1291.
13. Kumpel BM, Goodrick MJ, Pamphilon DH et al. Human RhD monoclonal antibodies (BRAD-3 and BRAD-5) cause accelerated clearance of Rh D^+ red blood cells and suppression of RhD immunization in Rh D^- volunteers. Blood 1995; 86:1701-1709.
14. Rao N, Ferguson DJ, Lee S-F et al. Identification of human erythrocyte blood group antigens on the C3b/C4b receptor. J Immunol 1991; 146:3502-3507.
15. Fearon DT, Wong WW. Complement ligand-receptor interactions that mediate biological responses. Ann Rev Immunol 1983; 1:243-271.
16. Pruzanski W and Katz A. Cold agglutinins: antibodies with biological diversity. Clin Immunol Rev 1984; 3:131-150.
17. Roelcke D. Cold agglutination. Transfus Med Rev 1989; III2:140-166.
18. Hakamori S. Blood group ABH and II antigens of human erythrocytes: chemistry, polymorphism and their developmental change. Semin Hematol 1981; 18:39-62.
19. Silberstein LE. Natural and pathologic human autoimmune responses to carbohydrate antigens on red blood cells. Springer Semin Immunopath 1993; 15:139-153.
20. Costea M, Yakulis V, Heller P. Experimental production of cold agglutinins in rabbits. Blood 1965; 26:323-340.
21. Colling RG, Pearson TC, Brown JC. Association of bacterial carbohydrate-specific cold agglutinin antibody production with immunization by group C, group B Type III, and *Streptococcus pneumoniae* type XIV streptococcal vaccines. Infect Immun 1983; 41:205-213.
22. Wood E, Lecomte J Childs RA et al. Preparative affinity chromatography of blood group II active sheep gastric mucins and release of antigenically active oligosaccharides by alkaline borohydrate degradation. Carbohydr Res 1981; 90:269-282.
23. Kannagi R, Hakomori S. Monoclonal antibodies directed to carbohydrate antigens. In: Weir DM, ed. Handbook of Experimental Immunology, applications of immunological methods in biomedical sciences. Vol. 4, 4th ed. Oxford: Blackwell Scientific Publications, 1986:117.1-117.20.
24. Pascual V, Victor K, Spellerberg M et al. V_H restriction among human cold agglutinins. The V_H4-21 gene segment is required to encode anti-I and anti-i specificities. J Immunol 1992; 149:2337-2344.
25. Silberstein L, Jefferies L, Goldman J et al. Variable region analysis of pathologic human autoantibodies to the related i and II red blood cell antigens. Blood 1991; 78:2372-2386.
26. Pascual V, Victor K, Lelsz D et al. Nucleotide sequence analysis of the V regions of two IgM cold agglutinins. Evidence that the V_H4-21 gene segment is responsible for the major cross-reactive idiotype. J Immunol 1991; 146:4385-4391.
27. Leoni L, Ghiso J, Goni F et al. The primary structure of the Fab fragment of protein KAU, a monoclonal immunoglobulin M cold agglutinin. J Biol Chem 1991; 266:2386-2842.

28. Grillot-Courvalin C, Brouet J-C, Piller F et al. An anti-B cell autoantibody from Wiskott-Aldrich syndrome which recognizes i blood group specificity on normal human B cells. Eur J Immunol 1992; 22: 1781-1788.
29. Stevenson FK, Wringhham M, Glennie MJ et al. Antibodies to shared idiotypes as agents for analysis and therapy for human B cell tumours. Blood 1986; 68:430-436.
30. Stevenson FK, Smith GJ, North J et al. 1989. Identification of normal B cell counterparts of neoplastic cells which secrete cold agglutinins of anti-I and anti-i specificity. Brit J Haematol 1989; 72: 9-15.
31. Thompson KM, Sutherland J, Barden G et al. Human monoclonal antibodies against blood group antigens preferentially express a V_H4-21 variable region gene-associated epitope. Scand J Immunol 1991; 34: 509-518.
32. Logtenberg T, Schutte MEM, Ebeling SB et al. Molecular approaches to the study of human B cell and (auto)antibody repertoire generation and selection. Immunol Rev 1992; 128:23-47.
33. Williams RC Jr, Kunkel HG, Capra JD. Antigenic specificities related to the cold agglutinin activity of gamma M globulins. Science (Wash DC) 1968; 161:379-381.
34. Matsuda F, Shin EK, Nagoaka H et al. Structure and physical map of 64 variable segments in the 3' 0.8-megabase region of the human immunoglobulin heavy-chain locus. Nature Genet 1993; 3:88-94.
35. Cook GP, Tomlinson IM, Walter G et al. A map of the human immunoglobulin V_H locus completed by analysis of the telomeric region of chromosome 14q. Nature Genet 1994; 7:162-168.
36. Kraj P, Friedman DF, Stevenson F et al. Evidence for the overexpression of the *V_H4-34 (V_H4-21)* Ig gene segment in the normal adult human peripheral blood B cell repertoire. J Immunol 1995; 154: 6406-6420.
37. Pascual V, Capra JD. V_H4-21, a human V_H gene segment overrepresented in the autoimmune repertoire. Arth Rheum 1991; 34:11-18.
38. Stevenson FK, Spellerberg MB, Treasure J et al. Differential usage of an Ig heavy chain variable region gene by human B cell tumors. Blood 1993; 82: 224-230.
39. Omary MB, Trowbridge IS, Battifora HA. Human homologue of mouse T200 glycoprotein. J Exp Med 1980; 152:842-852.
40. Childs RA, Dalchau R, Scudder P et al. Evidence for the occurrence of O-glycosidically linked oligosaccharides of poly-N-acetyllactosamine type on the human leucocyte common antigen. Biochem Biophys Res Commun 1983; 110:424-431.
41. Childs RA, Feizi T. Differences in carbohydrate moieties of high molecular weight glycoproteins of human lymphocytes of T of B origins revealed by monoclonal autoantibodies with anti-I specificities. Biochem Biophys Res Commun 1981; 102: 1158-1164.
42. Justement LB, Campbell KS, Chien NC et al. Regulation of B cell antigen receptor signal transduction and phosphorylation by CD45. Science 1991; 252:1839-1842.
43. Sanders ME, Makgoba MW, Shaw S. 1988. Human naive and memory T cells: reinterpretation of helper-inducer and suppressor-inducer subsets. Immunol Today 1988; 9:195-199.
44. George A, Rath S, Shroff KE et al. Ligation of CD45 on B cells can facilitate production of secondary Ig isotypes. J Immunol 1994; 152:1014-1021.
45. Feizi T. The blood group II system: A carbohydrate antigen system defined by naturally monoclonal or oligoclonal autoantibodies of man. Immunol Commun 1981; 10:127-156.
46. Adinolfi M. Anti-I antibody in normal human newborn infants. Immunol 1965; 9:43-52.
47. Chapman CJ, Spellerberg MB, Smith GA et al. Autoanti-red cell antibodies synthesized by patients with infectious mononucleosis utilize the V_H4-21 gene segment. J Immunol 1993; 151:1051-1061.
48. Feizi,T. Monotypic cold agglutinins in infection by *Mycoplasma pneumoniae.* Nature 1967; 215:540-542.
49. Schwartz RS. Autoimmunity and autoimmune diseases. In: Paul WE, ed. Fundamental Immunology. Third edition. New York: Raven Press, Ltd., 1993: 1033-1097.

50. Jefferies LC, Carchidi CM, Silberstein LE. Naturally occurring anti-i/I cold agglutinins may be incoded by different V_H3 genes as well as the V_H4-21 gene segment. J Clin Invest 1993; 92:2821-2833.
51. Schutte MEM, van Es JH, Silberstein LE et al. $V_H4.21$ encoded natural autoantibodies with anti-i specificity mirror those associated with cold hemagglutinin disease. J Immunol 1993; 151:6569-6576.
52. Pascual V, Victor K, Randen II et al. Nucleotide sequence analysis of rheumatoid factors and polyreactive antibodies derived from patients with rheumatoid arthritis reveals diverse use of V_H and V_L gene segments and extensive variability in CDR-3. Scand J Immunol 1992; 36:349-362.
53. Ng VL, Hurt MH, Fein CL et al. IgMs produced by two acquired immune deficiency syndrome lymphoma cell lines: Ig binding specificity and V_H gene putative somatic mutation analysis. Blood 1994; 83:1067-1078.
54. van Es J, Meyling FHJG, van de Akker W et al. Somatic mutations in the variable regions of a human IgG anti-double-stranded DNA autoantibody suggest a role for antigen in the induction of sytemic lupus erythematosus. J.Exp Med 1991; 173: 461-470.
55. Spellerberg M, Chapman C, Hamblin T, Stevenson F. Dual recognition of lipid A and DNA by human antibodies encoded by the V_H4-21 gene. Ann New York Acad Sci 1995; 764:694-705.
56. Hirabayashi Y, Munakata Y, Takai O et al. Human B cell clones expressing lupus nephritis-assoociated anti-DNA idiotypes are preferentially expanded without somatic mutation. Scand J Immunol 1993; 37: 533-540.
57. Bhat NM, Bieber MM, Chapman CJ et al. Human antilipid A monoclonal antibodies bind to human B cells and the i antigen on cord red blood cells. J Immunol 1993; 151:5011-5021.
58. Victor K, Pascual V, Williams C et al. Human monoclonal striational autoantibodies isolated from thymic B lymphocytes of patients with myasthenia gravis use V_H and V_L gene segments associated with the autoimmune repertoire. Eur J Immunol 1992; 22:2231-2236.
59. Bye JM, Carger C, Hui Y et al. Germline variable region gene segment derivation of human monoclonal anti-Rh(D) antibodies. Evidence for affinity maturation by somatic hypermutation and repertoire shift. J Clin Invest 1992; 90:2481-2490.
60. Borretzen M, Chapman C, Stevenson FK et al. Structural analysis of V_H4-21 encoded human IgM allo- and autoantibodies against red blood cells. Scand J Immunol 1995; 42:90-97.
61. Sanz I, Casali P, Thomas JW et al. Nucleotide sequences of eight human natural autoantibodies V_H regions reveals apparent restricted use of V_H families. J Immunol 1989; 142: 4054-4061.
62. Ikematsu H, Kasaian MT, Schettino EW et al. Structural analysis of the V_H-D-J_H segments of human polyreactive IgG mAb. J Immunol 1993; 151:3604-3616.
63. Thompson K, Barden G, Sutherland J et al. Human monoclonal antibodies to C, c, E, e and G antigens of the Rh system. Immunol 1990; 71:323-327.
64. Thompson KM, Sutherland J, Barden G et al. Human monoclonal antibodies specific for blood group antigens demonstrate multispecific properties characteristic of natural autoantibodies. Immunol 1992; 76:146-157.
65. Marks JD, Ouwehand WH, Bye JM et al. Human antibody fragments specific for human blood group antigens from a phage display library. Bio/Technology 1993; 11:1145-1149.
66. Siegel DL, Silberstein LE. Expression and characterization of recombinant anti-Rh(D) antibodies on filamentous phage: a model system for isolating human red blood cells antibodies by repertoire cloning. Blood 1994; 83:2334-2344.
67. Blancher A, Roubinet F, Oksman F et al. Polyreactivity of human monoclonal antibodies: human anti-Rh monoclonal antibodies of IgM isotype are frequently polyreactive. Vox Sang 1991; 61:196-204.
68. Roelcke D. Cold agglutination. Antibodies and antigens. Clin Immunol Immunopathol 1974; 2:266-280.

69. Roelcke D, Ebert W, Giesen H. Anti-Pr_3: serological and immunochemical identification of new anti-Pr subspecificity. Vox Sang. 1976; 30:122-133.
70. Pruzanski,W, Roelcke D, Armstrong M et al. Pr and Gd antigens on human B of T lymphocytes and phagocytes. Clin Immunol Immunopathol 1980; 15:631-641.
71. Romer W, Seelig H, Lenhard V et al. The distribution of I/i, Pr, and Gd antigens in mammalian tissues. Invest Cell Pathol 1979; 2:157-162.
72. Silberstein LE, Robertson GA, Hannam Harris AC et al. Etiological aspects of cold agglutinin disease: evidence for cytogenetically defined clones of lymphoid cells and the demonstration that anti-Pr cold autoantibody is derived from a chromosomally aberrant B cell clone. Blood 1986; 67: 1705-1709.
73. Silberstein LE, Litwin S, Carmack CE. Relationship of variable region genes expresseed by a human B cell lymphoma secreting pathologic anti-Pr_2 erythrocyte autoantibodies. J Exp Med 1989; 169:1631-1643.
74. Reidl LS, Friedman DF, Goldman J et al. Structural basis of a conserved idiotype expressed by an autoreactive human B cell lymphoma: evidence that a V_H CDR3 mutation alters idiotypy and specificity. J Immunol 1991; 147:3623-3631.
75. Wang AC, Fudenberg HH, Wells JV et al. A new subgroup of the kappa chain variable region associated with anti-Pr cold agglutinins. Nature 1973; 243:126-128.
76. Friedman DF, Cho EA, Goldman J et al. The role of clonal selection in the pathogenesis of an autoreactive human B cell lymphoma. J Exp Med 1991; 174:525-537.
77. Cartron JP, Rahuel C. Human erythrocyte glycophorins: protein and gene structure analyses. Transpl Med Rev 1992; 6:63-92.
78. Chasis JA, Mohandas N. Red blood cell glycophorins. Blood 1992; 80:1869-1879.
79. Blackall DP, Ugorski M, Pahlsson P et al. A molecular biologic approach to study the fine specificity of antibodies directed to the MN human blood group antigens. J Immunol 1994; 152: 2241-2247.
80. Judd WJ, Issitt PD, Pavone BG et al. Antibodies that define NANA-independent MN-system antigens. Trans 1979; 19:12-18.
81. Bigbee WL, Langlois RG, Vanderlaan M et al. Binding specificities of eight monoclonal antibodies to human glycophorin A-studies with M^cM and $M^kEn(UK)$ variant human erythrocytes and M-and MN^v-type chimpanzee erythrocytes. J Immunol 1984; 133:3149-3155.
82. Dahr W. Miltenberger subsystem of the MNSs blood group system: Review and outlook. Vox Sang 1992; 62:129-135.
83. Rearden A, Frandson S, Carry JB. Severe hemolytic disease of the newborn due to anti-Vw and detection of glycophorin A antigens on the Miltenberger II sialoglycoprotein by Western blotting. Vox Sang 1987; 52:318-321.
84. Roelcke D, Riesen W, Geisen H,et al. Serological identification of the new cold agglutinin specificity anti-Gd. Vox Sang 1977; 33:304-306.
85. Angel de la Fuente M, Coumaran E, Pereira A et al. Characterization of a monoclonal IgMK (IgMGAS) anti-Gd cold agglutinin (CA). Its existence with a monoclonal IgG3K (IgGGAS) without CA activity that might be clonally related to IgMGAS. Blood 1994; 83:1310-1322.
86. Potter KN, Li Y-C, Pascual V et al. Molecular characterization of a cross-reactive idiotope on human immunoglobulins utilizing the V_H4-21 gene segment. J Exp Med 1993; 178:1419-1428.
87. Victor KD, Randen I, Thompson K et al. Rheumatoid factors isolated from patients with autoimmune disorders are derived from germline genes distinct from those encoding the Wa, Po and Bla cross-reactive idiotypes. J Clin Invest 1991; 87: 1603-1613.
88. Victor KD, Pascual V, Lefvert AK et al. Human anti-acetylcholine receptor antibodies use variable gene segments analogous to those used in autoantibodies of various specificities. Mol Immunol 1992; 29:1501-1506.
89. Sanz I, Capra JD. V_κ and J_κ gene segments of A/J ars-A antibodies: somatic recombination generates the essential arginine at the junction of the variable and joining regions. Proc Natl Acad Sci USA 1987; 84:1085-1089.

90. Saul FA, Amzel LM, Poljak RJ. Preliminary refinement and structural analysis of the Fab fragment from human immunoglobulin New at 2.0 A resolution. J Biol Chem 1978; 253:585-597.
91. Riboldi P, Gaidano G, Schettino EW et al. Two acquired immunodeficiency syndrome-associated Burkitt's lymphomas produce specific anti-i IgM cold agglutinins using somatically mutated V_H4-21 segments. Blood 1994; 83:2952-2961.
92. Li Y-C, Spellerberg MB, Stevenson FK et al. The II binding specificity of human V_H4-34 (V_H4-21) encoded antibodies is determined by both V_H framework region 1 and complementarity determining region 3. J Mol Biol 1996; 256:577-589.
93. Vazquez-Abad D, Pascual V, Zanetti M et al. Analysis of human antitopoisomerase-I idiotypes. J Clin Invest 1993; 92: 1302-1313.
94. Jefferies LC, Silverman GJ, Carchidi CM et al. Idiotypic heterogeneity of V_kIII autoantibodies to red blood cell antigens. Clin Immunol Immunopath 1992; 65:119-128.
95. Capra JD, Kehoe JM, Williams RC Jr et al. Light chian sequences of human IgM cold agglutinins. Proc Natl Acad Sci USA 1972; 69:40-43.
96. Cisar J, Kabat EA, Dorner MN et al. Binding properties of immunoglobulin combining sites specific for terminal or nonterminal antigenic determinants in dextran. J Exp Med 1975; 142:435-459.
97. Furukawa K, Welt S, Yin BWT et al. Analysis of the fine specificities of 11 mouse monoclonal antibodies reactive with type 2 blood group determinants. Mol Immunol 1990; 27:723-732.
98. Lloyd KO, Old LJ. Human monoclonal antibodies to glycolipids and other carbohydrate antigens: dissection of the humoral immune response in cancer patients. Can Res 1989; 3445-3451.
99. Shikham AR, Greenspan NS, Cunningham MW. Cytokeratin peptide SFGSGFGGGGY mimics N-acetyl-b-D-glucosamine in reaction with antibodies and lectins, and induces in vivo anti-carbohydrate response. J Immunol 1994; 153:5593-5606.
100. Schlomichik MJ, Nemazee DA, Sato VL et al. Variable region sequence of murine IgM anti-IgG monoclonal autoantibodies (Rheumatoid Factor). A structural explanation for the high frequency of IgM anti-IgG B cells. J Exp Med 1986; 164:407-427.
101. Sheriff S, Dilverton EW, Padlan EA et al. Three-dimensional structure of an antibody-antigen complex. Proc Natl Acad Sci USA 1987; 84:8075-8079.
102. Panka DJ, Mudgett-Hunter M, Parks DR et al. Variable region framework differences result in decreased or increased affinity of variant anti-digoxin antibodies. Proc Natl Acad Sci USA 1988; 85:3080-3084.
103. Scott BB, Sadigh S, Andrew EM et al. Affinity maturation and isotype switch in clonally related anti-erythrocyte autoantibodies. Scand J Immunol 1994; 40:16-21.
104. Kabat EA, Wu TT. Identical V region amino acid sequences and segments of sequences in antibodies of different specificities. Relative contributions of V_H and V_L genes, minigenes, and complementarity-determining regions to binding of antibody-combining sites. J Immunol 1991; 147: 1709-1719.
105. Parr TB, Johnson TA, Silberstein LE et al. Anti-B cell autoantibodies encoded by V_H4-21 genes in human fetal spleen do not require in vivo somatic selection. Eur J Immunol 1994; 24:2941-2949.
106. Cartron J-P, Agre P. Rh blood group antigens: protein and gene structure. Sem Hematol 1993; 30:193-208.
107. Moore S, Green C. The identification of specific rheusus-polypeptide-blood-group-ABH-active -glycoprotein complexes in the human red cell membrane. Biochem J 1987; 244:735-741.
108. Matsubara K, Tanabe K, Akane A et al. A novel assay for typing Rh antigens in bloodstains using a lectin specific to the bisecting N-acetyl-D-glucosamine side chain of glycoprotein. J Immunol Methods 1994; 173:175-180.
109. Crews S, Griffin J, Huang H et al. A single V_H gene segment encodes the immune response to phosphoylcholine: somatic mutation is correlated with the class of the anitbodies. Cell 1981; 25:59-66.
110. Clafin JL, Cubberley M. Clonal nature of

the immune response to phosphorylcholine. IV. Hybridoma representation of group II (T-15-like) and group II (non-T15-like) antibodies utilized distinct V_H genes. Immunol 1980; 132:1550-1558.

111. Klinman NR, Pickard AR, Sigal NH et al. Assessing B cell diversification by antigen receptor and precursor cell analysis. Annales d'Imunologie 1976; 127:489-502.

112. Briles DE, Forman C, Crain M. Mouse antibody to phosphocholine can protect mice from infection with mouse-virulent human isolate of *Streptococcus pneumoniae*. Infect Immun 1983; 60:1957-1965.

113. Limpanasithikul W, Ray S, Diamond B. Cross-reacative antibodies have both protective and pathogenic potential. J Immunol 1995; 155:967-973.

114. Rathbun G, Otani F, Milner ECB et al. Molecular characterization of the A/J J558 family of heavy chain variable region gene segments. Mol Biol 1988; 202:383-395.

115. Shin EK, Akamizu T, Matsuda F et al. Variable regions of Ig heavy chain genes encoding antithyrotropin receptor antibodies of patients with Graves' Disease. J Immunol 1994; 152:1485-1492.

116. Pascual V, Cha S, Gershwin M.E et al. Nucleotide sequence analysis of natural and combinatorial anti-PDC-E2 antibodies in patients with primary biliary cirrhosis. Recapitulating immune selection with molecular biology. J Immunol 1994; 152: 2577-2585.

117. Isenberg DA, Ehrenstein MR, Longhurst C et al. The origin, sequence, structure, and consequences of developing anti-DNA antibodies. Arth Rheum 1994; 37:169-180.

118. Andris JS, Capra JD. The molecular structure of human antibodies specific for the human immunodeficiency virus. J Clin Immunol 1995; 15:17-26.

119. Andris JS, Ehrlich PH, Ostberg L et al. Probing the human antibody repertoire to exogenous antigens. Characterization of the J and L chain V region gene segments from anti-hepatitis B virus antibodies. J Immunol 1992; 149:4053-4059.

120. Andris JS, Brodeur BR, Capra JD. Molecular characteization of human antibodies to bacterial antigens: utilization of the less frequently expressed V_H2 and V_H6 heavy chain variable region gene families. Mol Immunol 1993; 30:1601-1616.

121. Adderson EE, Shackelford PG, Quinn A et al. Restricted Ig H chain V gene usage in the human antibody response to *Heamophilus influenzae* type b capsular polysaccharide. J Immunol 1991; 147:1667-1674.

122. Ikematsu H, Ichiyoshi Y, Schettino EW et al. V_H and $V\kappa$ segment structure of anti-insulin IgG autoantibodies in patients with insulin-dependent diabetes mellitus. Evidence for somatic selection. J Immunol 1994; 152:1430-1441.

123. Thomas JW. V region diversity in human anti-insulin antibodies. Preferential use of a V_HIII gene subset. J Immunol 1993; 150:1375-1382.

CHAPTER 17

CD4-Immunoglobulin Interaction: A Proposal for a Novel Self-Regulatory Circuit

Petar Lenert and Maurizio Zanetti

INTRODUCTION

CD4-Distribution and Structure

The CD4 receptor, previously called T4 in human and L3T4 in the mouse, is a glycoprotein expressed on helper/inducer T cells and, to a lesser degree, on monocytes/macrophages, some B cells as well as other hematopoietic and non-hematopoietic cells.[1-4] CD4 consists of several domains: an N-terminal extracellular region containing a leader sequence and four immunoglobulin (Ig)-like domains; a transmembrane region; and a cytoplasmic region that is highly charged.[5] Resolution of the crystal structure of the first two extracellular human domains (D1 and D2)[6-8] and of rat D3/D4 domains[9] has allowed the visualization and better understanding of the spatial arrangement of the molecule and it similarities with the light (L) chain of Ig. CD4 is an rod-like protein about 125 Å long and 25-30 Å wide. The first two extracellular domains of CD4 contain the principal HIV-binding site and also mediate the interaction with major histocompatibility complex (MHC) class II molecules on target cells.[7,8,10] Within the D1 domain the C'-C'' loop is extended by several residues in relation to the complementarity-determining region (CDR2) loop in the Ig molecule and appears to be crucial for the high-affinity binding of human immunodeficiency virus (HIV) gp120. By contrast, loops involved in dimerization in Ig-like domains, e.g., in Ig and CD8, are several residues shorter in CD4 then in Ig. This may explain why CD4 under normal conditions is monomeric.[10] Both D1/D2 and D3/D4 domains in CD4 are intimately connected forming rigid rods, while the segment between the D2 and D3 junction appears to be quite flexible relative to one another.

Human B Cell Superantigens, edited by Moncef Zouali. © 1996 R.G. Landes Company.

CD4—A MULTIFUNCTIONAL RECEPTOR MOLECULE

CD4 at the surface of T lymphocytes plays important roles in thymic development and T cell activation through specific recognition of MHC class II molecules.[11] Although of low intrinsic affinity (< 10^{-4} M for CD4/Ia interaction and ~$10^{-5}/10^{-6}$ M for human CD4/HLA class II),[12-13] this interaction contributes to T cell activation and cytokine secretion.[11] The coreceptor function of CD4 appears to be important in light of the fact that the T cell receptor (TcR) possesses low affinity for the peptide/MHC complex.[14,15] The costimulatory effect of CD4 is mediated by binding to MHC class II β2 region via its extracellular D1 and D2 domains,[12,16,17] but may also involve interactions with the TcR/CD3 complex and with CD45.[18-22] Co-aggregation of CD4 is followed by activation of the cytoplasm-associated $p56^{lck}$ protein-tyrosine kinase and subsequent phosphorylation of a number of intracellular substrates. $p56^{lck}$ activation is viewed as the one crucial early event following the CD4/TcR coengagement.[18]

Ligands that bind CD4 with high-affinity induce T cell downregulation, both in vitro and in vivo.[23-28] This occurs when their binding to CD4 precedes TcR/CD3 engagement. For example, the administration of monoclonal antibodies to CD4 was shown to induce profound immunosuppression in vivo if this preceded antigenic challenge.[28] Similar treatment also resulted in long term acceptance of foreign grafts[29] and induced an apparent switch towards the Th2 response.[29,30] Experiments in vitro using monoclonal antibodies to CD4 or cross-linked gp120 glycoproteins of HIV showed that if these high-affinity ligands interact with CD4 prior to T cell activation by antigen immunosupression follows.[23,27,31] In peripheral blood T cells and T cell lines, high-affinity CD4 ligands promote spontaneous cell death and enhance activation-induced apoptosis,[32,33] although it is unclear whether the Fas/Fas-ligand pathway is involved.[34-36] Even though CD4-ligation upregulates Fas-receptor expression and apoptosis,[37] CD4 crosslinking may not be restricted to the induction of Fas.[38]

In conclusion, a myriad of CD4-promoted effects could be dependent on a number of factors, including the localization of the CD4 epitope recognized by a particular ligand, CD4 density at the cell surface, activation of different intracellular signaling pathways, and expression of CD4 on accessory cells.

CD4 AND ITS LIGANDS

Over the last 10-15 years a number of structurally diverse molecules have been implicated as possible CD4-ligands: (1) MHC class II molecules,[39] (2) HIV-gp120 glycoprotein,[40] (3) sulfated dextrans and other polyanions, e.g., alkylated oligonucleotides, aurintricarboxyllic acid, heparin,[41-44] (4) immunoglobulins,[45] (5) human seminal plasma glycoprotein and equivalent molecules, e.g., seminal actin binding protein; gross cystic disease fluid protein and prolactin inducible protein,[46] (6) gangliosides (e.g., GM1),[47] (7) lectins (e.g., Jacalin),[48] and (8) lymphocyte chemoattractant (IL-16).[49] Whereas the molecular aspects of the interaction between CD4 molecule and its best known ligands (MHC class II molecules and HIV-gp120) has been a subject of several recent reviews,[18,40,50] little has been reported on other ligands, e.g., human seminal plasma glycoprotein, gangliosides, Jacalin and IL-16. In this review we will focus only on the CD4/Ig interaction and its possible implication in immune function.

CD4/IMMUNOGLOBULIN INTERACTION

A few years ago we and others provided evidence that both recombinant and native CD4 could interact with immunoglobulins.[45,51-53] Under experimental conditions that favored low-affinity binding, we demonstrated reactivity with CD4 in 39 out of 50 human myeloma proteins of various isotypes.[45] This interaction was documented using a variety of techniques including ELISA, radioimmunoassay, Western blot and flow cytometry. Human myeloma proteins and polyclonal IgG all bound CD4, regardless of their heavy (H) and light (L) chain isotypes. The interaction's avidity varied even among myeloma proteins of the same IgG subclass and light chain isotype. A notable exception was encountered with myeloma proteins of the IgG4 subclass, which did not bind. However, binding was restored in some of them when their F(ab')2 fragments were tested,[54] suggesting that CD4 binding may be dependent on the overall Ig structure (T versus Y shape) and that the binding site for CD4 on an Ig molecule can be hindered sterically.

Saturation of the Ig binding to rCD4 in ELISA performed for 3 hours at 22°C was reached at ~40 μg/ml for IgM, IgG, IgD and IgE, and at ~80 μg/ml for IgA. By comparison, the murine anti-CD4 molecule antibody Leu 3a reached a plateau at 3-4 μg/ml.[45] Competitive inhibition studies further demonstrated that the CD4/Ig interaction could be inhibited by a number of polyanionic substances, e.g., high molecular weight dextran sulfates, heparin, aurintricarboxyllic acid, due to their direct effect on CD4.[49,55-57]

Initial mapping studies to characterize the CD4/Ig interaction were carried out on CD4 and on Ig, independently. With respect to CD4, studies took advantage of the fact that electrophoresis of CD4 under reducing conditions did not affect the subsequent binding to Ig in Western blot (Fig. 17.1). We interpreted this to suggest that the principal Ig-binding site on CD4 was independent of the three-dimensional conformation of the molecule. Consequently, we considered using synthetic peptides for mapping purposes. Second, we observed that recombinant HIV gp120 was able to block the binding of Ig to rCD4. Since HIV gp120 binds to residues of the CDR2 loop of the first extracellular domain,[50,58,59] evidence was provided that the CD4/Ig interaction involved a conserved region of the receptor close to, or overlapping with, the virus-binding site. Our studies focused, therefore, on the first and second extracellular domains (D1 and D2) of CD4.

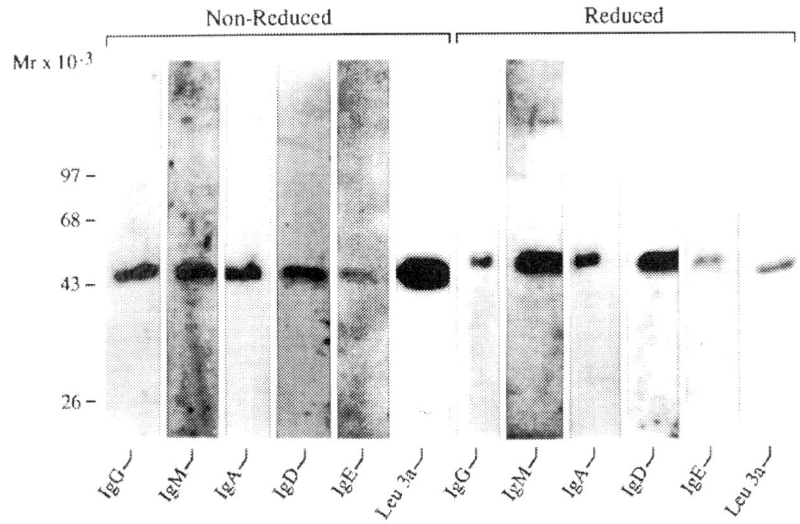

Fig. 17.1. Western blot analysis of the CD4/Ig interaction. ^{125}I-labeled human myeloma proteins bind to rCD4 electrophoresed under reducing and nonreducing conditions in a 10% SDS-PAGE. Monoclonal antibody Leu3a was used as the positive control.

In experiments in which synthetic peptides of human CD4 were used, we found that peptides corresponding to amino acid residues 16-49 and 21-49 (p16-49 and p21-49) bound human Ig in a way comparable to that of recombinant CD4 (rCD4). Interestingly, p16-49 had been shown to inhibit HIV infection in vitro,[60] further indicating that the binding site for Ig and for the virus were very close. In competitive inhibition experiments p21-49 significantly blocked the binding of Ig to rCD4.

Mapping studies further included the use of a panel of truncated synthetic peptides. Since a synthetic peptide spanning residues 21-38 had an Ig-binding activity almost identical to that of the longer peptide 21-49, truncated peptides comprised this region only. Using this approach we determined that the binding activity could reside in two discrete stretches of amino-acid residues (25-58 and 35-38). When this information was plotted against the X-ray coordinates of CD4,[7,8] it became evident that the residues 25-28 (QFHW) and 35-38 (KILG) are located on two juxtaposed antiparallel β strands (C and C'), within a same β sheet in the Ig-like fold of the molecule (Fig. 17.2).

The possible existence of at least two sub-sites within the first extracellular domain of CD4 was recently confirmed in a series of experiments in which rCD4 and CD4-derived synthetic peptides mediated agglutination of human Ig-coated polystyrene particles.[57] Agglutination of Ig-coated particles occurred only in cases when both stretches of amino acid residues (i.e., 25-28 and 35-38) were simultaneously present. In turn, peptides containing only one sub-site caused little (if any) inhibition of agglutination.

Taken together, these studies indicated that CD4 residues found to be involved in Ig-binding are located within the D1 do-

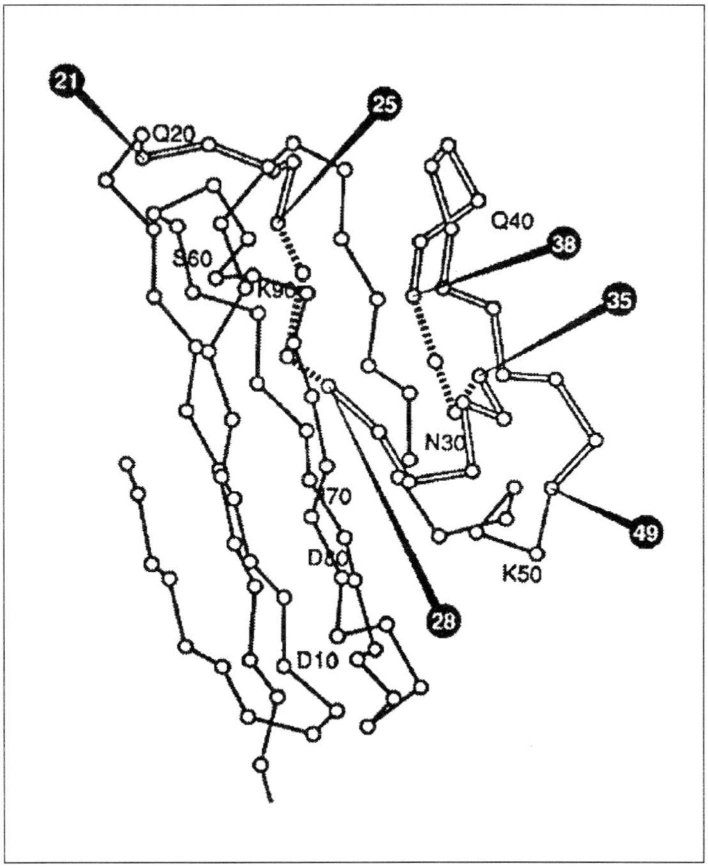

Fig. 17.2. Alpha carbon trace of the first extracullular domain of human CD4 from Wang et al and Ryu et al.[7,8] Key residues are identified. Tram-track line identifies the portion of the receptor spanning from residue 21 through 49. Interrupted segments identify the two subsite described in the text.

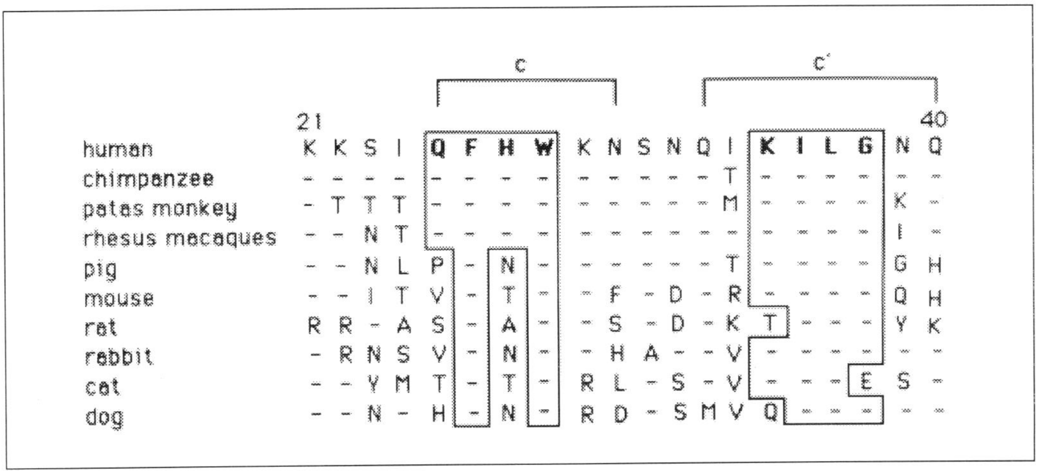

Fig. 17.3. Amino acid homology between CD4 sequences of various species in the region corresponding to amino acid residue 21 through 40. The composite underline the sequence conservation in the two subsites in the C and C′ loops, respectively.

main and are proximal to those residues mediating HIV-gp120 binding. Moreover, CD4/Ig interaction depends on relatively invariant residues on CD4, suggesting their conservation in evolution. We analyzed this issue from two different perspectives. First by directly comparing the sequences of various mammalian CD4 molecules between residues 21 and 40 (Fig. 17.3). It can be seen that six out of eight residues involved in Ig-binding (i.e., F26, W28, K35, I36, L37 and G38) were identical in evolutionary distant species such as rodents and primates. Second, since the structure of CD4 was found to be similar to that of an Ig L chain,[5] we aligned the sequences of human and murine CD4, with those of the Ig L chain and of the REI myeloma protein, a Bence-Jones protein whose three-dimensional structure had been solved by X-ray crystallography.

As shown in Figure 17.4, there exists great conservation among the CD4 and the Ig L chain. Most strikingly, those residues characterized as being part of the Ig-binding site reside in a region of high conservation of the L chain, precisely where most residues involved in V-V packing are located. Therefore, it is intriguing to speculate that the Ig-binding peptide 21-49 may be mimicking the natural domain association between V_H and V_L. Indeed, in analogy with the low affinity characteristics of the CD4/Ig interaction, the relative affinity of interaction between V_H and V_L is also low (~10^6-10^7 M^{-1}).[61] Taken together, our data imply that the CD4/Ig interaction best corresponds to a domain-domain type interaction between two molecules with a characteristic Ig-fold. This interaction is traditionally regarded as being noncovalent.

CD4 BINDING IS MEDIATED BY THE V_H DOMAIN OF THE IG MOLECULE

Mapping studies on the Ig molecule indicated that CD4 binding depends on the V_H portion of the Ig molecule. As mentioned above, CD4 binding was independent of the Ig H and L chain isotypes. We found that isolated H chains, but not L chains, bound CD4. In a chain recombination experiment in which the same H chain was associated with a κ or a λ L chain, respectively, we obtained unequivocal demonstration that the CD4 binding is mediated by the H chain.[45] When several human myeloma proteins and polyclonal IgG were subjected to enzymatic treatment, only F(ab')2 and Fab fragments bound to rCD4 and synthetic peptide 21-49. The binding of these Ig fragments was comparable to that of intact Ig molecules. On the other hand, heavy chain disease proteins, i.e., natural deletion mutants consisting of isolated H chains which lack major portions of the V_H regions and complete C_H1 domains, did not bind rCD4. Moreover, since binding to rCD4 of a natural C_H1 deletion mutant of murine myeloma protein MOPC 21 was the same as MOPC 21.[62] Therefore, we concluded that the Ig V_H domain is critical in mediating CD4 binding. This does not rule out that other Ig domains may contribute to the overall avidity of the CD4/Ig interaction possibly by stabilizing the conformation and accessibility of the Fab region to CD4.

In the V_H region, loops corresponding to the complementarity-determining regions (CDR) play a major role both in antigen binding and idiotype expression. Therefore, we were interested to verify if these functions of the Ig molecule were blocked by CD4. We first observed that various murine monoclonal antibodies could bind to the synthetic peptide 21-49 irrespective of their antigen specificity. Second, we observed that antibodies having the same isotype and fine epitope specificity varied in binding to synthetic peptide 21-49. Taken together these facts suggest that residues within CDR loops do not contribute significantly to the CD4/Ig interaction. Similarly, soluble p21-49 and rCD4 did not block, and in certain instances even enhanced, the interaction between idiotype and anti-idiotype antibodies.[54] Thus, considering the facts that neither conventional antigen:antibody nor idiotype:anti-idiotype interactions were blocked by CD4 or CD4-derived synthetic peptides, we concluded that CDR loops of the Ig molecule were not involved in the interaction between V_H and CD4.

IMMUNOCHEMISTRY OF THE CD4-IG INTERACTION

Because Fab fragments proved sufficient to mediate binding to CD4, we decided to investigate binding of antibody (Ab) complexed with antigen (Ag). We began these studies using two Ab:Ag systems: (1) A conventional hapten,

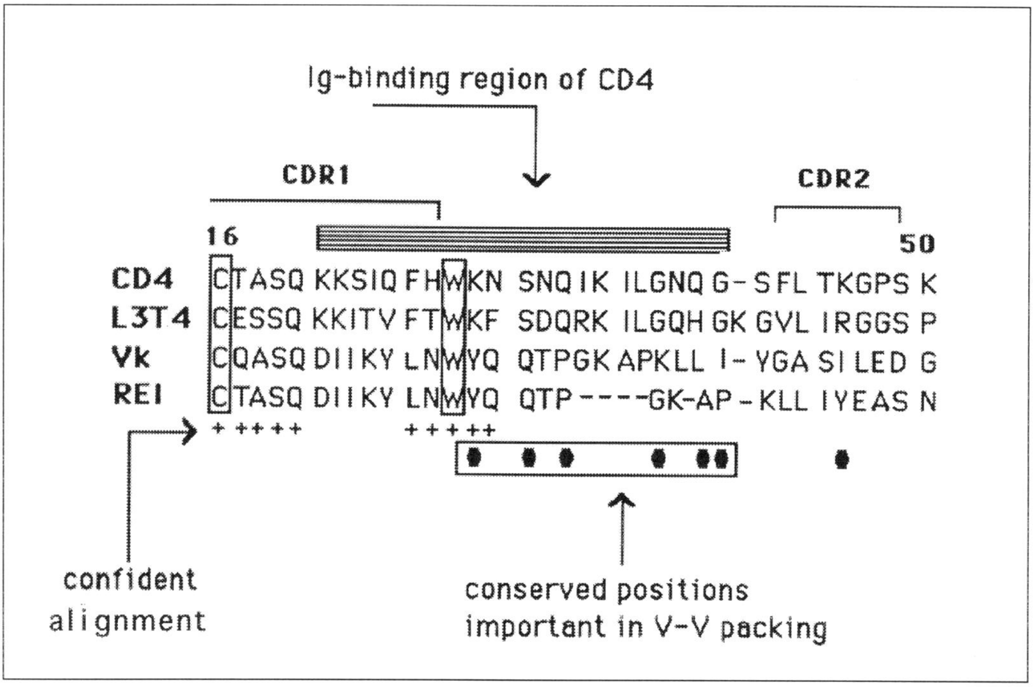

Fig. 17.4. Analysis of the Ig-binding region of human CD4 and comparison with murine CD4 (L3T4), mouse Vk and human light chain REI. Confident alignment and conserved positions important in V-V packing are indicated.

dinitrophenyl (DNP), conjugated to bovine serum albumin ($DNP_{37}BSA$) and a murine monoclonal antibody to DNP (IgG1, κ),[63] and (2) a prototype protein antigen, thyroglobulin, and a murine monoclonal antibody to thyroglobulin (IgG1, κ)[64] Ab:Ag complexes formed in vitro by adding constant amounts of Ab to varying amounts of antigen were transferred to microtiter plates coated with either rCD4 or synthetic peptide 21-49 (and their respective controls). Binding of the complexed material was revealed by an enzyme-conjugated rabbit antibody to mouse Ig. In the thyroglobulin system, binding of the Ab:Ag complexes increased progressively as a function of the amount of Ag. A maximum binding was reached when the Ab:Ag ratio was < 1, that is a value characteristic of soluble complexes. A quantitative analysis of the affinity of interaction between rCD4 or synthetic peptide 21-49 and Ab:Ag (anti-DNP:$DNP_{37}BSA$) complexes vs. monomeric or heat-aggregated anti-DNP monoclonal antibody is shown in Table 17.1. Enhancement of CD4 binding also occurred when $F(ab')_2$ fragments were used instead of the intact antibody. Collectively, in 5 out of 6 Ab:Ag systems tested we observed that Ab:Ag complexes bound CD4 with higher affinity than monomeric Ig. While the affinity of interaction of several murine monoclonal antibodies was found to be in the order of $< 10^{-5}$ M, preformed Ab:Ag complexes bound to CD4 with 50- to 100-fold higher affinity.[45] High epitope density (e.g., DNP_{37}-BSA vs DNP_{15}-BSA) further enhanced the binding of Ab:Ag complexes to CD4.

UPERANTIGEN FUNCTION OF CD4

The realization that the CD4/Ig interaction does not involve residues within the CDR loops of V_H or VL regions, and by analogy with the proposed Ig superantigen binding property of *Staphylococcus* protein A,[65-70] it is tempting to speculate that the autoantibodies to CD4 described in ~10-20% of HIV-infected patients[71-76] and in a subset (~20%) of SLE patients,[77] may in fact reflect a CD4/Ig interaction of the type described above rather than a conventional reactivity via the antigen-binding site. Preliminary evidence obtained through computer modeling studies indicates that CD4 binding involves residues within a relatively invariant region of the V_H domain. Whether or not these V_H residues are the same also involved in binding *Staphylococcus* protein A, remains to be defined.

Table 17.1. Enhanced binding of Ab:Ag complex to CD4

Wells Coating	Equivalent nM of an anti-DNP antibody				Ratio Ab:Ag/Ab
	Monomeric* Ig	Aggregated** Ig	Ab:Ag*** complex	$F(ab)_2$	$F(ab')_2$:Ag complex
rCD4	156·	312	15	312	20
~10:1					
*p*16-49	156	156	0.8	156	1.1
~150:1					
*p*39-60	$>10^4$	$>10^4$	$>10^4$	$>10^4$	$>10^4$
BSA	$>10^4$	$>10^4$	$>10^4$	$>10^4$	$>10^4$

*Monoclonal antibody to DNP (109.3; IgG1, K) was used diluted in PBSA buffer.
**Aggregtion was done by heating at +63°C for 30 minutes a solution of 28 mg/ml of mAb 109.3.
***Ab:Ag complex were formed in vitro by mixing at a molar ratio of 1:6 the $DNP_{37}BSA$ conjugate with anti-DNP antibody 109.3 for 12 hours at 4°C. After preincubation the mixture was transferred to microtiter wells.
·Values refer to equivalent amount (nM) of Ab to give an O.D. A_{492} of 0.5.

Implications for B Cell Antigen-Presenting Function and Signal Transduction

Functionally, a CD4/Ig interaction could play a role in both antigen-presenting function of B cells and in B cell receptor (BcR)-dependent signal transduction.[78-82] It is well established that the essential function of antigen presenting cells (APC), including B cells, is the conversion of a foreign protein into antigenic peptides by proteolysis and the formation of peptide-MHC complexes which are expressed at the cell surface. B cells function as APC primarily (but not exclusively) by concentrating and endocytosing antigen via the BcR. B cells can in fact trigger antigen-specific T cell proliferation at a 1000-fold lower concentration of antigen compared with professional APC.[83] As CD4 has higher affinity for antibodies complexed with antigen, one could assume that CD4, on T cells and monocytes, may enhance the APC function of B cells.

It is firmly established that antigen binding to the BcR induces internalization of the membrane (m)Ig/Ag complex, an event which could proceed with or without triggering signal transduction. CD4 may facilitate the whole process by augmenting the affinity of interaction between mIg and antigen (particularly if the latter is complexed to an antibody). Whether or not the outcome of the cross-linking of the BcR-Ag complex by CD4 is activation or anergy can only be speculated and may depend on various factors. In turn, these events may have an impact on activation or anergy of T cells. For instance, resting B cells may play a critical role in anergizing antigen-specific T cells if the antigen can not cross-link the BcR,[84] and resting B cells primed with monovalent antigen do not upregulate costimulatory molecules (e.g., B7) as they do when they encounter multivalent antigens.[85-87] Thus, cross-linking of the BcR/antigen complex by CD4 may lead to B cell activation and bypass induction of T cell anergy.

Role of the CD4/Ig Interaction in Shaping the B Cell Repertoire

BcR occupancy by antigen or superantigen could result not only in clonal expansion of the antigen-specific B lymphocyte pool, but also in anergy or clonal deletion of self-reactive B cell clones. It is possible that a threshold density of surface receptors determines whether a cellular interaction will generate positive or negative signals. In immature B cells ($mIgM^+/mIgD^-$) ligation of the BcR usually results in clonal deletion via programmed cell death. Similarly, one could envision that most B cell clones expressing Ig receptors with high affinity for CD4, particularly those recognizing immunodominant epitopes on CD4, will undergo apoptosis. Only those B cells expressing mIg receptors with relatively low affinity for CD4 would have a chance to survive. Since the residues involved in CD4 binding may have variable surface accessibility and this may increase following antigen binding, the possibility exists that in the absence of antigen these clones are positively selected. Thus, CD4 on T cell-monocytes could be one of the key factors (possibly with some other endogenous superantigens) involved in shaping the B cell repertoire, both during fetal and postnatal development. An analogy can be seen with another proposed superantigen, HIV gp120, which binds Ig V_H regions and was found to induce expansion and subsequent marked decrease of human B cells that rearrange V_H3 gene products[88,89] At the present time, we do not know which among the multiple human V_H gene products bind CD4. However, even in the absence of precise genetic information one can predict that, similar to what reported for *Staphylococcus* protein A,[67-70] somatic hypermutation in the V_H region could either abrogate binding to CD4 or generate B cells having higher affinity for CD4. We speculate that this may be the case in SLE.[77]

HYPOTHESIS AND CONCLUSIONS

We propose that the interaction between CD4 and certain V_H gene family products could regulate T and B cell activation events. After recognizing peptide/MHC complex T cells drive the expansion not only of antigen-specific B cells but also of B cells expressing a BcR with higher affinity for CD4. CD4 at the surface of activated T cells will directly select such B cell subsets and promote cross-linking of mIg, thus initiating BcR-dependent signaling. Consequently, CD4-binding clones will undergo clonal expansion and differentiation, events resulting in an increased secretion of CD4-binding antibodies. In turn, these may bind CD4 on T cells and monocytes and prevent their further activation by inducing clonal anergy and/or apoptosis. Consequently, B cells will be deprived of T cell help and become anergic. This biphasic model of positive selection followed by negative selection could play a role in the balance between T of B lymphocytes and could be at play in pathological conditions such as in AIDS and SLE.

In conclusion, much of our earlier theoretical predictions about possible functional implications of the CD4/Ig interaction have been experimentally validated over the last few years. Future experiments will have to determine the exact CD4-binding site within a Ig-V_H region. Progress in this field may further help our understanding of the role of Ig on T cell development, and vice versa, the potential role of CD4 T cells in shaping the B cell repertoire.

ACKNOWLEDGMENTS

This manuscript was supported in part by a grant from the Medical Research Council of Canada-Invited Scientist Grant to P.L. and in part by grant NIH PO1 AI33204 to M.Z. M.Z. is a Faculty Member of the Biomedical Sciences Graduate Program.

REFERENCES

1. Lucey DR, Dorsky DI, Nicholson-Weller A et al. Human eosinophils express CD4 protein and bind human immunodeficiency virus 1 gp120. J Exp Med 1989; 169: 327-32.
2. Stewart SJ, Fujimoto J, Levy R. Human T lymphocytes and monocytes bear the same Leu-3(T4) antigen. J Immunol 1986; 136:3773-78.
3. Wood GS, Warner NL, Warnke RA. Anti-Leu-3/T4 antibodies react with cells of monocyte/macrophage and Langerhans lineage. J Immunol 1983; 131:212-16.
4. Tourvieille B, Gorman SD, Field SD et al. Isolation and sequence of L3T4 complementary DNA clones: Expression in T cells and brain. Science 1986; 234:610-14.
5. Maddon PJ, Littman DR, Godfrey M et al. The isolation and nucleotide sequence of a cDNA encoding the T cell surface protein T4: A new member of the immunoglobulin gene family. Cell 1985; 42:93-104.
6. Kwong PD, Ryu S-E, Hendrickson WA et al. Molecular characteristics of recombinant human CD4 as deduced from polymorphic crystals. Proc Natl Acad Sci USA 1990; 87:6423-27.
7. Wang J, Yan Y, Garrett TPJ et al. Atomic structure of a fragment of human CD4 containing two immunoglobulin-like domains. Nature 1990; 348:411-18.
8. Ryu S-E, Kwong PD, Truneh A et al. Crystal structure of an HIV-binding recombinant fragment of human CD4. Nature 1990; 348:419-26.
9. Brady RL, Dodson EJ, Dodson GG et al. Crystal structure of domains 3 and 4 of rat CD4: Relation to the NH2-terminal domains. Science 1993; 260:979-83.
10. Leahy DJ. A structural view of CD4 and CD8. FASEB J 1995; 9:17-25.
11. Gay D, Maddon P, Sékaly R et al. Functional interaction between human T cell protein CD4 and the major histocompatibility complex HLA-DR antigen. Nature 1987; 328:626-29.
12. Cammarota G, Scheirie A, Takacs B et al. Identification of a CD4 binding site on the

beta2 domain of HLA-DR molecules. Nature 1992; 356:799-801.
13. Weber S and Karjalainen K. Mouse CD4 binds MHC class II with extremely low affinity. Int Immunol 1993; 5:695-98.
14. Matsui K, Boniface JJ, Reay PA et al. Low affinity interaction of peptide-MHC complexes with T cell receptors. Science 1991; 254:1788-91.
15. Weber S, Traunecker A, Oliveri F et al. Specific low-affinity recognition of major histocompatibility complex plus peptide by soluble T cell receptor. Nature 1992; 356:793-95.
16. Konig R, Shen X, Germain RN. Involvement of both major histocompatibility complex class II alpha and beta chains in CD4 function indicates a role for ordered oligomerization in T cell activation. J Exp Med 1995; 182:779-87.
17. Fleury S, Thibodeau J, Croteau G et al. HLA-DR polymorphism affects the interaction with CD4. J Exp Med 1995; 182:733-41.
18. Janeway Jr CA. The T cell receptor as a multicomponent signalling machine: CD4/CD8 coreceptors and CD45 in T cell activation. Annu Rev Immunol 1992; 10:645-74.
19. Dianzani U, Shaw A, al-Ramadi BK et al. Physical association of CD4 with the T cell receptor. J Immunol 1992; 148:678-88.
20. Emmrich F, Kanz L, Eichmann K. Crosslinking of the T cell receptor complex with the subset-specific differentiation antigen stimulates interleukin 2 receptor expression in human CD4 and CD8 T cells. Eur J Immunol 1987; 17:529-34.
21. Anderson P, Blue ML, Schlossman SF. Comodulation of CD3 and CD4. Evidence for a specific association between CD4 and approximately 5% of the CD3:T cell receptor complexes on helper T lymphocytes. J Immunol 1988; 140:1732-37.
22. Dianzani U, Bragardo M, Buonfiglio D et al. Modulation of CD4 lateral interaction with lymphocyte surface molecules induced by HIV-1 gp120. Eur J Immunol 1995; 25:1306-11.
23. Bank I, Chess L. Perturbation of the T4 molecule transmits negative signal to T cells. J Exp Med 1985; 162:1294-303.
24. Diamond DC, Sleckman BP, Gregory T et al. Inhibition of CD4[+] T cell function by the HIV envelope protein gp120. J Immunol 1988; 141:3715-17.
25. Mann DL, Lasane F, Popovic M et al. HTLV-III large envelope protein (gp120) suppresses PHA-induced lymphocyte blastogenesis. J Immunol 1987; 138: 2640-44.
26. Rosoff PM, Burakoff SJ, Greenstein JL. The role of the L3T4 molecule in mitogen and antigen-activated signal transduction. Cell 1987; 49:845-53.
27. Mittler RS, Hoffmann MK. Synergism between HIV gp120 and gp120-specific antibody in blocking human T cell activation. Science 1989; 245:1380-82.
28. Tomer Y, Blank M, Shoenfeld Y. Suppression of experimental antiphospholipid syndrome and systemic lupus erythematosus in mice by anti-CD4 monoclonal antibodies. Arthritis Rheum 1994; 37:1236-44.
29. Mottram PL, Han WR, Purcell LJ et al. Increased expression of IL-4 and IL-10 and decreased expression of IL-2 and interferon-gamma in long-surviving mouse heart allografts after brief CD4-monoclonal antibody therapy. Transplantation 1995; 59:559-65.
30. Stumbles P, Mason D. Activation of CD4[+] T cells in the presence of nondepleting monoclonal antibody to CD4 induces a Th2-type response in vitro. J Exp Med 1995; 182:5-13.
31. Wang J, Yan T, Simmer B et al. The effect of anti-CD4 on helper function of CD4, 45RA[+] versus CD4, 45RO[+] T cells. Clin Exp Immunol 1994; 95:128-34.
32. Newell MK, Haughn LJ, Maroun CR et al. Death of mature T cells by separate ligation of CD4 and the T cell receptor for antigen. Nature 1990; 347:286-89.
33. Banda NK, Bernier J, Kurahara DK et al. Crosslinking CD4 by human immunodeficiency virus gp120 primes T cells for activation-induced apoptosis. J Exp Med 1992; 176:1099-106.
34. Wang Z-q, Dudhane A, Orlikowsky T et al. CD4 engagement induces Fas antigen-dependent apoptosis of T cells in vivo. Eur J

Immunol 1994; 24:1549-52.

35. Di Somma MM, Nuti S, Telford JL et al. p56lck plays a key role in transducing apoptotic signals in T cells. FEBS Let 1995; 363:101-04.
36. Howie SE, Sommerfield AJ, Gray E et al. Peripheral T lymphocyte depletion by apoptosis after CD4 ligation in vivo: selective loss of CD44- and 'activating' memory T cells. Clin Exp Immunol 1994; 95: 195-200.
37. Oyaizu N, McCloskey TW, Than S et al. Cross-linking of CD4 molecules upregulates Fas antigen expression in lymphocytes by inducing interferon-gamma and tumor necrosis factor-alpha secretion. Blood 1994; 84:2622-31.
38. Zerbib AC, Reske-Kunz AB, Lock P et al. CD4-mediated enhancement or inhibition of T cell activation does not require the CD4:p56lck association. J Exp Med 1994; 179:1973-83.
39. Doyle C, Strominger JL. Interaction between CD4 and class II MHC molecules mediates cell adhesion. Nature 1987; 330:256-59.
40. Capon DJ, Ward RHR. The CD4-gp120 interaction and AIDS pathogenesis. Annu Rev Immunol 1991; 9:649-78
41. Baba M, Pauwels R, Balzarini J et al. Mechanism of inhibitory effect of dextran sulfate and heparin on replication of human immunodeficiency virus in vitro. Proc Natl Acad Sci USA 1988; 85:6132-36.
42. Mitsuya H, Looney DJ, Kuno S et al. Dextran sulfate suppression of viruses in the HIV-family: inhibition of virion binding to $CD4^+$ cells. Science 1988; 240:646-49.
43. Szabo Jr G, Pine PS, Weaver JL et al. CD4 changes conformation upon ligand binding. J Immunol 1992; 149:3596-604.
44. Yakubov L, Khaled Z, Zhang L-M. Oligonucleotides interact with recombinant CD4 at multiple sites. J Biol Chem 1993; 268:18818-23.
45. Lenert P, Kroon D, Spiegelberg H et al. Human CD4 binds immunoglobulins. Science 1990; 248:1639-43.
46. Autiero M, Cammarota G, Friedlein A et al. A 17-kDa CD4-binding glycoprotein present in human seminal plasma and in breast tumor cells. Eur J Immunol 1995; 25:1461-64.
47. Morrison WJ, Offner H, Vandenbark AA. Ganglioside (GM1)-treated T cells shed CD4. Immunopharmacology 1991; 22:77-84.
48. Blasco E, Barra A, Nicolas M et al. Proliferative response of human $CD4^+$ T lymphocytes stimulated by the lectin jacalin. Eur J Immunol 1995; 25:2010-18.
49. Center DM, Berman JS, Kornfeld H et al. The lymphocyte chemoattractant factor. J Lab Clin Med 1995; 125:167-72.
50. Miceli MC, Parnes JR. Role of CD4 and CD8 in T cell activation and differentiation. Adv Immunol 1993; 53:59-122.
51. Lederman S, Yellin MJ, Cleary AM et al. Recombinant, truncated CD4 molecule (rT4) binds IgG. J Immunol 1990; 144: 214-20.
52. Berneman A, Ternynck T, Avrameas S. Natural mouse IgG reacts with self antigens including molecules involved in the immune response. Eur J Immunol 1992; 22:625-33.
53. Kazatckine MD, Dietrich G, Hurez V et al. V region-mediated selection of autoreactive repertoires by intravenous immunoglobulin (i.v.Ig). Immunol Rev 1994; 139:79-107.
54. Lenert P, Zanetti M. CD4/immunoglobulin interaction: implications for immune physiology and autoimmunity. Int Rev Immunol 1991; 7:237-44.
55. Lenert P, Mehta RL, Zanetti M. Synthetic peptides of human CD4 enhance binding of Ig to monocyte/macrophage cells. I. Characterization and mapping studies. J Immunol 1992; 148:1759-63.
56. Mehta RL, Lenert P, Zanetti M. Synthetic peptides of human CD4 enhance binding of immunoglobulins to monocyte/macrophage cells. II. Mechanisms of enhancement. Cell Immunol 1994; 156:146-54.
57. Lenert P, Lenert G, Zanetti M. Human recombinant CD4 and CD4-derived synthetic peptides agglutinate immunoglobulin-coated latex particles. Evidence that residues 25-28 and 35-38 of human CD4 form two separate immunoglobulin binding sites. Mol Immunol in press.
58. Lamarre D, Ashkenazi A, Fleury S et al. The MHC-binding and gp120-binding functions

of CD4 are separable. Science 1989; 245:743-46.

59. Clayton LK, Sieh M, Pious DA et al. Identification of human CD4 residues affecting class II MHC versus HIV-1 gp120 binding. Nature 1989; 339:549-51.
60. Jameson BA, Rao PE, Kong LI et al. Location and chemical synthesis of a binding site for HIV-1 on the CD4-protein. Science 1988; 240:1335-39.
61. Horne C, Klein M, Polidoulis II et al. Noncovalent association of heavy and light chains of human immunoglobulins. III. Specific interactions between V_H and V_L. J Immunol 1982; 129:660-64.
62. Adetugbo K, Milstein C, Secher DS. Molecular analysis of spontaneous somatic mutants. Nature 1977; 265:299-304.
63. Liu FT, Bohn JW, Ferry EL, et al. Monoclonal dinitrophenyl-specific murine antibody: Preparation, isolation and characterization. J Immunol 1980; 124:2728-37.
64. Sollazzo M, Castiglia D, Billetta R et al. Molecular characterization of the VH region of murine autoantibodies from neonatal and adult BALB/c mice. Eur J Immunol 1989; 19:453-457.
65. Inganas M. Comparison of mechanisms of interaction between protein A from *Staphylococcus aureus* and human monoclonal IgG, IgA and IgM in relation to the classical Fcγ and the alternative $F(ab')_2\varepsilon$ protein A interactions. Scand J Immunol 1981; 13:343-52.
66. Romagnani S, Giudizi MG, Del Prete G et al. Demonstration on protein A of two distinct immunoglobulin-binding sites and their role in the mitogenic activity of Staphylococcus aureus Cowan II on human B cells. J Immunol 1982; 129:596-602.
67. Silverman GJ, Sasano M, Wormsley SB. Age-associated changes in binding of human B lymphocytes to a VH3-restricted unconventional bacterial antigen. J Immunol 1993; 151:5840-55.
68. Sasano M, Burton DR, Silverman GJ. Molecular selection of human antibodies with an unconventional bacterial B cell antigen. J Immunol 1993; 151:5822-39.
69. Hillson JL, Karr NS, Oppliger IR et al. The structural basis of germline-encoded V_H3 immunoglobulin binding of staphylococcal protein A. J Exp Med 1993; 178:331-36.
70. Roben PW, Salem AN, Silverman GJ. V_H3 family antibodies bind domain D of staphylococcal protein A. J Immunol 1995; 154:6437-45.
71. Kowalski M, Ardman B, Basiripour L et al. Antibodies to CD4 in individuals infected with human immunodeficiency virus type 1. Proc Natl Acad Sci USA 1989; 86: 3346-50.
72. Wilks D, Walker LC, Habeshaw JA et al. Anti-CD4 autoantibodies and screening for anti-idiotypic antibodies to anti-CD4 monoclonal antibodies in HIV-seropositive people. AIDS 1990; 4:113-18.
73. Sekigawa I, Groopmen, JE, Allan JD et al. Characterization of autoantibodies to the CD4 molecule in human immunodeficiency virus infection. Clin Immunol Immunopathol 1991; 58:145-53.
74. Corre J-P, Fevrier M, Chamaret S et al. Anti-idiotypic antibodies to human anti-gp120 antibodies bind recombinant and cellular human CD4. Eur J Immunol 1991; 21: 743-51.
75. Chams V, Idziorek T, Klatzmann D. Biological properties of anti-CD4 autoantibodies purified from HIV-infected patients. AIDS 1991; 5:565-69.
76. Callahan LN, Roderiquez G, Mallinson M et al. Analysis of HIV-induced autoantibodies to cryptic epitopes on human CD4. J Immunol 1992; 149:2194-202.
77. Lenert G, Lenert P. Human CD4-reactive antibodies from SLE patients induce reversible inhibition of polyclonal T lymphocyte proliferation. Hum Immunol 1996, in press.
78. Chesnut RW, Grey HM. Antigen presentation by B cells and its significance in T-B interactions. Adv Immunol 1986; 39:51-94.
79. Ashwell JD. Are B lymphocytes the principal antigen-presenting cells in vivo? J Immunol 1988; 140:3697-700.
80. Lassila O, Vainio O, Matzinger P. Can B cells turn on virgin T cells? Nature 1988; 334:253-55.
81. Myers CD. Role of B cell antigen processing and presentation in the humoral immune response. FASEB J 1991; 5:2547-53.
82. Parker DC. T cell-dependent B cell activation. Annu Rev Immunol 1993; 11:331-60.

83. Lanzavecchia A. Receptor-mediated antigen uptake and its effect on antigen presentation to class II-restricted T lymphocytes. Annu Rev Immunol 1990; 8:773-93.
84. Eynon EE, Parker DC. Small B cells as antigen-presenting cells in the induction of tolerance to soluble protein antigens. J Exp Med 1992; 175:131-38.
85. Constant S, Schweitzer N, West J et al. B lymphocytes can be competent antigen-presenting cells for priming $CD4^+$ T cells to protein antigens in vivo. J Immunol 1995; 155:3734-41.
86. Koulova L, Clark EA, Shu G et al. The CD28 ligand B7/BB1 provides costimulatory signal for alloactivation of $CD4^+$ T cells. J Exp Med 1991; 173:759-62.
87. Lenschow DJ, Sperling AI, Cooke MP et al. Differential upregulation of the B7-1 and B7-2 costimulatory molecules after Ig receptor engagement by antigen. J Immunol 1994; 153:1990-97.
88. Berberian L, Goodlick L, Kipps TJ et al. Immunoglobulin V_H3 gene products: natural ligands for HIV gp120. Science 1993; 261:1588-91.
89. Zouali M. B cell superantigens: implications for selection of the human antibody repertoire. Immunol Today 1995; 16:399-405.

INDEX

Items in italics denote figures (f) or tables (t).

A

B

C

D

E

F

G

H

I

J

K

L

M

N

O

P

R

S

T

V

W

Z